Textbook of
Dental Radiography

Revised Second Printing

TEXTBOOK OF DENTAL RADIOGRAPHY

By

Olaf E. Langland, D.D.S., M.S., F.A.C.D.

Professor and Head
Department of Oral Diagnosis/Medicine/Radiology
School of Dentistry
Louisiana State University
New Orleans, Louisiana

and

Francis H. Sippy, B.S., M.Ed.

Instructor
Division of Dental Radiology
College of Dentistry
University of Iowa
Iowa City, Iowa

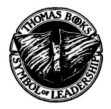

CHARLES C THOMAS · PUBLISHER
Springfield · Illinois · U.S.A.

Published and Distributed Throughout the World by

CHARLES C THOMAS • PUBLISHER

Bannerstone House

301-327 East Lawrence Avenue, Springfield, Illinois, U.S.A.

© *1973, by* CHARLES C THOMAS • PUBLISHER

ISBN 0-398-02746-3

Library of Congress Catalog Card Number: 72-93219

First Printing, 1973
Revised Second Printing, 1977

With THOMAS BOOKS careful attention is given to all details of manufacturing and design. It is the Publisher's desire to present books that are satisfactory as to their physical qualities and artistic possibilities and appropriate for their particular use. THOMAS BOOKS will be true to those laws of quality that assure a good name and good will.

Printed in the United States of America

C-1

THIS TEXTBOOK IS DEDICATED TO
OUR STUDENTS, IN PARTIAL PAYMENT OF
THE DEBT WE OWE OUR TEACHERS

PREFACE

THIS TEXTBOOK was written to serve four purposes:

First, to serve as a reinforcement of the learning acquired in lectures in dental radiography;

Second, to serve as a reference guide for the clinical application of the radiographic procedures learned in lectures in dental radiography;

Third, to serve as a reference after completion of courses in dental radiography;

Fourth, and to serve as a source of information for the dental assistant, dental hygienist, registered X-ray technologist and dentist.

Specifically, it is hoped that this textbook will aid the student in dental radiography to develop competence in the skills and understandings of dental radiography; provide an orderly progression of learning for the student of dental radiography; arouse the spirit of curiosity in the student of dental radiography; stimulate the student of dental radiography to become more responsive to the changing needs of dental radiography; and to promote the dentist's awareness of his responsibility to his patient to use dental radiographic procedures intelligently.

This textbook represents a compilation of information based for the most part on publications of our contemporaries and predecessors.

In order to present the material in an informal manner, continuous references to these sources have been deleted. However, the reader will find a list of suggested references at the end of each chapter. We realize that this textbook could not have been written without the ideas, data, observations and conclusions of others. Therefore, this textbook is dedicated to our contemporaries and predecessors who have made this textbook a reality.

INTRODUCTION

R ADIOGRAPHIC EXAMINATION is as essential for diagnostic purposes in dentistry as it is in medicine. A clinical examination of the oral cavity without the aid of radiographs is restricted to the exposed surfaces of the teeth and associated soft tissues. Therefore, dental radiography offers the only preoperative means of inspecting the hidden structures of the oral cavity, namely, the roots and internal structures of the teeth, the approximal surfaces of the teeth and the surrounding alveolar bone. It is obvious, then, that a general radiographic examination of the oral structures is essential to the diagnosis of dental and oral conditions.

Kurt H. Thoma,* well known authority in medicine and dentistry, had this to say concerning dental radiographic examination.

> "Radiographic examination is useful to discover, to confirm, to classify, to define, and to localize a lesion. It is helpful in establishing an early diagnosis, in finding the origin of symptoms and cause of disease, and in discovering the extent of tissue involvement. It is of great value in establishing a differential diagnosis between inflammatory processes and benign and infiltrating tumors. Finally, radiographic examination is a valuable aid in checking the progress of treatment."

The purpose of dental radiography is to provide the dentist with a radiograph of the best diagnostic quality. The requisites of any good diagnostic radiograph, regardless of technic used, are (1) proper contrast and density of the tissues radiographed, (2) maximal definition and minimal distortion of the anatomical structures involved, (3) anatomical accuracy and (4) coverage of the boundaries of the anatomical region under consideration. Of course, to attain these requisites every step in the radiographic procedure must be thoroughly understood and carried out. The equipment must be adequate; the projection, exposure, and processing technics must be correct; and the operator must be completely competent.

Although radiography is defined as the art and practice of making radiographs, it is much more than a series of procedures—it is both a *science* and an *art*. It is a *science* in that it embodies the sciences of physics, mathematics, and chemistry; it is an *art* in that it requires practice, study, experience and judgement to attain the desired skill.

Those that desire to become competent in dental radiography must possess the following abilities:

---

* Thoma, Kurt H.: *Oral and Dental Diagnosis*, 3rd edition. Philadelphia, W. B. Saunders Co., 1949.

1. Understand the scientific principles that govern radiographic technics;
2. Understand the means by which those principles are applied;
3. Be able to produce an acceptable diagnostic radiograph consistently;
4. Determine common radiographic errors that cause poor radiographs and to be able to correct these errors;
5. Appreciate and guard against the dangers of x-radiation;
6. Manage dental patients correctly under difficult situations.

It is important to remember that the slightest inaccuracy in a dental radiograph may nullify its possible assistance in oral diagnosis. Any misconception of the images on the radiograph by the dentist may cause an interpretative error that in turn may cause the dentist to arrive at an incorrect diagnosis. Thus, the ability to master dental radiography is as equally important as the ability to interpret the radiograph. These abilities go "hand-in-hand" because a poor radiograph could not be accurately read by the best dental diagnostician, and a quality radiograph is useless unless read properly.

ACKNOWLEDGMENTS

IT IS DIFFICULT to acknowledge every individual and manufacturer who has assisted us in the writing of this textbook.

We are indebted to our administrators of the University of Iowa and Louisiana State University for providing the facilities and opportunity to complete this project. Special appreciation is due Dean Edmund E. Jeansonne of Louisiana State University, School of Dentistry.

We are particularly grateful to Mr. Raymond Calvert, L.S.U. Dental Illustrator, for his excellent art work; Mr. William Stallworth, L.S.U. Photographer, for his excellent photography; and Mr. Claude Mahaffey, R.T., L.S.U. School of Dentistry, for his skillful radiography.

We are indebted to several of our colleagues and predecessors for their publications, which served as a valuable source of reference. Included in this group are Professor Albert Richards of the University of Michigan; Dr. J. Meschan of Bowman Gray School of Medicine; Mr. William Bloom of General Electric; Dr. William Updegrave of Temple University; Dr. Lincoln Manson-Hing of University of Alabama; Dr. Harrison Berry, Jr. of the University of Pennsylvania; Arthur Fuchs (deceased) of Rochester, New York; Dr. Michel Ter-Pogossian of Washington University (St. Louis); Mr. F. Jaundrell-Thompson of London, England; and Mr. Herman Seeman, Rochester, New York.

Special mention should be made of the following publishers and manufacturers for permission to use illustrations and to quote from articles in which these illustrations appeared: W. B. Saunders Company; C. V. Mosby Company; Charles C Thomas, Publisher; General Electric Medical Systems; B. F. Wehmer Company; Eastman Kodak Company; Rinn Corporation; Pennwalt Corporation; and Siemens Medical of America.

We are very grateful to our associates who in our discussions gave us pertinent advice concerning the manuscript: Dr. Robert Fleming, the University of Iowa; Dr. A. Peter Fortier of L.S.U.; Dr. Charles H. Boozer, L.S.U.; and Dr. Ronald Barrett of L.S.U.

It is with sincere appreciation that we acknowledge the superb secretarial work of Mrs. Judy Carriere, Miss Carol Pagragan, and Miss Linda Lotz in the preparation of the manuscript. Their loyalty and patience is without peer.

We are indebted to Mr. Payne Thomas for his encouragement, guidance, and patience. He is truly an understanding and astute editor.   O. E. L.

F. H. S.

ADDITIONAL ACKNOWLEDGMENTS

A CKNOWLEDGMENT is made to the following individuals and their publishers, whose illustrations have been the source for drawings and
other illustrations prepared for this text.

Figure 2-2: Michel M. Ter-Pogossian: *The Physical Aspects of Diagnostic Radiology.*
New York, Hoeber Medical Division, Harper and Row, 1967, p. 16.

Figure 2-3: William R. Hendee: *Medical Radiation Physics.* Chicago, Year Book Medical
Publishers, 1970, p. 37.

Figure 2-6: Michel M. Ter-Pogossian: *The Physical Aspects of Diagnostic Radiology.*
New York, Hoeber Medical Division, Harper and Row, 1967, p. 29.

Figure 2-7: F. Jaundrell-Thompson, and W. J. Ashworth: *X-Ray Physics and Equipment,*
2nd ed. Philadelphia, F. A. Davis, 1970, p. 725.

Figure 2-8: F. Jaundrell-Thompson, and W. J. Ashworth: *X-Ray Physics and Equipment,*
2nd ed. Philadelphia, F. A. Davis, 1970, p. 728.

Figure 2-9: Michel M. Ter-Pogossian: *The Physical Aspects of Diagnostic Radiology.*
New York, Hoeber Medical Division, Harper and Row, 1967, p. 34.

Figure 2-10: *Dental X-Ray Generation and Radiographic Principles.* Milwaukee, General
Electric Company, p. 1.

Figure 2-11: *X-Rays in Dentistry.* Rochester, New York, Eastman Kodak Company, 1964,
p. 2.

Figure 2-12: *Dental X-Ray Generation and Radiographic Principles.* Milwaukee, General
Electric Company, p. 6.

Figure 2-13: *X-Rays in Dentistry.* Rochester, New York, Eastman Kodak Company, p. 3.

Figure 2-14: *The Fundamentals of Radiography,* 10th ed., Rochester, New York, Eastman
Kodak Company, 1960, p. 10.

Figure 2-15: *Dental X-Ray Generation and Radiographic Principles.* Milwaukee, General
Electric Company, p. 5.

Figure 2-16: *Dental X-Ray Generation and Radiographic Principles.* Milwaukee, General
Electric Company, p. 5.

Figure 2-17: *Dental X-Ray Generation and Radiographic Principles.* Milwaukee, General
Electric Company, p. 5.

Figure 2-20: *The Fundamentals of Radiography,* 10th ed. Rochester, New York, Eastman
Kodak Company, 1960, p. 8.

Figure 3-2: Herman E. Seeman: *Physical and Photographic Principles of Medical Radiography.* New York, John Wiley and Sons, 1968, p. 6.

Figure 3-3: *The Fundamentals of Radiography,* 10th ed. Rochester, New York, Eastman
Kodak Company, 1960, p. 13.

Figure 3-4: *X-Rays in Dentistry.* Rochester, New York, Eastman Kodak Company, p. 5.

Figure 3-8: Arthur W. Fuchs: *Principles of Radiographic Exposure and Processing,* 2nd
ed. Springfield, Illinois, Charles C Thomas, 1969, p. 7.

Figure 3-9: Arthur W. Fuchs: *Principles of Radiographic Exposure and Processing,*
2nd ed. Springfield, Illinois, Charles C Thomas, 1969, p. 7.

Figure 3-10: *The Fundamentals of Radiography,* 10th ed. Rochester, New York, Eastman
Kodak Company, 1960, p. 43.

Figure 6-48: Updegrave, William: *New Horizons in Periapical Radiography*. Elgin, Illinois, Rinn Corporation, 1966, p. 27.

Figure 6-54: Ennis, LeRoy M., and Berry, Harrison M.: *Dental Roentgenology*, 5th ed. Philadelphia, Lea & Febiger, 1959, p. 106.

Figure 6-57: Richards, Albert: New concepts in dental x-ray machines. *J Am Dent Assoc*, 73:69, 1966.

Figure 8-1: *X-rays in Dentistry*. Eastman Kodak Company, 1969, p. 67.

Figure 8-4: Porter, A., and Sweet, S.: Safelights reconsidered. *Dent Radiol Photo*, 35, No. 2, 1962, Figure 5.

Figure 8-5: Ibid., Figure 6.

Figure 8-6: Ibid., Figure 7.

Figure 8-7: Ibid., Figure 8.

Figure 8-8: Ibid., Figure 9.

Figure 8-9: Ibid., Figure 10.

Figure 8-11: *X-rays in Dentistry*. Eastman Kodak Company, 1969, p. 71.

Figure 8-21: Wainwright, William W., and Villanyi, Andrew A.: The simplest radiographic analyzer: The x-ray checker, *J So Calif State Dent Assoc*, 28:124, April, 1960.

Figure 9-15: *Radiodontic Pitfalls*. Eastman Kodak Company, Figure 18.

Figure 9-25: *Darkroom Procedures to Assure Diagnostic Quality Results*, Taped-slide Series, Rinn Corporation, Slide No. 70, reticulation.

Figure 11-1: Bloom, William L., Hollenback, John L., and Morgan, James A.: *Medical Radiographic Technic*, 3rd ed. Springfield, Illinois, Charles C Thomas, 1969, p. 195.

Figure 11-2: Updegrave, William J.: Panoramic Radiography, *Dental Rad & Photo*, Eastman Kodak Company, Vol. 36, No. 4, 1963.

Figure 11-5: Ibid.

Figure 11-12: Ibid.

CONTENTS

Textbook of
Dental Radiography

CHAPTER 1

HISTORICAL BACKGROUND OF DENTAL RADIOLOGY

The Discovery of X-Rays

X-RAYS WERE DISCOVERED on November 8, 1895 by Wilhelm Conrad Roentgen, Professor of Physics and Director of the Physical Institute of the University of Wurzburg. X-rays rank with anesthesia as one of the two greatest discoveries that have revolutionized the medical and dental professions. Today, it is extremely difficult to imagine practicing either profession without the aid of these discoveries.

One must remember that the apparatus used by Roentgen in his discovery represented the labor of many ingenious investigators. Various European investigators twenty-five years before the discovery of x-rays began intensive experimentation with vacuum tubes and the production of fluorescence. The first vacuum tubes used were called Geissler tubes after Geissler, an ingenious mechanic of Bonn, Germany. Later on they were called by the names of investigators that modified the original Geissler tubes (for example—the Hittorf & Crookes Tubes). During these twenty-five years between 1870 and 1895, Hittorf, Hertz, Goldstein, and Plucker of Germany, Sir William Crookes of England, and Lenard of Hungary had revealed many new and interesting phenomena concerning the production of fluorescence in a vacuum tube. Their experiments suggested to Roentgen the probability that there were more problems in connection with these developments which were yet to be solved.

At the beginning of October, 1895, Roentgen decided to make some experiments with this fluorescence phenomena which seemed to be coming from the cathode electrode. This fluorescence had already been called "cathode rays" by Goldstein. During the course of determining whether the cathode fluorescence or cathode rays could pass through the thick glass of the vacuum tube, he covered a Hittorf-Crookes tube with black paper and darkened the room completely (See Figure 1-1). At this very instant an electric discharge was passed through the tube, he noticed a faint greenish glowing object coming from a table near the tube. Roentgen struck a match and discovered the mysterious light was a piece of barium platinocyanide screen, which is fluorescent.

After further investigation of this phenomenon, he concluded that the effect was caused by the generation of new invisible rays capable of penetrating opaque materials and producing visible fluorescence in certain chemicals. By interposing his hand between the source of the rays and a luminescent cardboard, Roentgen was the first to see the bones of a living hand projected in silhouette

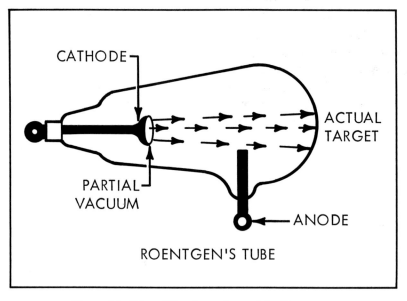

CATHODE

ACTUAL
TARGET

PARTIAL
VACUUM

ANODE

ROENTGEN'S TUBE

Figure 1-1. Hittorf-Crookes tube used by Roentgen.

upon the screen. The replacing of the fluorescent screen with a recording photographic plate was the next important discovery. This discovery enabled Roentgen to take the first radiograph ever taken of the human body—it was a radiograph of his wife Bertha's hand.

Roentgen's name and the news of his discovery became known throughout the whole world, and the modest discoverer spoke for the first time on his "New Kind of Ray" before the Physical Medical Society of the University of Wurzburg on January 23, 1896. At this meeting Roentgen demonstrated numerous successful experiments with the x-rays and exhibited various x-ray pictures and they, of course, excited the greatest interest. After the lecture and demonstration, the scientists rose as one and declared that henceforth these rays should be known as roentgen rays.

The Beginning of Dental Radiology

Two weeks after the announcement of Roentgen's discovery, Dr. Otto Walkhoff of Braunschweig, Germany, had completed the first radiograph of the jaws. The exposure time for Walkhoff's first radiograph of the jaws was twenty-five minutes. He used a regular photographic glass plate, placed on the outside of the jaws. The glass plate was quite insensitive to x-rays.

Dr. W. G. Morton, New York physician, has the distinction of taking the first dental radiograph in America in 1896. This was accomplished by use of dry human skulls. He read a paper on this subject before the New York Odontological Society on April 24, 1896, and it was published in the June, 1896 issue of *Dental Cosmos*. He also was the first to take a whole-body x-ray which was accomplished in 1897 by use of a 3 x 6 feet sheet of film. The exposure time was thirty minutes. The subject was a thirty-year-old female.

Dr. C. Edmund Kells of New Orleans was the first dentist in the United States to take an intraoral radiograph of a living patient. He also originated the technique of placing diagnostic wires in the roots of pulpless teeth (May, 1899). Dr. Kells presented the first clinic on the use of x-rays in dentistry at a meeting of the Southern Dental Association at Asheville, North Carolina in July, 1896. Exposures of five to fifteen minutes were used with a developing time of thirty to sixty minutes. As an indication of the intensive work on x-ray tubes and high-voltage sources can be revealed by the fact that Kells read a paper at the meeting of the National Dental Association in 1899 which records the fact that he had reduced exposure times to one to five minutes in three years.

Dr. Kells' contribution to the development of x-rays in dentistry finally cost him his life. Nothing was known about the hidden dangers lurking in the strange penetrating rays. The early x-ray machines were very crude. The variations in the quality of the x-rays was adjusted by a method called "setting the tube." One hand held the fluoroscope (hand type) and the other hand was placed between the tube and the fluoroscope. The rheostat of the x-ray machine was adjusted according to how sharp the bones in the hand would show up on the fluoroscope. The hand was exposed to a few seconds of x-radiation every time the tube was set. No harmful effects were noticed for at least five to ten years of this continued exposure to small amounts of radiation. Then the hands of the early pioneers started to show evidences of malignant growths. Dr. Kells first lost three fingers, later his whole hand was removed, and then his arm had to be amputated. But even this did not help. Preferring death to long and continuous suffering, Kells committed suicide—another unsung hero who gave his life for humanity.

Many of these early researchers in radiation, unaware of its effect on living tissue, gave their very lives to science. We today, who use and benefit from x-radiation in many ways, owe these men a debt of gratitude.

The Development of the Dental X-Ray Machine

At the turn of the century x-ray pictures were taken with very long exposure times (one to five minutes for a single exposure). *Why were such long exposure times necessary?*

For three reasons: (1) Direct Current was the only available source of power (A.C. power was not yet in universal use), (2) the poor efficiency of gas tubes, and (3) extreme lack of emulsion sensitivity of films used.

A transformer cannot transform low-voltage current into high-voltage current from a direct current source. To overcome this obstacle electrical interrupters were developed to change direct current into alternating current. The most common interrupter was a "vibrator" type that *made* and *broke* the primary circuit by vibrating a thin steel strip within the magnetic field of the metal core of the transformer. This strip had to be thin and lightweight if it was

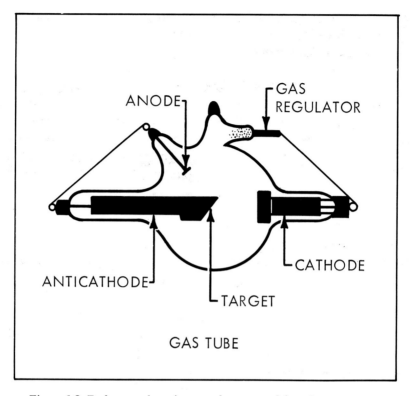

Figure 1-2. Early gas tube using metal target and focusing structures.

to vibrate, which limited its current capacity, and thus made for long exposure times.

X-rays were produced in the gas tube used by Roentgen (See Figure 1-1) by the bombardment of the glass by electrons developed by ionization of the residual gas in the tube. Later a target of metal was inserted into the tube to replace the glass as an area of electron bombardment (See Figure 1-2). Focusing structures within the tube served to focus the electrons on the target. The real obstacle to duplication of results was the variability of the vacuum within the tube. Under continued use, the vacuum changed, and hence the number of electrons available to produce x-rays.

Every worker had a whole series of gas tubes to "fit" the occasion. All sorts of pressure regulators were devised to regulate the vacuum in the tube. This variability of the vacuum tube made for long exposure times.

This was the state of affairs when Clyde Snook became interested in x-rays in 1903. Alternating current was just becoming available in some cities and even where direct current was in use, it could be used to produce alternating current by means of a converter. Snook saw that the use of alternating current to energize the primary made the electrical interrupter unnecessary. This solved the problem of power limitations always imposed by the interrupter systems. In 1907, Clyde Snook installed his first commercially available x-ray machine for his company in the Jefferson Hospital in Philadelphia. It was rated at 110 kVp and 200 mA. This machine solved the problem of the high-voltage source needed in the production of x-rays, but the gas tube still needed much improvement.

It was about this time (1907) that a team of researchers at the General Electric Research Laboratory began their work on high vacuum technics. In 1913, Dr. W. D. Coolidge, an electrical engineer with General Electric, described his first high-vacuum tube with contained tungsten targets filaments. He had found a way to make brittle tungsten workable. It was in 1917 that Dr. Coolidge developed an x-ray tube especially designed for dental application. It was a radiator-type of tube (air-cooled) in the shape of a right-angle to better enable the dentist to project intraoral exposures. This tube operated in a self-rectified circuit and was rated at a three-inch spark gap or sixty-three kVp. This gave rise to the so-called three inch dental unit, a voltage which influenced the design of dental x-ray units from 1917 to 1956 when the ninety kVp machines were first developed.

The final link in the chain of developments toward complete safety came in 1921 with Coolidge's development of the General Electric CDX unit. This x-ray unit placed the self-rectified x-ray tube with all its exposed electrical elements in a grounded, oil-filled metal housing. This development was made possible by the discovery of refined oils that could be used to dissipate the excessive heat produced at the anode of the x-ray tube.

History of Dental X-Ray Film

The first x-ray films had to be handled with extreme care since they were made of an emulsion on a glass plate, enclosed in black paper and sheets of rubber dam. Later, flexible celluloid was used as a film base, but it was difficult to work with because it had to be cut into the proper sizes and wrapped individually in protective materials to keep the film base and emulsion free from light and moisture. The early celluloid films were temperamental and dangerous because they contained cellulose in nitrate which is highly inflammable and under certain conditions explosive. Modern x-ray film employs a celluose acetate base because acetate is slow burning and much safer to use.

The Eastman Kodak Company produced the first pre-packaged intraoral film and thereby increased the acceptance and use of x-rays in dentistry. The present day high speed films are a great improvement over the older slower speed films in that the exposure time can be greatly decreased which in turn reduces radiation exposure to both the operator and the patient.

History of Intraoral Radiographic Technics

Since rays in the useful beam are divergent rather than parallel, inherent distortions are produced in the film image unless an intraoral projection technic is used to overcome this obstacle. This has led to the establishment of two technics, each based on a different principle, the bisecting-of-the-angle principle and the paralleling principle.

In 1904, Dr. Weston Price proposed a projection technic based on the age-old "rule of isometry." Ciesznski, a Polish engineer, also applied the "rule of isometry" to intraoral radiography in 1907. This technic became known as the bisection-of-the-angle technic and has been the intraoral projection technic of choice of the dental profession for several years. Dr. Raper of Indiana University refined the original technic by the introduction of average projection angles for the different regions of the dental arches. Dr. Clarence O. Simpson of Washington University of St. Louis later modified these original angles proposed by Raper.

One of the first advocates of the paralleling technic was Franklin W. McCormack, who first wrote on this subject in the *British Dental Journal* in 1920. His fervor for accurate shadow casting by the use of the paralleling technic fell on deaf ears of the dental profession because of its impracticability in the dental office. McCormack recommended the use of five- and six-foot target-film distances with the patient's body supine and the head stabilized with sandbags. This was hardly the method that would attract a dentist's attention.

It took Dr. Gordon Fitzgerald of the University of California in the late 1940's to revive the interest of the paralleling technic as first recommended by McCormack. Fitzgerald developed and introduced a paralleling intraoral technic that had practicality in a dental office. Of course, we must remember, in all fairness to McCormack, that Fitzgerald was using modern dental x-ray equipment that had a small focal spot size that

allowed him to use shorter target-film distances. In 1920 McCormack was using x-ray equipment with a gas x-ray tube that had a large focal spot which in turn almost dictated the longer target-film distances.

Today, three men besides Dr. Fitzgerald stand above all others as leaders in the field of teaching of the paralleling technic. They are Dr. Donald T. Waggener of the University of Nebraska, Dr. William J. Updegrave of Temple University at Philadelphia, and Dr. Arthur H. Wuehrmann of the University of Alabama.

The Development of Dental Radiology

The development of dental radiology to its present important position in dentistry may be attributed to the research and investigation by hundreds of dental researchers, no one of whom has contributed more to its development as a branch of dental science than Dr. Howard R. Raper of Indiana University. Dr. Raper wrote the first textbook on the subject; read the first paper urging inclusion of the subject in the dental curriculum; established the first full-time course in a dental college (Indiana); and during 1924, crowned these achievements by originating and introducing the intraoral method of radiographing the crowns of both the upper and lower teeth upon a single film, now commonly called the bitewing film technic.

The dental profession owes a lasting debt to those pioneers in the practice of dental radiology who by their accomplishment distinguish themselves as benefactors of the dental profession. The following is a partial list of the outstanding members of the dental profession and allied professions that have shared in the establishment of dental radiology as an indispensable branch of dental science.

Dr. Holly Broadbent—Western Reserve University

Dr. LeRoy Ennis—University of Pennsylvania

Dr. Gordon Fitzgerald—University of California

Dr. Cline Fixott, Sr.—Oregon

Dr. C. Edmund Kells—New Orleans, Louisiana

Dr. LeRoy Main—St. Louis University

Dr. John McCall and Dr. Sam Wald—New York University

Dr. James McCoy, and Dr. Walter Thompson—University of Southern California

Dr. R. Ottolenqui—Buffalo, New York

Dr. Howard Raper—Indiana University

Dr. William Rollins—Massachusetts

Dr. Clarence Simpson—Washington University at St. Louis

Dr. Edward Stafne—Mayo Clinic, Rochester, Minnesota

Dr. Kurt Thoma—Boston, Massachusetts

Dr. H. M. Worth—Guy's Hospital, London, England

REFERENCES

Andrews, Cuthbert: Half a century of shadows. *Radiography*, 22:250-254, 1956.

Beck, Carl: *Roentgen Ray Diagnosis and Therapy.* New York, D. Appleton, 1904, p. 75.

Bremner, M. D. K.: *The Story of Dentistry*, 3rd ed. Brooklyn, Dental Items of Interest Publishing, 1959, pp. 298-304.

Brown, Percy: *American Martyrs to Science Through the Roentgen Rays.* Springfield, Charles C Thomas, 1936.

Coolidge, W. D., and Carlton, E. E.: Roentgen-ray tubes, *Radiology*, 45:449-466, 1945.

Ennis, LeRoy, and Berry, Harrison M., Jr.: *Dental Roentgenology.* Philadelphia, Lea & Febiger, 5th ed. 1959, pp. 11-15.

Fitzgerald, Gordon M.: Dental roentgenography I. Control of geometric unsharpness. *J Am Dent Assoc*, 34:1-20, January, 1947.

Fitzgerald, Gordon M.: Dental roentgenography II. Vertical angulation. *J Am Dent Assoc*, 34:160-170, February, 1947.

Fitzgerald, Gordon M.: Dental roentgenography III. Upper molar region. *J Am Dent Assoc*, 38:293-303, March, 1949.

Fitzgerald, Gordon M.: Dental roentgenography IV. Voltage factor. *J Am Dent Assoc*, 41:19-28, July, 1950.

Glasser, Otto: *The Science of Radiology*, Springfield, Illinois, Charles C Thomas, 1933, pp. 1-14.

Glasser, Otto: *Wilhelm Conrad Roentgen*, Springfield, Illinois, Charles C Thomas, 1934.

Glasser, Otto: Fifty years of roentgen rays. *Dent Radiogr Photogr*, 19, No. 1, 1946.

Kells, C. Edmund: Protection for the roentgen ray. *Dental Items of Interest,* 24:805, 1912.

Kells, C. Edmund: *Three Score Years and Nine.* New Orleans, C. Edmund Kells, 1926, p. 404.

McCall, John Oppie, and Wald, Samuel S.: *Clinical Dental Roentgenology*, 4th ed. Philadelphia, W. B. Saunders, 1957, pp. 1-4, 35-38, and 82.

McCormick, Franklin W.: A plea for standardized oral radiography. *Br Dent J*, 41: 1162, 1920, abstracted *J Dent Res*, 11:496, September, 1920.

McCormick, Don W.: Dental roentgenology: A technical procedure for furthering the advancement toward anatomical accuracy. *J Calif State Dent Assoc*, May-June, 1937, pp. 89-116.

McCormick, Don W.: Mechanical aids for obtaining accuracy in dental roentgenology. *J Am Dent Assoc*, 40:144-153, February, 1950.

McCoy, James: *Dental and Oral Radiography.* St. Louis, C. V. Mosby, 1925, pp. 17-22.

Nitske, W. Robert: *The Life of Wilhelm Con-*

rad Roentgen. Tucson, Ariz., University of Arizona Press, 1971.

Peterson, Shailer: *Clinical Dental Hygiene*. St. Louis, C. V. Mosby, 1959, pp. 199-200.

Pollio, J. A.: Fundamental principles of alveolodental radiography. *Dental Items of Interest,* 47:405, 1925.

Preece, John W.: Roentgen alchemy, part I and part II. *Oral Surg,* 28:680, November, 1969; 28:830, December, 1969.

Raper, Howard: *Radiodontia*. Brooklyn, Dental Items of Interest Publishing, 1925, pp. 17-18.

Raper, Howard: Critical analysis of three radiodontic technics introduction. *Dent Surv,* June, 1955, p. 731.

Raper, Howard: Mathematical angulation technic. *Dent Surv,* July, 1955, p. 863.

Raper, Howard: Criticism of mathematical angulation technic, *Dent Surv,* August, 1955, p. 986.

Raper, Howard: Advantages and disadvantages of three radiodontic technics, *Dent Surv,* November, 1955, p. 1404.

Satterlee, F. LeRoy: *Dental Radiology*. New York, Swenarton Stationery, 1914.

Sweet, A. Porter: William Herbert Rollins, D.D.S., M.D. dentistry's forgotten man. *Dent Radiogr Photogr,* 33:3, 1960.

Sweet, A. Porter: Some historical aspects of radiodontics. *Dent Radiogr Photogr,* 15:9-11, 1942.

Thoma, Kurt H.: *Oral Roentgenology*. Boston, Ritter, 1917, pp. 11-15.

Thoma, Kurt H.: *Oral and Dental Diagnosis,* 3rd ed. Philadelphia, W. B. Saunders, 1949, p. ix.

Thompson, Walter S.: *Operative and Interpretive Radiodontia*. Philadelphia, Lea & Febiger, 1936, pp. 2-20.

Trout, E. Dale, and Kelley, John: The evolution of equipment for dental radiography. *J Ontario Dent Assoc,* 35:10-18, September, 1958.

Wuehrmann, Arthur: The long cone technic. *Prac Dent Monogr,* July, 1957, pp. 3-4.

CHAPTER 2

X-RAYS
AND THEIR
PRODUCTION

Definition of Terminology

W HEN WILHELM CONRAD ROENTGEN announced to the world the discovery of a new kind of ray, he called it the x-ray after the algebraic symbol for an unknown quantity. The scientific world for the most part called it the "roentgen ray" in honor of the discoverer.

Radiology: A broad term meaning the science of ionizing radiations, encompassing radium and other radioactive materials as well as x-rays. *Radi* means radiation and *ology* means the study of or science of. It is a branch of the medical sciences that deals with the use of radiation in the diagnosis and treatment of disease.

Roentgenology: A science of roentgen rays (or x-rays) solely and includes the taking of x-ray pictures, their interpretation, and the use of x-rays in the treatment of disease (therapeutic use).

Radiograph: A shadow picture produced by x-rays or roentgen rays on a photographic film. The word can be used as a verb or a noun. Some of the synonyms used for the word "radiograph" are roentgenograph, roentgenogram, radiogram, skiagraph, skiagram, shadowgram. The authors prefer term, "radiograph," because it has more

common usage and is less cumbersome than "roentgenogram."

Radiography: The art and science of making radiographs. Synonyms used for "radiography" are actinography, roentgenography, and skiagraphy. The authors prefer the words "radiography" and "radiographic" rather than "roentgenography" and "roentgenographic" for the same reasons as given above.

Dental Radiography

Dental radiography, for the most part, deals with projection, exposure, and processing technics. These technics are based on the knowledge of the fundamentals of ionizing radiation, its production, and the potential hazards involved. Therefore, it is important that the student of dental radiography be familiar with the nature of x-rays, their production, and methods for protection in order to better inable himself to operate and maintain dental x-ray equipment with precision, safety and confidence. In this way, the student will better prepare himself to produce quality radiographs routinely.

The Structure of the Atom

In order to understand the nature of x-rays, it is important to be familiar with the structure of the atom.

Matter is defined as a physical manifestation possessing mass (occupies space and has weight). All matter is composed of atoms. There are at present 103 known types of atoms. The structure of the atom can be described as a miniature solar system. Each atom consists of a small dense *nucleus,* which has a positive electric charge, and with a number of lighter particles with negative charges called *electrons* moving around the nucleus in definite orbits.

The atom is said to be neutral when the net number of positive charges of the nucleus equals the negative charges of the orbital electrons. The electrons are kept in their orbits by the balance between (1) the electrostatic attraction of unlike charges and (2) the centrifugal forces of the fast moving electrons.

The nucleus is composed of protons and neutrons. These particles are called nucleons. Protons carry a positive charge, which is equal to in magnitude, but opposite in size to the charge carried by the electrons. The neutrons carry no electrical charge (See Figure 2-1).

The mass of the atom is derived mainly from the nucleons. The mass of a proton or a neutron is approximately 1,836 times that of an electron. Although the electrons have very little mass, they do occupy a great deal of space within the atom. For example, if the atom was increased to the size of a convention hall, the nucleus would occupy the center of the hall with the size of a pinhead.

Orbital Electrons

The electron of the atom revolves around the nucleus in well-defined shells or specific areas that exist at varying distances from the nucleus. A maximum number of seven potential electron-containing shells exist. No known atom contains more than seven shells. These seven shells are designated as K, L, M, N, O, P, Q in order of increasing distance from the nucleus. Each orbit or shell holds only a certain maximum number of electrons (See Figure 2-2).

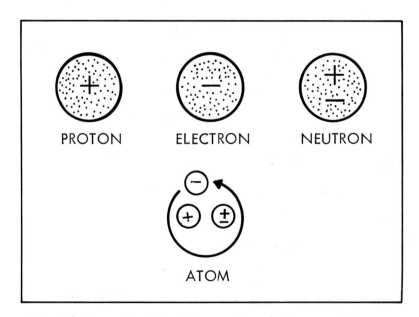

Figure 2-1. Upper: Particles of the atom. Bottom: Structure of the atom.

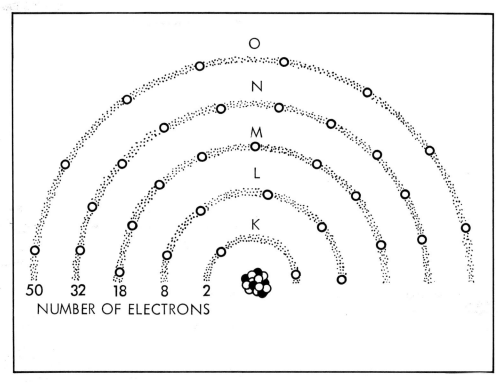

Figure 2.2. Schematic representation of a tungsten atom. (Courtesy of Dr. Michel Ter-Pogossian.)

K-shell	2 electrons
L-shell	8 electrons
M-shell	18 electrons
N-shell	32 electrons
O-shell	50 electrons
P-shell	72 electrons
Q-shell	98 electrons

Each shell has a different energy level. Electrons are bound to the nucleus by an electrostatic force of attraction resulting from the positive electrical charge of the nucleus and the negative charge of the electrons. The attractive force is dependent upon the atomic number of the atom and the distance the electron is from the nucleus. This is referred to as the binding energy of an electron in a particular shell. It is a negative energy because it is the amount of energy required to remove an electron from a shell. The binding energy is greatest nearest the nucleus and diminishes with increasing distances away from the nucleus.

Energy is measured by the amount of work it does or the amount of work it is capable of doing. The most useful unit of energy for our purposes is the *electron-volt*. It is the kinetic energy of an electron accelerated through a potential difference of 1 volt (1 eV = 1.6 × 10^{-19} joule).*

For example, the binding energies of

_____

* 1 KeV = 1,000 eV, 1 MeV = 1 million eV.

the K, L, and M shells of tungsten are 70 KeV, 11 KeV, and 2.5 KeV respectfully. In order to remove a K shell electron from tungsten it would require an energy of 70 KeV.

Since the electrons in the inner shells have greater binding energies, it takes x-rays, gamma rays or high-energy particles to remove electrons from these shells. Electrons in the outer shells are not held so tightly to the nucleus, and therefore, can be affected by lesser energies, such as visible light rays and ultraviolet rays.

Ionization

Normally, the atom contains the same number of electrons and protons, and therefore, the positive and negative charges balance and the atom is said to be "electrically neutral."

However, many of the elements have incompletely filled outer shells, which tend to capture electrons quite readily from adjacent atoms. Of course, when this occurs, the atom has more electrons than it should, and it becomes a negative atom. When atoms lose electrons, they become deficient in negative charges and, therefore, will behave as a positively charged atom. An atom which is not electrically balanced is called an ion.

In any ionization process, ion pairs are formed, and it is this process that elicits chemical changes in matter.

Isotopes

The total number of nucleons (protons and neutrons) in the nucleus is called the mass number (Symbol A). The number of protons in the nucleus as well as the number of electrons outside the nucleus defines the element and is referred to as its atomic number (Symbol Z). All atoms of a given element have the same atomic number (Z). However, atoms may have different mass numbers (A). These different forms of an element are called isotopes. They are composed of nuclei with the same number of protons (Z) but with a different number of neutrons. By subtracting the atomic number (Z) from the mass number (A) the neutrons in the nucleus of an isotope may be calculated.

Isotopes of a given element have identical chemical properties; however, they differ in their physical properties. Various isotopes of an element are separated by means of a mass spectrometer. For example, the atomic weight of zinc (atomic number 30) is 65.38. This is an average of the mixture of proportions of the isotopes of zinc with masses (A) of 64, 66, 67, 68, and 70.

Nature of X-Rays

Radiation can be defined as the propagation and emission of energy through space or a material medium.

All radiations can be divided into two groups (1) corpuscular or particulate radiations and (2) electromagnetic radiations.

Corpuscular radiations are actually minute particles of matter that travel in straight lines at high speeds from their sources. Although incredibly small, they possess mass. All are charged electrically, except the neutrons, and they all move extremely fast, in fact, sometimes almost as fast as light. Examples of corpuscular radiation are:

1. *Electrons*
   a. *Beta rays:* negative electrons or

positive electrons (positron) which arise from radioactive nuclei.

Beta radiation is more penetrating than alpha radiation and has an average path of penetration in tissues from a few millimeters up to a centimeter or more before they are absorbed.

b. *Cathode rays* are streams of electrons passing from the hot filament of the cathode to the target or anode in an x-ray tube. Their speed is one third the speed of light, more or less, depending on the impressed voltage.

2. *Alpha Rays* are accelerated helium nuclei $(Z = 2, A = 4)$. They have little ability to penetrate tissues, and they give up their large energies within a very short distance in the air.

3. *Protons* are accelerated hydrogen nuclei (weight of 1 and a charge of $+ 1$).

4. *The neutron* is the other subatomic particle in the atom nucleus. It carries no electrical charge and the mass of hydrogen atom. The characteristic of being electrically neutral has proved of great importance in nuclear physics since such a particle can penetrate into the nucleus of an atom without being subjected to the enormous forces of repulsion that resist the entrance of a positively charged particle.

Electromagnetic Radiation

Electromagnetic radiation is the propagation of the wave-like energy (which has no mass) through space or matter. It is called electromagnetic radiation because the energy which is radiated is accompanied by oscillating electric and magnetic fields.

Each field is in phase with and perpendicular to each other and perpendicular to the direction of wave propagations (See Figure 2-3).

Examples of electromagnetic radiation are:

1. The radio waves that we hear.
2. The light waves we see.
3. The infrared waves that can take pictures in the dark.
4. The ultraviolet rays that we use to treat skin diseases and that also cause sunburn.

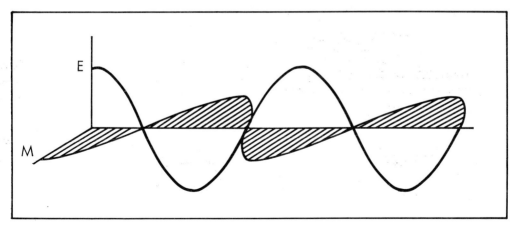

Figure 2-3. Simplified diagram of an electromagnetic wave. The electric (e) and magnetic fields (m) are at right angles to each other. (Courtesy of Dr. William Hendee.)

5. The x-rays that you will be studying.
6. The gamma rays of the atomic bomb.
7. The cosmic rays, which at the moment, hinder our travel in space.

Wave Motion

We shall first consider wave motion since x-rays, light, radiowaves and gamma rays are all propagated by means of wave motion.

All waves are associated with *wavelength, frequency,* and *velocity.* The *wavelength* (λ) is the distance between the crest of one wave to the crest of the next, measured in Angstrom (Å) units ($1\text{Å} = 10^{-8}$ cm) for the short waves and centimeters or meters for the longer waves. The *frequency* of a wave (n) is the number of vibrations the wave makes per second or the number of times the wave rises to its crest and falls to its trough in a second. Frequencies are usually given in hertz (hz). A hertz equals one cycle per second.

All electromagnetic waves travel with a *velocity* of 3.0×10^8 m/sec or 186,000 miles per second in a vacuum. The velocity is usually referred to as c. (See Figure 2-4).

For electromagnetic waves the following relationship exists:

Wavelength (in meters) × Frequency (in cycles per second) = velocity (meters per second). $\lambda \, n = c$ (3×10^8 m/sec).

Since the velocity is always known, the wavelength of the radiation can be determined if the frequency is known, and conversely, the frequency if the wavelength is known. Also, it holds true that if the frequency of the wave is high, the wavelength will be short, and if the frequency is low the wavelength will have to be long (See Figure 2-4).

When the wavelengths change, the properties change. For example, the longer waves of the electromagnetic spectrum are utilized for communication (e.g. radar, television, and radiowaves).

The distance from the crest of one wave to the crest of another wave in the

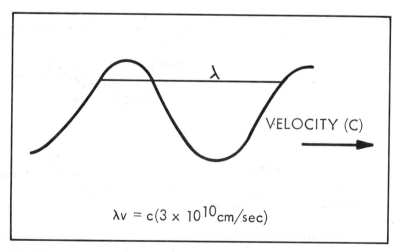

Figure 2-4. Diagram of an electromagnetic wave illustrating the meaning of wavelength.

standard broadcast portion of radio waves is as long as a football field. The length of television waves is approximately one to five yards. The electromagnetic waves in which we are interested are very short in wavelength and it is convenient to express their length in Angstrom units, where $1Å = 10^{-8}$ cm. Whenever the eye receives a certain wavelength within the visible portion of the spectrum (from 3,800 Å to 8,000 Å) we have been trained to call it a certain color: red, orange, yellow, green, blue, indigo, or violet (Roy G. Biv). If the wavelength is longer than 8,000 Å, the human eye cannot detect it and we refer to the radiation as infrared. If the wavelength is shorter than 3,800 Å, the radiation is again invisible to the eye and is called ultraviolet. The useful range in medical and dental radiography comprises wavelengths of between 0.1Å to 0.5Å.

The Electromagnetic Spectrum

X-rays constitute a portion of the electromagnetic wave spectrum, which is a series of radiant energies arranged in order of their wavelengths (See Figure 2-20). It should be noted that regions of the spectrum overlap, and that there is no sharp change in properties as we change from one region to another. Also, it should be emphasized that there is essentially no difference between the properties of Gamma rays and x-rays. The only difference is that x-rays are produced by events outside the nucleus of the atom, and gamma rays arise within the nucleus.

All of the energies of the electromagnetic spectrum possess certain properties which they have in common. They are listed below:

1. They have no mass (weight) or electrical charge (neutral polarity).
2. They travel with the speed or velocity of light waves in a vacuum (186,000 miles/second or 3×10^{10} centimeters/second).
3. They all travel with wave motion.
4. As they travel through space, they propagate an electric field at right angles to their path of travel. At right angle to this electric field, a magnetic field is formed; hence the name—electromagnetic wave.

Dual Nature of X-Rays

As the wavelength becomes very short and the corresponding frequency very high it is necessary to consider the *quantum* nature of x-radiation. Although we consider electromagnetic radiations as traveling in waves, we must also think of the x-rays as particles traveling with a velocity (c) and each carrying a certain amount of energy. This bundle of energy is called a quantum or photon. By combining the electromagnetic wave theory with the quantum theory, x-rays can be thought of as small particles of energy called quanta or photons existing in waveform. The dual nature of x-rays is inseparable. For instance, to know the energy in a single quantum or photon, it is necessary to know the frequency of the wavelength. One quantum is equal to the product of the frequency and a constant, represented by the letter *h*, called "Planck's constant," after the originator of the quantum theory of radiation. The quantum is the fundamental unit of x-ray energy and is measured in joules.* The equation for the energy of a quantum is as follows:

E   =   h   x   n

Energy   Planck's   Frequency
in   constant   (1/sec.)
joules   (joule sec.)

(h = 6.61 × 10^{-34} joule sec.)

In radiology, it is preferred to express the energy of electromagnetic radiation in electron volts† rather than in joules.

This can be done by use of the following conversion formula:

$$E \text{ (electron volts)} = \frac{12,400}{\lambda \text{ (wavelength in angstroms)}}$$

What Are X-Rays?

X-rays, then, are weightless packages of pure energy (photons) that are without electrical charge that travel in waves with a specific frequency at a speed of 3 × 10^{10} cm/sec. Their energies depend upon the frequency of their wavelengths. The greater the frequency of the wavelength, the greater will be the energy of the photon.

Properties of X-Rays

To gain still more understanding of x-rays, it is necessary for you to know a little more of how they act and what they do. Fundamentally, x-rays obey all of the laws of light, but among their special properties certain ones are of interest to the student of dental radiography.

---

* The fundamental unit of work is the joule. It is the product of the force exerted and the distance through which the force acts.

† The electron volt is the amount of energy released when an electron falls through a potential difference of one volt. For many purposes, a unit 1,000 times as large, the KEV, is useful.

1. X-rays are invisible and weightless. You cannot see, hear, feel, or smell them.

2. X-rays travel in straight lines. They can be deflected from their original direction, but the new trajectory is linear.

3. X-rays travel at the speed of light (186,000 miles/second).

4. X-rays have a wide range of wavelengths between 0.8 Å to 0.5 Å in length.

5. X-rays cannot be focused to a point.

6. X-rays have extremely short wavelengths which enables them to penetrate opaque substances that absorb or reflect visible light.

7. X-rays are differentially absorbed by matter. This absorption depends on the atomic structure of the matter and the wavelength of the x-rays.

8. X-rays can ionize gases. They do this by increasing the electrical conductivity of a gas through which they pass. This effect is brought about by the rays actually disrupting the atoms and the molecules of the air by the process of dissociation.

9. X-rays cause certain substances to fluoresce, that is to emit radiation in longer wavelengths, e.g. visible light and ultraviolet light.

10. X-rays affect photographic film emulsions, similar to the action of light, producing a latent image that can be made visible by film processing.

11. X-rays cause biologic changes (somatic and genetic), a fact that

necessitates caution in the use of x-radiation.

How Are X-Rays Produced?

X-rays are produced by the sudden deceleration or stoppage of a rapidly moving stream of electrons at a metal target in a high vacuum tube (See Figure 2-5). The most efficient method of generating x-rays is by an x-ray tube. An x-ray tube in principle is a simple electronic tube, highly evacuated, containing a positive and a negative electrode, with a filament in relation to the negative electrode (cathode) to supply electrons. When high voltage is applied to the tube, electrons leave the cathode and are accelerated at high speed toward the anode (positive electrode). Because of the vacuum the electrons are not impeded by collisions with air atoms. The

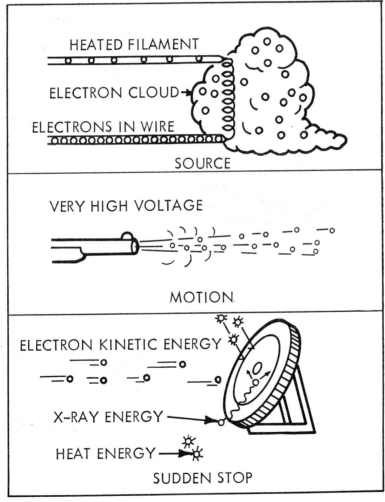

Figure 2-5. The production of x-rays by the sudden stoppage or deceleration of rapidly moving electrons.

high energy electrons strike the anode, are suddenly arrested, and their kinetic energy is transformed into heat with the exception of a small portion which appears as the electromagnetic energy of x-rays. For ordinary medical and dental units, this fraction is very small, usually being less than 1 percent of the total energy.

Two types of x-rays are produced by the conventional diagnostic x-ray tube. They are:

1. Bremsstrahlung or General Radiation
2. Characteristic Radiation

Bremsstrahlung or General Radiation

Most of the x-rays produced are called bremsstrahlung, white, or general radiation. Bremsstrahlung is derived from two

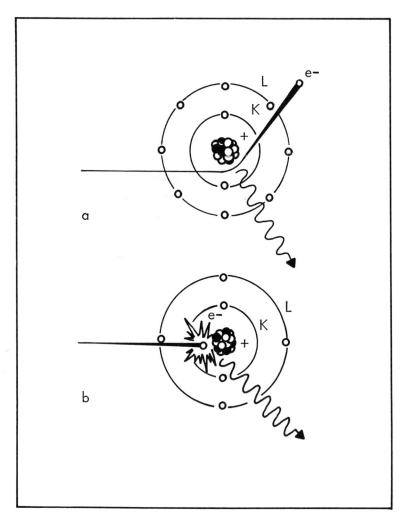

Figure 2-6. Generation of general or white radiation. (Bremsstrahlung) by interaction of electron of the nucleus: (a) impinging electron deflected and decelerated, (b) total kinetic energy of impinging electron is converted into x-radiation. (Courtesy of Dr. Michel Ter-Pogossian.)

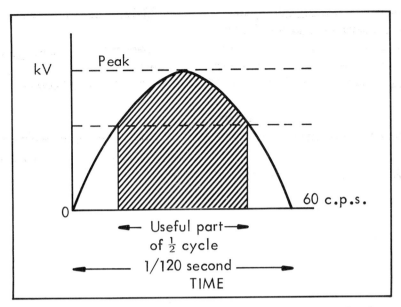

Figure 2-7. Variation in voltage which occurs during a single half-cycle of current in a typical x-ray generator. (Courtesy of F. Jaundrell-Thompson.)

German words: *bremse* meaning "brake" and *strahl* meaning "ray." It is called "braking radiation" because the radiation is produced by deceleration or braking high-speed electrons. When a negatively charged cathode electron travels close to the nucleus of a tungsten atom, the positively charged nucleus will deflect the electron, and consequently, decelerate it. This, in time, will produce a loss of energy, which is given off in the form of electromagnetic radiation. Sometimes, there will be a collision between a cathode electron and the nucleus of a tungsten atom. In this case, the energy given off is equal to the total kinetic energy of the cathode electron (See Figure 2-6).

Bremsstrahlung radiation is often referred to as continuous or white radiation because like white light, it consists of a continuous range of wavelengths.

The x-ray beam produced by the x-ray tube has a wide distribution of wavelengths which is due for the most part to a combination of two factors:

1. The cathode electrons have different energies when they arrive at the tungsten target. One of the reasons for this is that there is a variation in the voltage in a conventional x-ray tube. The x-ray tube is not energized by a constant potential. Since the energies of the cathode electrons are dependent on the kilovoltages of the x-ray tube, the resultant energies of the cathode electrons will vary accordingly (See Figure 2-7).

2. Cathode electrons lose their energies in a random fashion when they interact with tungsten atom nuclei. A very few of them lose all their energy in one interaction. Most of them lose their energies gradually in stages, which produces x-rays of

lower energy than maximum. This gives use to a wide range of x-rays having energies forming a continuous wavelength spectrum (See Figure 2-8).

Characteristic or Line Radiation

Characteristic or line radiation is produced when cathode electrons of sufficient energy collide with electrons of one of the innermost shells and ejects the electron from the atom. This leaves a hole or vacancy within this shell or energy level. Almost immediately this vacancy is filled by an electron from one of the shells farther from the nucleus. As the vacancy is filled, electromagnetic radiation is given off. This radiation is called characteristic because the radiation given off is characteristic of differences in binding energies of electrons in a specific atom. For example, binding energy of the K shell of tungsten is approximately 70 keV. It will take a cathode electron of at least 70 keV in order to get an electron of the K shell out of

the tungsten atom. Once an electron from the K shell is removed, any electron from one of the L, M, or outer shells of the atom may drop into the K-shell vacancy. If an electron of the M-shell (2.8 keV) moves into the vacancy, the characteristic radiation given off would be equal to the difference between the binding energies of the K-shell and the M-shell or 68.2 keV (70 keV − 2.8 keV = 68.2 keV). There are various other transitions that may take place when the K-shell is removed by a cathode electron. See Figure 2-9 for illustration of these various transitions. Hardly any characteristic radiation is produced below 70 kVp, and relatively few characteristic x-rays are produced under 100 kVp.

Usually, the wavelengths of characteristic radiation are relatively long in comparison to the greater part of the general spectrum. This type of radiation is easily absorbed by the glass walls of the tube, the aluminum filter, or living tissue. See Figure 2-8 for illustration of the intensity and wavelengths of charac-

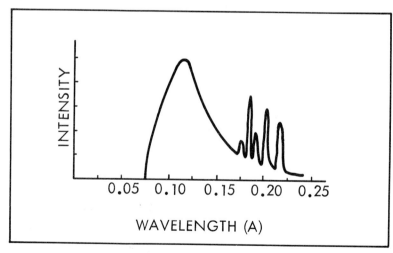

Figure 2.8. Illustration of the intensity and wavelengths of characteristic radiation on comparison to the general spectrum of radiation. (Courtesy of F. Jaundrell-Thompson.)

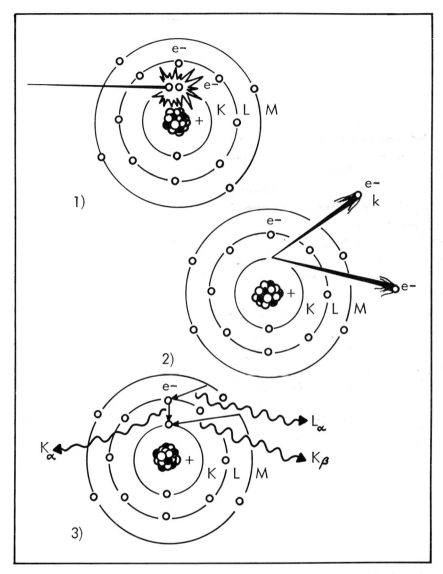

Figure 2-9. Generation of characteristic radiation. (1) collision of impinging electron with K-electron. (2) Removal of K-electron from atom by impinging electron. (3) Generation of three photons of characteristic radiation (Courtesy of Dr. Michel Ter-Pogossian).

teristic radiation in comparison to the general spectrum of radiation.

X-Ray Tube

The x-ray tube used in dental radiography is called the "hot cathode" or Coolidge tube. The tube is sealed in a lead glass envelope, from which air has been pumped, which contains two important parts—the cathode and the anode. The air is removed from the tube to prevent ionization of gas molecules during electron movement toward the tungsten target. The basic principles of the "hot cathode" tube are as follows:

1. The filament must be heated for a source of electrons. The higher the temperature, the more electrons freed by *thermionic* emission (See Figure 2-10).
2. When the kilovoltage is applied, electrons are driven from the filament (cathode) to the target (anode).
3. When no kilovoltage is supplied, electrons will form a cloud around the filament of the tube.

4. If the kilovoltage supplies the electrons with enough speed, x-rays will be produced when the electrons hit the target.

Cathode

The cathode of an x-ray tube is the negative side of the tube. It consists of a tungsten wire (filament) wound in the form of a spiral set in a molybdenum cup-shaped holder (called a focusing cup). The cathode has two separate circuits (See Fig. 2-11).

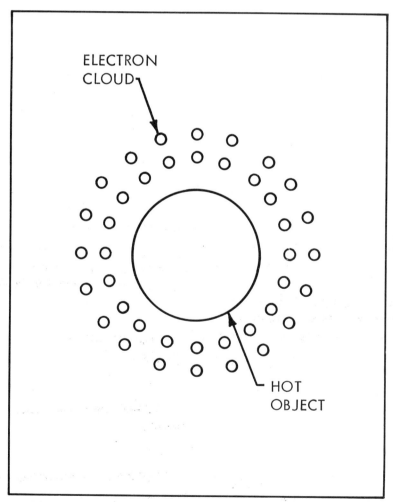

ELECTRON CLOUD

HOT OBJECT

Figure 2-10. Electron emission from hot object. (Courtesy of General Electric Co.)

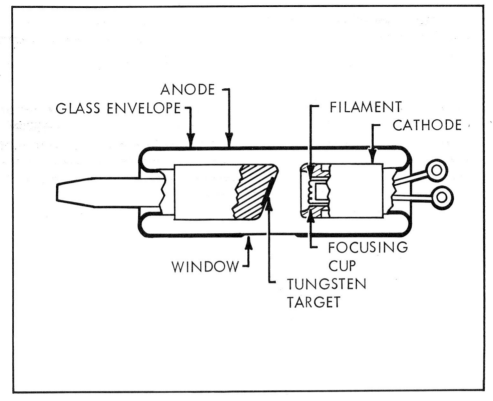

Figure 2-11. The stationary-anode tube. (Courtesy of Eastman-Kodak Co.)

Tungsten is used for the filament because it can stand a great deal of heat without melting. The filament is heated by a low voltage circuit. It also is connected to one end of the step-up transformer which provides the high voltage necessary to set electrons in motion. The molybdenum focusing cup is negatively charged and focuses the electron stream so that it will hit only a tiny area on the target of the anode (See Figure 2-12).

The filament uses 8 to 12 volts and from 3 to 5 amperes when in operation to heat the filament and boil off the electrons. The electrons are then accelerated across a 1″ or so gap to the target of the anode by the electrical field which the high potential gradient (60-100 kilo-

volts) produces. Bombardment of the target of the anode by these high-speed electrons produces x-rays. The voltage applied across the tube determines the maximum energy of the x-rays produced.

Anode

The anode is the positive side of the x-ray tube. You will find that there are two types of anodes—the stationary anode and the rotating anode. The stationary anode is used in dental x-ray machines and the rotating anode is employed in the larger medical x-ray machines.

The stationary anode is usually formed of copper and extends from one end of the tube to the center. A small block of

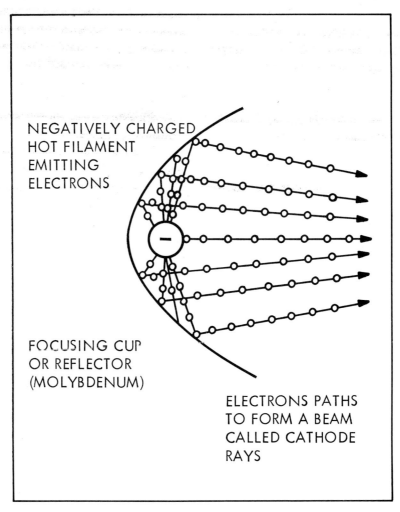

NEGATIVELY CHARGED
HOT FILAMENT
EMITTING
ELECTRONS

FOCUSING CUP
OR REFLECTOR
(MOLYBDENUM)

ELECTRONS PATHS
TO FORM A BEAM
CALLED CATHODE
RAYS

Figure 2-12. The formation of electron beam by focusing device. (Courtesy of General Electric Co.)

tungsten is set in the anode face. This is called the *target*. Tungsten is used for the target since it is a metal relatively efficient in x-ray production and one that will withstand a great amount of heat. Copper is used because it is a good conductor of heat. Although tungsten can withstand a great amount of heat, it can be damaged if it receives too much heat. When electrons hit the target only about .2 percent of their kinetic energy is con-

verted into x-rays, and the other 99.8 percent is converted into heat. (Ionization in the outermost shells of tungsten produces only heat.) Copper conducts the heat away from the tungsten target dissipating it into air, water, gas, or most often into oil. Most of the x-ray manufacturers at the present time use oil-immersed tubes. If the heat is not removed, the tungsten target will melt or become "pitted." This destroys the usefulness of the tube. The small area of the target that most of the electrons strike is called the *focal spot,* and is the source of the x-radiation. The size of the focal spot has a very important effect upon the sharpness of the x-ray film image. The smaller the focal spot, the sharper the x-ray image. However, the smaller the focal spot becomes the less heat the focal spot will be able to absorb at one time. Some method had to be found to obtain a practical size of the focal spot which would provide image detail. The *Benson line focus* principle is such a method and is employed in the stationary anode tubes (See Figure 2-13).

The target face is made at an angle of 20° to the cathode as shown in the diagram. When the rectangular focal spot is viewed from below—in the position of the film—it appears more nearly

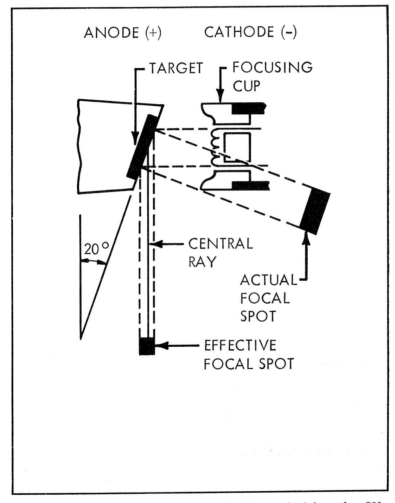

Figure 2-13. Diagram showing how use of the line-focus principle and a 20° angle of target face (anode) provides a small effective focal spot. (Courtesy of Eastman Kodak Co.)

square. This is called the "effective focal spot." Thus, the projected focus or "effective focal spot" is only a fraction of the actual focal spot. By using x-rays that emerge at this angle, *radiographic definition* is improved while the *heat capacity* of the anode is increased because the electron stream is spread over a greater area. The "effective focal spot" of most dental x-ray tubes measures approximately 1 mm to 1.5 sq mm depending upon the manufacturer.

Rotating Anode

The *rotating anode* was developed to allow for greater exposures on the target. This type of anode has the tungsten target rotating during the bombardment of the electrons. In this way the electrons are still focused to a certain small area, but the surface that they are striking is always new. Because of this the heat is not concentrated in one particular area but is spread over a much larger area.

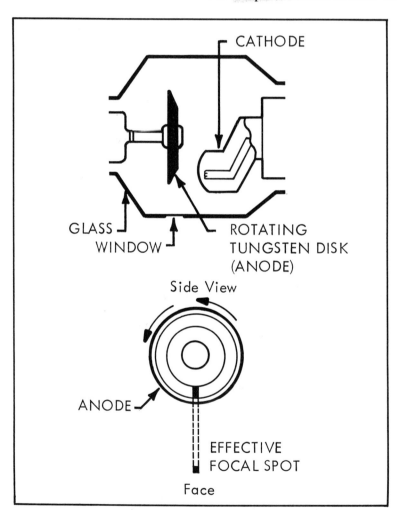

Figure 2-14. Diagram of side view (upper) and face of rotating anode (bottom). (Courtesy of Eastman Kodak Co.)

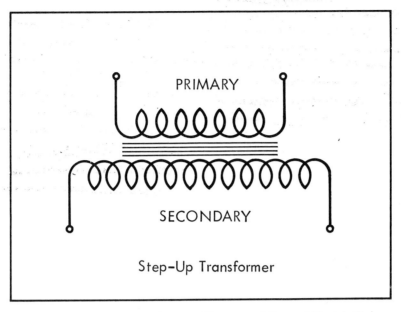

Figure 2-15. Step-up transformer. (Courtesy of General Electric Co.)

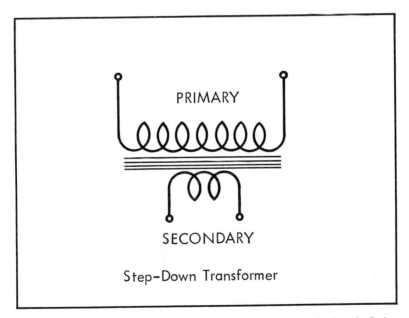

Figure 2-16. Step-down transformer. (Courtesy of General Electric Co.)

The larger medical diagnostic x-ray machines use the rotating anode principle (See Figure 2-14).

X-Ray Generating Apparatus

To complete the story of the production of x-rays, a brief description of the generating apparatus is needed. The devices, aside from the x-ray tube, are:

1. A high-voltage or step-up transformer
2. A step-down transformer
3. An autotransformer

A *transformer* is an electromagnetic device for changing an alternating current voltage to a higher or lower alternating curent voltage. This is made possible by the principles of "mutual induction." Voltage is induced in the secondary winding when energy is applied to the primary winding. The voltages in the two windings are directly proportional to the number of turns of wire in each—assuming a theoretical 100 percent efficiency. The transformer that has more turns of wire in the secondary coil or winding than in the primary coil is known as a *step-up transformer* (See Figure 2-15).

A transformer which has more turns in the primary than in the secondary coil or winding is called a *step-down transformer* (See Figure 2-16).

The step-up or high-voltage transform-

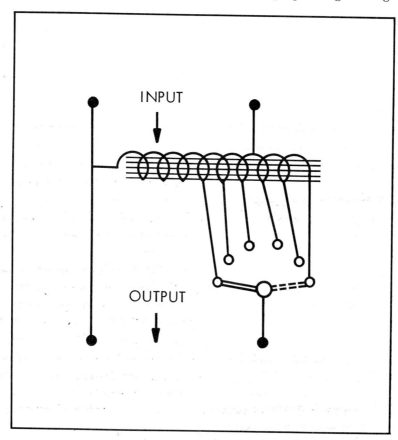

INPUT

OUTPUT

Figure 2-17. Autotransformer. (Courtesy of General Electric Co.)

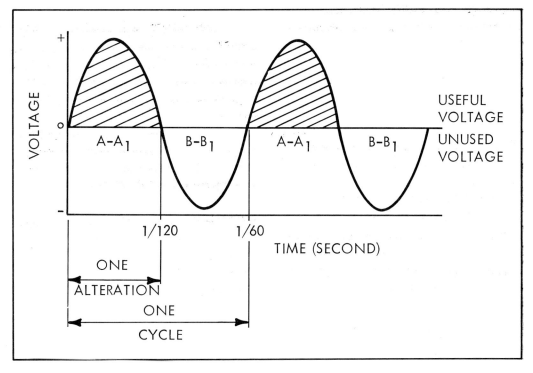

Figure 2-18. Voltage is applied to the tube electrodes in an alternating or pulsating manner.

er is used to produce very high voltages which will drive the electrons across the tube to the target. Dental x-ray machines can use either 110 or 220 line voltages. The 220 voltage is preferred. Voltages of between 60,000 to 100,000 volts can be induced in the secondary circuits of the step-up transformers depending upon the machine.

A *step-down transformer* is used to reduce the line voltage to 8 to 12 volts which results in a higher current (amperes) to heat the filament.

Since dental radiographic technics require a wide variety of kilovoltages, another type of transformer, the *autotransformer* is used. The autotransformer adjusts the line voltage so that the primary of the step-up or high-voltage transform-

er has a variable and predetermined supply. The result is that the kilovoltage can be preselected at the autotransformer before the x-ray exposure is actually made. The device is called an autotransformer because the primary and secondary windings are combined in one winding (See Figure 2-17).

Rectification is the process of changing alternating current into a pulsating direct current. Alternating current is a 60-cycle current—it flows first in one direction and then it flows in the opposite direction—changing directions every 1/120 of a second. It makes a complete cycle—back and forth—every 1/60 of a second, and makes 60 cycles every second (See Figure 2-18).

Since the electrons must flow in only

one direction from the cathode to the anode within the x-ray tube, some means of rectification is necessary. There are two types of rectification:

1. self-rectification
2. value-tube rectification

Self-rectification is the type used in dental x-ray machines and the valve-tube type is found in the larger medical x-ray units.

Self-Rectification

In this type the x-ray tube acts as its own rectifier. The anode is positive first and then negative with respect to the cathode during each half-cycle (every 1/120th of a second). When the anode is positive, the electrons are attracted to the anode from the negative cathode, conversely, when the anode is negative, there is no attraction for the electrons. Hence, there is no current in the tube—no electron stream—and no x-radiation. The unused half-cycle is called inverse voltage. The x-ray tube acts as its own rectifier, and the tube produces x-rays in a series of pulses or bursts (See Figure 2-19).

Valve-Tube Rectification

As it becomes necessary for x-ray tubes to carry more power, as in the larger

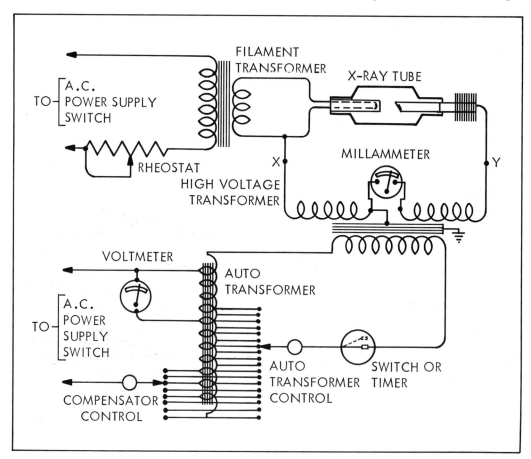

Figure 2-19. Typical dental x-ray circuit: Self rectified circuit for generation of x-rays.

medical x-ray units, it is desirable to prevent them from operating as self-rectifiers and to find some means of preventing the inverse voltage from being applied to the x-ray tube. This is accomplished by introducing valve tubes into the high-voltage circuit. This results in maximum efficiency of the equipment.

X-Ray Timers

There are several types of timers that may be found in an x-ray machine. Exposure time is the amount of time that you are impressing the high voltage across the x-ray tube. This time may be controlled in several ways:

(1) The mechanical timer is the hand timer found on the older dental x-ray units. When the button is pushed it closes the circuit and allows the voltage to flow. When the exposure time is expended, the circuit is broken. These timers are usually inaccurate under one second exposure time.

(2) The *synchronous timer* uses a synchronous motor. It is called a synchronous timer because the motor which runs it must rotate at the same speed as the alternating current or generator which supplies the power. It is limited because of this fact and cannot be faster than the generator running it.

(3) The *impulse timer* gets down to 1/120th of a second but it is used more commonly at 1/60th of a second. Remember that alternating 60 cycle current has two impulses or alterations each cycle. If you are using 1/60th of a second you would be impressing the voltage across the tube for the time it takes to produce two impulses of the current.

(4) The *electronic timer* is a device that enables the operator to use 1/30th of a second on up. Most of the modern dental x-ray units use this type of timer. The electronic timer has two electronic circuits—one called the *time delay circuit* to delay the start of the exposure for about .5 of a second in order to preheat the x-ray tube and one called the *timing circuit* which stops the x-ray exposure at the end of the time preselected by the operator. The x-ray tube filament is preheated in order to obtain full electron emission at the start of the exposure.

Comparison of Roentgen Rays, Gamma Rays and Cosmic Rays

As pointed out previously, roentgen rays occupy roughly the same portion of the electromagnetic spectrum as gamma rays and in many ways are identical to them (See Figure 2-20). Like x-rays, gamma radiation can pass through solid material and the mode of interaction of both roentgen rays and gamma rays with matter is the same. The biological and photographic effects are also identical. Roentgen rays and gamma rays differ only in their origin. Roentgen rays are man-made and are produced artificially in x-ray tubes, whereas gamma rays emanate from radioactive naturally-occurring substances such as radium.

Continuing up the spectrum one encounters the shortest known waves—cosmic waves. These are extremely penetrating forms of radiation of unknown origin (probably coming from interstellar space) and continuously bombard the earth's population with small but measurable amounts of both particulate and electromagnetic forms of radiation. Cos-

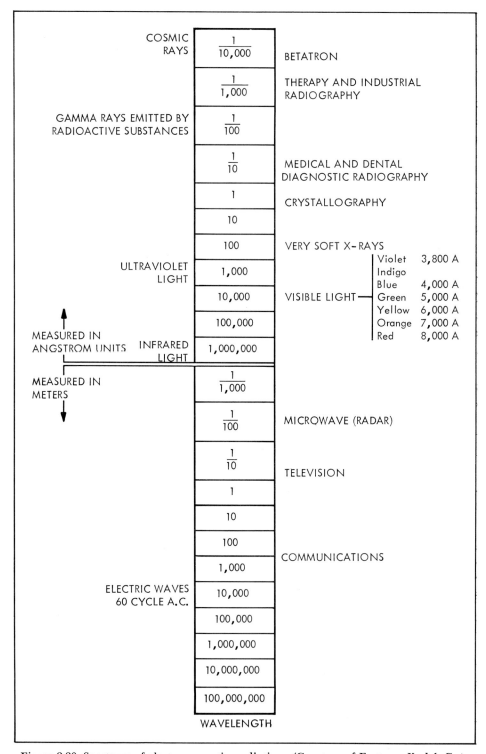

Figure 2-20. Spectrum of electromagnetic radiation. (Courtesy of Eastman Kodak Co.)

mic rays are a source of background radiation.

These rays have extraordinarily high penetrating power and will pass through at least 200 feet of water—so great is their penetrating power that it may be detected readily through 36 inches of lead. Cosmic radiation poses a major problem in space travel for the future, but much information is being obtained by earth satellites.

REFERENCES

Beck, James O.: *Syllabus of Oral Radiology.* University of Minnesota, School of Dentistry, 1970.

Fundamentals of Radiography, 10th ed. Rochester, N. Y., Eastman Kodak Co., 1960.

Goodwin, Paul N., Quimby, Edith H., and Morgan, Russell H.: *Physical Foundations of Radiology,* 4th ed. New York, Harper & Row, 1970.

Heidersdorf, S. D.: X-ray fundamentals. *Dental Radiological Health Course Manual.* Cincinnati, Robert A. Taft Sanitary Engineering Center, U. S. Dept. of Health, Education and Welfare, January, 1961.

Hendee, William R.: *Medical Radiation Physics.* Chicago, Year Book Medical Publishers, 1970.

Herz, R. H.: *The Photographic Action of Ionizing Radiations.* New York, John Wiley & Sons, 1969.

Hodges, F. J., Lampe, I., and Holt, J. F.: *Radiology for Medical Students,* 3rd ed. Chicago, Year Book Medical Publishers, 1961.

Johns, Harold E.: *The Physics of Radiology,* 3rd ed. Springfield, Ill., Charles C Thomas, 1969.

Muncheryan, H. M.: *Modern Physics of Roentgenology.* Los Angeles, Wetzel, 1940.

Peterson, Shailer: *Clinical Dental Hygiene.* St. Louis, C. V. Mosby, 1959.

Radiology Specialist. Department of the Air Force, Washington, D. C., 1958.

Seemann, Herman: *Physical and Photographic Principles of Medical Radiology.* London, John Wiley & Sons, New York, 1968.

Stewart, Oscar M.: *Physics.* Chicago, Ginn and Co., 1931.

Ter-Pogossian, Michel M.: *The Physical Aspects of Diagnostic Radiology.* New York, Hoeber Medical Div., Harper & Row, 1967.

Thompson, Jaundrell, F.: *X-ray Physics and Equipment.* 2nd ed. Philadelphia, F. A. Davis, 1970.

X-Ray Generation and Radiographic Principles in Dentistry. General Electric X-ray Department, Milwaukee.

CHAPTER 3

THE X-RAY BEAM AND IMAGE FORMATION

Intensity of X-Ray Beam

THE ABILITY to control independently both the *quality* and *intensity* of radiation makes the x-ray unit an invaluable tool in modern dental radiography.

Intensity can be described, as in the case of light, as the brightness or brilliance of the x-ray beam. It is the rate that energy is propagated through a unit area perpendicular to the beam. Intensity always involves a quantity per unit of time ($I = \frac{Q}{t}$).

The *intensity* of the x-ray beam at a particular kilovoltage depends on the *number of electrons* emitted by the cathode filament. The temperature of this filament is controlled by the current which flows through it, thereby enabling one to control the available number of electrons which are accelerated to the target. This, then, indirectly controls the number of x-rays produced. The hotter the filament, the more electrons that are emitted and become available to form the electron stream.

Therefore, if all of the other factors remain constant, the *rate* at which x-rays are produced at the anode focus is directly proportional to the tube current, usually expressed in milliamperes (1 mA = 1/1000 ampere).

When we use milliamperage to describe intensity of the beam, it follows, then, that the quantity of the x-ray beam will be expressed in milliampere/seconds ($Q = It$). The unit of exposure in diagnostic radiography is the milliampere/second (mA/s). The higher the exposure in milliampere/seconds, the greater the quantity of the x-ray beam. Sometimes in diagnostic radiography, x-ray quantity or radiographic exposure is expressed in roentgens per second or roentgens per minute. The roentgen is a unit of x-ray quantity based on the ionization of air. We will discuss the roentgen more fully in Chapter 5.

Quality of X-Ray Beam

The quality of the x-ray beam describes the ability of the x-ray beam to penetrate matter.

The voltage applied across the cathode and anode of the x-ray tube will determine the quality or effective energy of the resultant x-ray beam. This higher voltage is usually expressed in terms of peak kilovolts (1 kilovolt = 1,000 volts). Kilovoltages between 55-100 kilovolts are used in dental radiography. Kilovoltage controls the *speed* of each electron which in turn has very important effects upon the x-rays produced. Radiation produced in the higher kilovoltage range has *greater energy, higher frequency, and shorter wavelengths*. Such x-rays are much more penetrating and are called "hard" x-rays. Radiation produced in the lower kilovoltage range has *less energy, lower frequency, and longer*

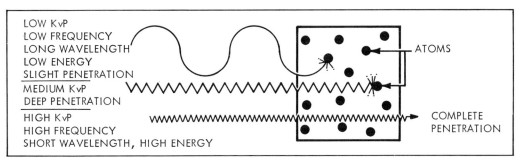

Figure 3-1. Penetration of x-rays.

wavelengths. Such x-rays are less penetrating and are called "soft" x-rays.

It must be understood, though, that the x-ray beam is heterogenous; it consists of x-rays of *different* wavelengths and, thus, different penetrating power. Of course, radiation produced by higher kilovoltages will have a greater percentage of the "hard" x-rays in its primary beam. This will give the primary beam more penetrating power (See Figure 3-1).

By increasing the kilovoltage and holding the milliamperage constant, the radiation spectrum of wavelengths will change. New wavelengths are added, which are shorter, and therefore increase the penetrating power of the x-ray beam (See Figure 3-2).

The quality of an x-ray beam can also be described by its *half-value layer (HVL)* or *half-value thickness (HVT).* The HVT of a beam is that thickness of

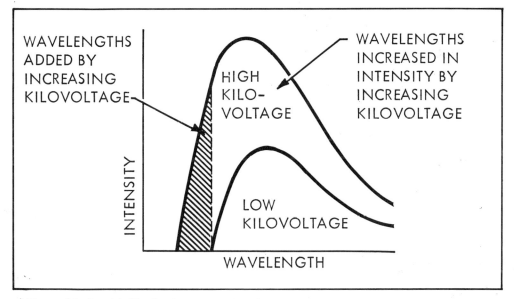

Figure 3-2. Special distribution curves showing the effect of a change in kilovoltage on the intensity and special composition of an x-ray beam. (Courtesy of Herman E. Seeman.)

some specified material (usually Al or Cu) which will attenuate (decrease in intensity) the beam to one-half of its original intensity. The higher the HVT, the more penetrating the beam.

Primary Beam

X-rays that are created at the focal spot come off the face of the tungsten target in all directions. They act like visible light waves in that they *radiate from the source in all directions* unless stopped by an absorber. For this reason the x-ray tube is enclosed in a heavy metal housing that stops most of the x-radiation—only the *useful rays* are permitted to leave the metal housing through an aperture or "window." Radiation which leaks through the metal housing is usually very slight and is called *leakage radiation*. The *useful rays* that pass through the metal housing at the "window" form the *primary beam*. That pencil of radiation at the geometric center of the *primary beam* is called the *central ray*. The aperture in the metal housing that the primary beam passes through is covered by a permanent seal, usually of aluminum or glass, to seal in the oil which surrounds the tube (See Figure 3-3).

Inverse-Square Law

The x-rays of the primary beam emerge from the protective housing *not* as parallel waves but as divergent rays

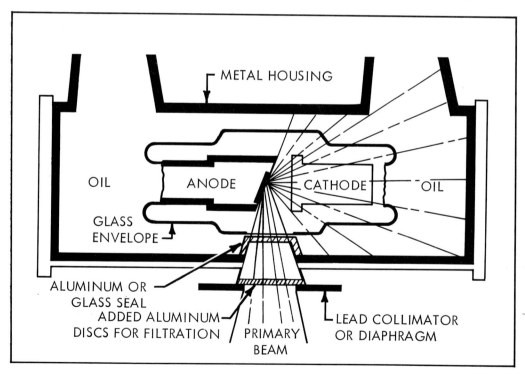

Figure 3-3. Since x-rays radiate in straight lines in all directions from the source, there is a need for a metal housing for the tube. (Courtesy of Eastman Kodak Co.)

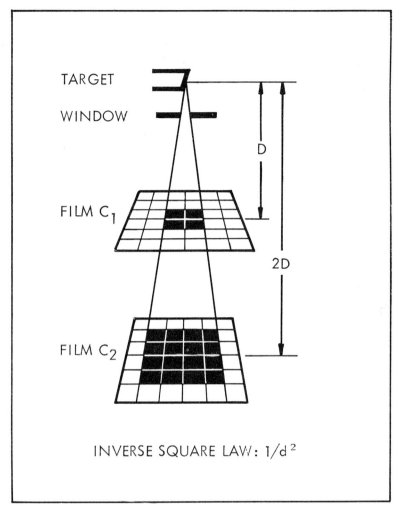

TARGET

WINDOW

D

FILM C$_1$

2D

FILM C$_2$

INVERSE SQUARE LAW: $1/d^2$

Figure 3-4. Diagram showing how the x-ray intensity is altered by changing the source-film distance. (Courtesy of Eastman Kodak Co.)

having a cone shape. Therefore, the intensity of the beam decreases as the distance from the target increases since the same amount of radiation covers a larger area at greater distances. You can prove this to yourself by a simple demonstration. With no other "light on" in the room, move a single light nearer to and farther away from a printed page. As you move the lamp away from the page, the light falling on it is less and less bright. Exactly the same thing happens with x-rays—as the distance from the object to the source of radiation is *decreased,* the x-ray intensity at the object *increases;* as the distance is *increased,* the radiation intensity at the object *decreases.* This relation between distance and intensity of radiation is called the *inverse square law,* because the intensity of radiation varies inversely as the square of the source-film distance (See Figure 3-4).

A practical formula to use in adjusting the exposure factor is as follows:

$$\frac{\text{Original mAs}}{\text{New mAs}} = \frac{\text{Original SFD}^2}{\text{New SFD}^2}$$

SFD = Source-Film Distance
mAs = milliampere/seconds (Quantity of Beam)

For example: When the SFD distance is changed from 8″ to 16″ or twice the distance, the mAs value will have to be increased four times.

Original SFD = 8 inches
Original mAs = 2.5 ($\frac{1}{4}$ second at 10 mA)
New SFD = 16 inches

$$\frac{2.5}{X} = \frac{8^2}{16^2}$$
$$64\,X = 640$$
$$X = 10 \ (1 \text{ sec. at } 10 \text{ mA})$$

Interaction of X-Rays with Matter

When a beam of x-rays passes through matter, the radiation becomes attenuated, meaning that its intensity is reduced. Some of the x-rays pass through unaffected, and are attenuated only by the effect of the inverse square law. The remainder of the x-ray photons of the beam may become attenuated in various ways as they enter and transverse matter.

Photoelectric absorption and Compton (Incoherent) scattering are the most important methods of attenuating x-rays in dental radiography.

Absorption consists of transfer of the total energy of the x-ray photon to the medium, and scattering consists in the deflection of the x-ray photon from its original direction. Both absorption and scattering causes the weakening and depletion of the energy of the photons of the x-ray beam.

Photoelectric Absorption

This process involves the direct interaction of an x-ray photon with an electron of one of the tightly-bound shells of an atom of the absorbing medium. Eighty percent of the reactions take place in the K shell of the atom. This interaction causes the ejection if the electron, and the x-ray photon loses all of its energy by absorption (See Figure 3-5). When an electron is ejected from one of the inner shells, an electron from one of the outer shells fills the vacancy or "hole" with the emission of energy *characteristic* of the atom. The characteristic radiation is usually of a low-energy type (unless the absorbing medium is of a high atomic number) and is absorbed almost immediately by adjacent atoms.

The ejected electron is called a photoelectron. It will, in turn, cause further ionizations with adjacent atoms until all of its energy is depleted. The predominant energy absorption process for bone up to 100 keV is by way of photoelectric absorption.

Compton Scattering (Incoherent)

This is a type of interaction between the x-ray and either a free electron or an electron loosely bound in one of the outer shells of the atom of absorbing medium. The interaction was first described by A. H. Compton in 1923. In Compton

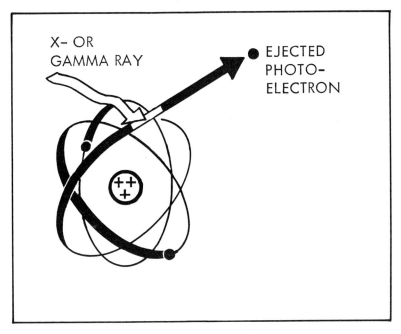

Figure 3-5. Photoelectric absorption.

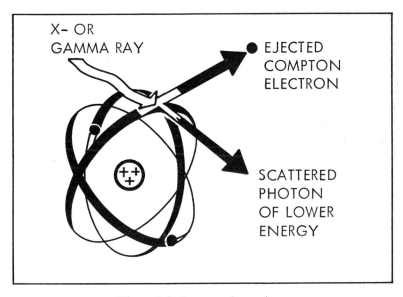

Figure 3-6. Compton Scattering.

scattering the photon ejects the electron from the orbit but gives up only a small portion of its energy in doing so.

The Compton interaction produces a scattered photon of lowered energy which has deflected from its original path and a high-speed electron (recoil or Compton) which has broken away from the atom (See Figure 3-6). Since the photon has given up part of its energy to the recoil electron, its total energy will be lower and its wavelength will be longer. The photon may be scattered in all directions, including backwards. Compton scattering usually takes place in soft tissue with x-ray energies between 30 keV and 30 MeV.

X-Ray Beam Absorption

Remember in listing the properties of x-rays, we stated that they are able to penetrate matter. That statement must be qualified, because not all the x-rays that enter an object penetrate it. Some are absorbed by photoelectric or Compton interactions. Those that do get through form the "latent" image—or "shadow" of the object radiographed.

The extent to which x-rays are absorbed by a material depends on four factors:

1. The wavelength or photon energy of the x-rays.
2. Thickness of the material.
3. Density (mass/unit volume) of the material.
4. Atomic number of the material.

The *wavelength* or photon energy of the x-radiation is indirectly determined by the kilovoltage applied to the x-ray tube. The higher kilovoltages produce shorter wavelength x-rays and they penetrate material more readily (See Figure 3-1).

The relation of x-ray absorption to *thickness* is simple—obviously a thick piece of any material absorbs more x-radiation than a thin piece of the same material. *Density* (wt/vol) of a material can be defined as the compactness of a material and is numerically equal to its specific gravity. It has the similar effect of *thickness*—for instance, an inch of water will absorb more x-rays than an inch of ice.

The atomic number (number of protons in nucleus) of an object usually has far more effect on x-ray absorption than thickness or density. The higher the atomic number of the material—the greater the absorption factor of the material. For example, a sheet of aluminum (Z = 13), being of lower atomic number than copper (Z = 29), absorbs a lesser amount of x-rays than does a sheet of copper of the same area and weight.

Dental X-Ray Absorption of Beam

In considering the dental use of x-rays, one must understand that the human jaws are complex structures made up of not only different thicknesses but of materials with different atomic numbers. These structures absorb x-rays in different degrees. That is, metallic restorations such as amalgam and gold absorb more x-rays than enamel does; enamel more than dentin does; dentin more than cementum does; cementum more than cortical bone; cortical bone more than cancellous bone; cancellous bone more than soft tissue such as the periodontal membrane, the pulp, and oral mucosa.

Teeth and bone contain large amounts of calcium and phosphorus with atomic numbers of 20 and 15 respectfully, whereas, the atomic number of muscle is approximately 7.4. Furthermore, diseased structures often absorb x-rays differently than normal dental structures. Even the age of the patient may have a bearing on absorption—for example, in the elderly, the bones of the jaws many times have less calcium content and hence, there is less x-ray absorption.

The variations in absorption depends for the most part upon the atomic number of the jaws and teeth, and, of course, the *quality* of the x-ray beam used. Materials that absorb or resist the passage of x-radiation to a degree are considered

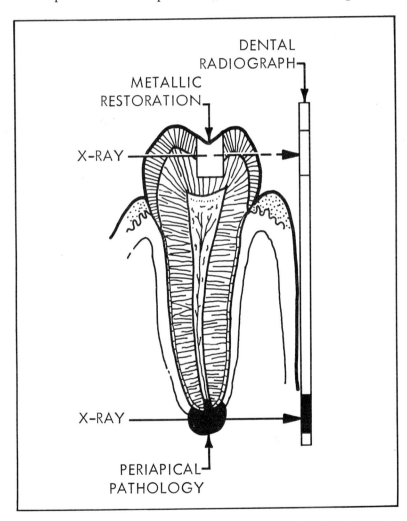

Figure 3-7. Diagram showing the variations of absorption in the human jaws. The *metallic restoration* absorbs the radiation resulting in a white or radiopaque area on the radiograph. The *periapical pathology* is easily penetrated by the x-radiation resulting in a dark or radiolucent area on the film.

radiopaque and appear within the range of light gray or white when recorded on a radiograph. This means that most of the energy of the x-rays have been absorbed and very little if any x-radiation has reached the surface of the radiograph. Radiopaque objects in the dental radiograph are metallic restorations, enamel, dentin, and compact or cortical bone.

Materials that are freely penetrated by the x-rays are called *radiolucent,* and appear within the range of dark gray to black on the radiograph. This means that the objects *do not* resist the passage of, or absorb the x-radiation to any great extent, and that most of the energy of the radiation freely passes through the object to the recording surface of the radiograph (See Figure 3-7).

Recording the X-Ray Beam

Remnant Radiation

The x-ray beam may be divided into

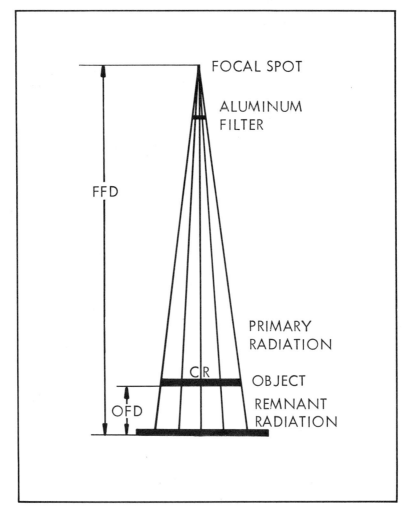

Figure 3-8. Components of x-ray beam with relation to object and x-ray film. (Courtesy of Mrs. Arthur W. Fuchs.)

two parts—the primary beam and the remnant beam (See Figure 3-8).

The *primary beam* is confined to that portion of the x-ray beam emitting from the focal spot of the x-ray tube and penetrating the object to be radiographed.

Before the x-ray beam reaches the object to be radiographed, the longer, useless wavelengths are absorbed out by selectively reducing the intensity of the primary beam by the process of filtration.

Filtration of the beam is accomplished by two methods: Inherent and Additional Filtration.

Inherent Filtration

Inherent Filtration takes place when the primary beam passes through the glass wall of the tube, a layer of oil, and the aperture window.

It is usually stated in terms of its *aluminum equivalent* which is defined as the thickness of aluminum (in mm) which will give the same filtration as the filtering material (glass and oil) of the x-ray head under the same conditions of irradiation. Usually, the inherent filtration of dental x-ray machines is between 0.5 to 1.0 mm aluminum equivalent.

The amount of filtration supplied by inherent filtration, in most cases, is not enough to meet the standards recommended by the National Council on Radiation Protection and Measurements. Therefore, *additional filtration* should be placed in the x-ray beam. It is usually in the form of a thin sheet of aluminum. The NCRP (1970) recommends that the aluminum equivalent of the total filtration (inherent plus added) of the

useful beam should be not less than that stated below:

Operating Potential	Minimum Total Filter (Inherent plus added)
Below 50 kVp	0.5 mm aluminum
50-70 kVp	1.5 mm aluminum
Above 70 kVp	2.5 mm aluminum

The aluminum filter absorbs those x-ray energies of low penetrating power which do not contribute to the information on the film, and therefore, expose the patient to useless radiation.

The *remnant radiation* is that portion of the x-ray beam that emerges from the body tissues to expose the x-ray film and record the radiographic image. The remnant radiation is the *image-forming* radiation. The image formed by the remnant radiation is called the *latent image*. Processing of the exposed film makes the latent image *visible* and permanent.

Scattered Radiation

The remnant radiation also contains scattered radiation emitted by the tissues. The amount of scatter radiation depends upon its wavelength and the manner in which it is controlled. When x-rays strike any form of matter, such as body tissue, *scattered x-rays* are produced that possess usually longer wavelengths than the primary radiation. Since scattered radiation is unfocused and may come from any direction, its action on the film is such that it may cover the entire image with a veil or fog unless it is controlled. Radiographically, this fog tends to make the visualization of the image details more difficult (See Figures 3-9).

The amount of scatter radiation present depends upon the kilovoltage used, as well as the thickness and density of the body part being radiographed. Bone

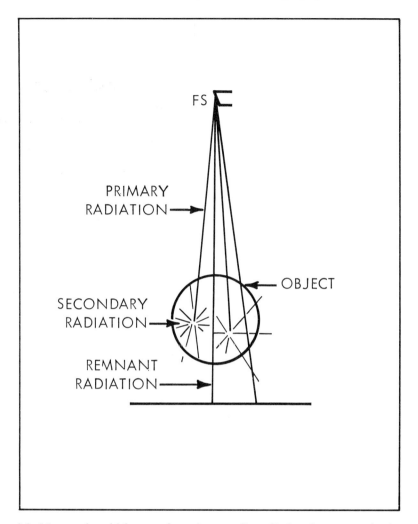

FS

PRIMARY
RADIATION→

OBJECT

SECONDARY
RADIATION→

REMNANT
RADIATION→

Figure 3-9. Manner in which secondary (scattered) radiation is generated when x-rays strike any form of matter. (Courtesy of Mrs. Arthur W. Fuchs.)

emits much less scatter radiation than soft tissue because it has a relatively high atomic weight. Scatter radiation is controlled by the use of proper exposure factors, grids, and collimators. We seldom use grids in dental radiography.

X-Ray Film

Let us consider the x-ray film itself. It consists of two important components:

1. A transparent blue-tinted *base* made of cellulose acetate or a plastic material.
2. An *emulsion,* coated on both sides of the base, containing silver bromide crystals suspended in gelatin.

If you could examine a cross section of x-ray film under a high-power microscope (See Figure 3-10), you would see the following:

1. At the center of the film, an optically blue-tinted base or support for the emulsion.
2. Substratum: adhesive material.
3. The *emulsion* (1/1000 inch in thickness) gelatin containing tiny crystals of silver bromide and covering both sides of base.
4. Emulsion coating: a very thin, transparent, nonabrasive layer to help protect the film surface from mechanical damage.

The base furnishes the proper support for the delicate emulsion. It is made from cellulose acetate or a plastic material which meets the safety requirements of the American Standards Association. The base is blue-tinted to emphasize contrast and thus make it easier to visualize the densities present in the image.

After the base is made, it is covered on both sides with a thin adhesive-type material so that the sensitive emulsion will adhere to the base. This is called the *subcoating* or *substratum* and prepares the base for emulsion coating.

The emulsion is composed of two constituents:

1. gelatin
2. silver bromide crystals

Gelatin is used because it can withstand the temperatures of the processing solution without interfering with the distribution of the silver bromide crystals.

The silver bromide crystals within the crystals or "grains" are so small it requires a microscope to see them. These silver bromide grains are sensitive to radiant energy such as light, x-rays, and gamma rays.

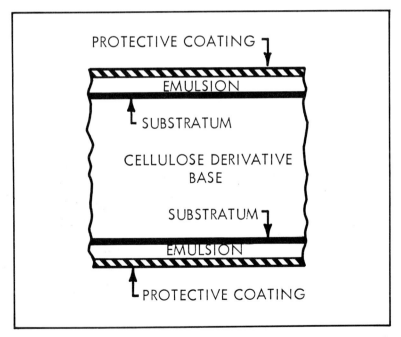

Figure 3-10. Cross section of an x-ray film showing its components. (Courtesy of Eastman Kodak Co.)

The purpose of the silver bromide crystals is to *absorb* radiation during an x-ray exposure and produce a latent image. The degree of exposure depends upon the intensity of the radiation emerging from the object radiographed which is between the source of the radiation and the film.

Latent Image Formation

The x-ray film is a delicate, sensitive product. It is sensitive to many things: to light, x-rays, and gamma rays; to various gases and fumes; to heat and moisture and even aging causes a gradual change in it. So you can see how important care in storage can be.

When x-rays strike the silver bromide crystals in the emulsion, minute amounts of metallic silver are formed on the surface of the crystal or grain and bromide is liberated. The degree of ionization within the crystal depends upon the amount of exposure received. When this situation is created, a *latent image* is produced in the film emulsion. The ionic equation can be written as follows:

$$AgBr + X\text{-}Rays = Ag^+ + Br^-$$

Silver Bromide Crystal   Silver Ion   Bromide Ion

The latent image formed by deposits of free silver cannot be seen or detected by any physical test devised as yet. It remains within the emulsion of the x-ray film until it is changed into a *visible silver image* by chemical processing procedures.

Intensifying Screens

There are two main groups of x-ray film:

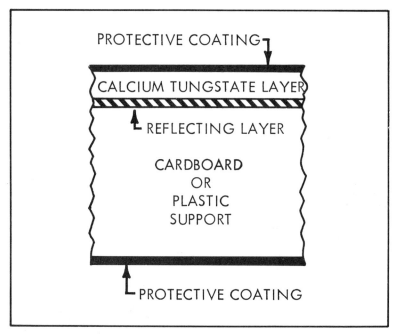

Figure 3-11. Schematic cross section of an intensifying screen. (Courtesy of Eastman Kodak Co.)

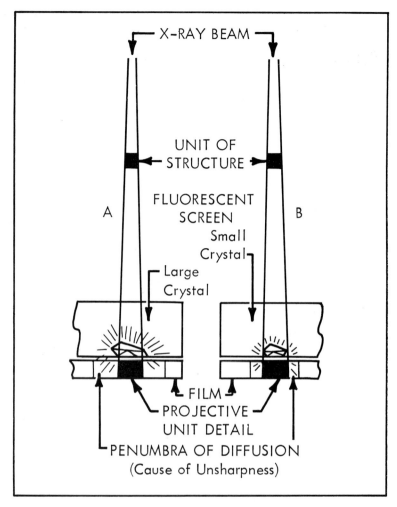

Figure 3-12. Effect of crystal size on sharpness of image. (A) Screen with large crystals. (B) Screen with small crystals. (Courtesy of Mrs. Arthur W. Fuchs.)

1. those films with emulsions which are sensitive to direct exposure of x-rays and,

2. those films with emulsions which are sensitive to bluish light emitted when x-rays strike salt intensifying screens.

When certain salts, such as calcium tungstate and barium lead sulfate, absorb x-rays, they fluoresce, or emit visible light. The ability for x-rays to cause fluorescence is the basis of fluoroscopy and the use of intensifying screens is extra-oral radiography.

The particles of calcium tungstate that fluoresce are called phosphors and they emit light in the blue region of the electromagnetic spectrum.

Intensifying screens usually contain calcium tungstate phosphors, which makes it possible to produce a radiographic image on the film with less radiation exposure than if x-rays alone were used. In other words, it intensifies the photographic effect on x-radiation. They have to be used in radiographing the deeper structures of the skull.

A screen consists of a thin layer of fluorescent calcium tungstate or other

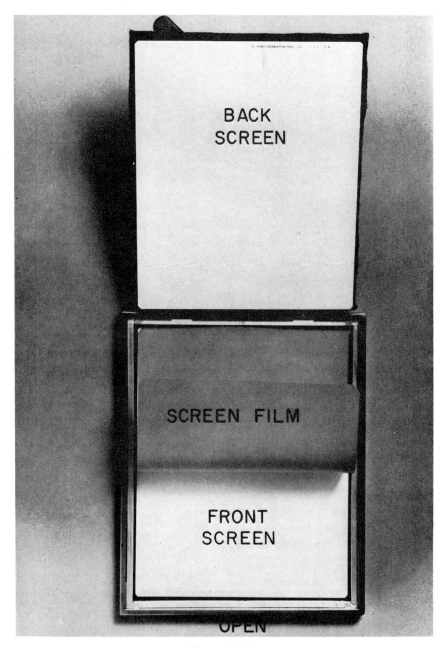

Figure 3-13A

Figure 3-13. Diagram of exposure cassette. Screen cassette (open, back and front).

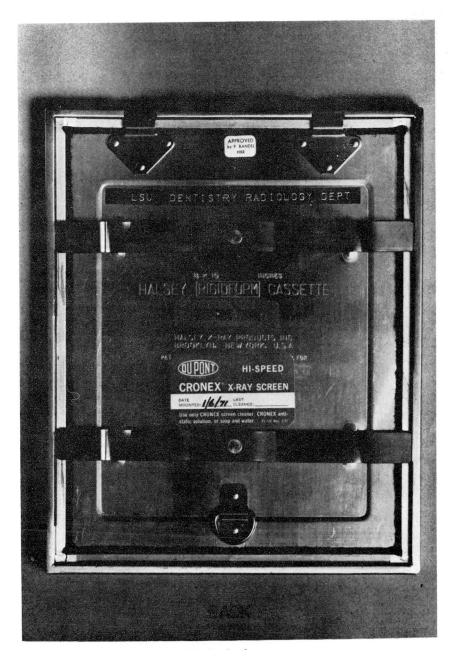

Figure 3-13B. Back of screen cassette.

phosphor crystals with a suitable lacquer and coated or plastic support (See Figure 3-11).

Each crystal of the screen emits bluish light while brightness is related directly to the intensity of the x-rays in that minute portion of the image. Thus, over the entire surface of the screen, differences in x-ray intensity are transformed into differences of blue-light brightness to which the film is highly sensitive (special screen type film). The entire image is thus "intensified" for recording by the film.

The thicker the fluorescent layer of a screen, the greater this intensification. The *size* of the crystals composing the layer also has an influence in this respect. The larger the crystals, the more light they produce and the greater the inten-

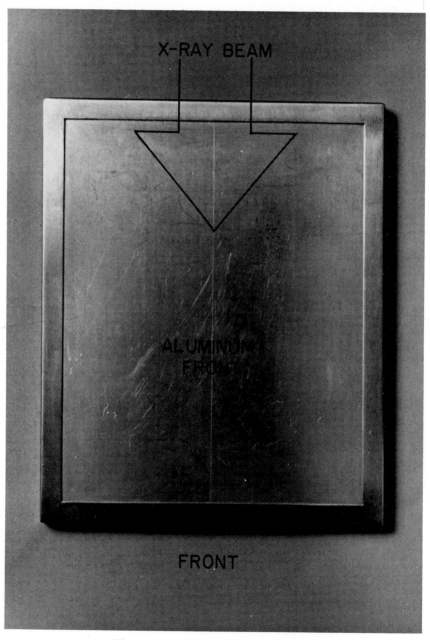

Figure 3-13C. Front of screen cassette.

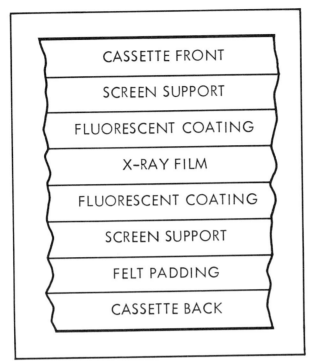

Figure 3-13D. Cross section of loaded cassette.

sification. However, because a thick fluorescent layer and larger crystals allow the light to spread more widely, the sharpness of the fluorescent image is decreased accordingly (See Figure 3-12).

A choice is usually available in the selection of intensifying screens:

1. *Fast Screens:* Thick layer and relatively large crystals used, maximum speed is attained but with some sacrifice in definition.

2. *Slow Screens or High Definition Screens:* A thin layer and relatively small crystals are used—definition is the best, but speed is slow. (*Definition* is the degree of distinctness with which radiographic details are recorded on the x-ray film.)

3. *Medium or Par Screens:* It has a medium thick layer of medium sized crystals in order to provide compromise between speed and definition.

In use, a pair of screens is enclosed in a hinged metal holder called a *cassette*. The film (special screen type film) is

INTENSIFYING SCREENS

Speed	Wolf	DuPont Patterson	Radelin	Ilford	Relative Speed	Average Unsharpness
Fast	Ultra	Hi-speed	+F	HV	1	.30
Medium	Rapid	Par-speed	T	Standard	2	.25
Slow		Detail	TD	Hi-resolution	8	.15

inserted between the screens so that the emulsion on each side of the film is in uniform contact with the screens (See Figure 3-13).

Four of the better-known commercially-available intensifying screens are listed on page 53, along with their relative speeds and average unsharpness measurements.

Types of X-Ray Film

Dental x-ray films are supplied in two forms—unwrapped sheets for *extraoral examinations* and in packets for *intraoral examinations.*

A. *Extraoral (Medical and Dental)*
1. Screen Type
2. No-Screen Type

B. *Intraoral Film (No-Screen Type)*
1. Periapical type
2. Bitewing type
3. Occlusal type

Extraoral Film

Screen-Type Film is particularly sensitive to the fluorescent light of x-ray intensifying screens. The visible fluorescent light from screens amplifies the direct action of the x-rays. Eastman Kodak Blue Brand® film is an example of a screen-type of film. For dental use the following sizes are available: 5 by 7 inches, 8 by 10 inches, and 10 by 12 inches.

No-Screen Film is a "direct-exposure" film. It is not as fast as the screen-type film with screens; it requires only one

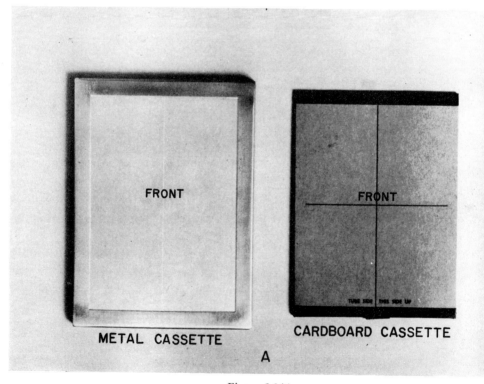

FRONT

FRONT

METAL CASSETTE

CARDBOARD CASSETTE

A

Figure 3-14A

Figures 3-14A & B. Comparison of metal cassette with cardboard cassette.

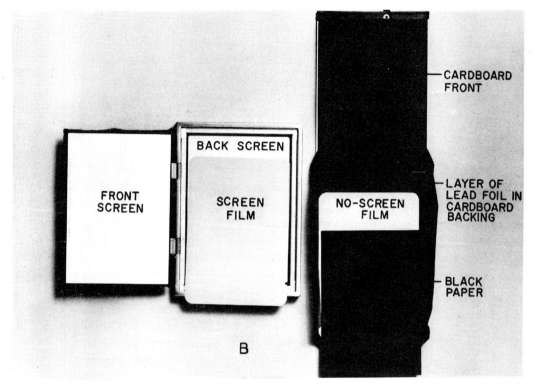

Figure 3-14B

fifth to one fourth the exposure time for screen-type as compared to no-screen films. This emulsion is sensitive to the direct exposure of x-radiation rather than to fluorescent light. It is used only for the thinner parts of the body such as the hands, feet, and jaws. No-screen film has a higher silver content and thus, a higher inherent contrast than screen film, but because of its thicker emulsion it must be processed 50 percent longer. The cardboard exposure holder is used to envelope the no-screen x-ray film during the exposure. The cardboard holder is composed of two pieces of x-ray-transparent paper board hinged together with binding cloth. One of the cardboard covers contains a thin layer of lead foil

which serves to absorb *back-scatter radiation* from tissues of the oral cavity (back-scatter radiation is secondary radiation that bounces back after penetrating an object) (See Figure 3-14).

Dental Intraoral X-Ray Film

Dental x-ray film is individually wrapped in packets of white, pebbled, moisture-resistant paper. Within it the film is further protected by black interleaving paper, and backed by lead foil. The sheet of lead foil placed in back of the film protects it from secondary radiation that may be backscattered by the tissues of the oral cavity during exposure. Also, the lead foil contributes to the rigidity of the packet. The Eastman

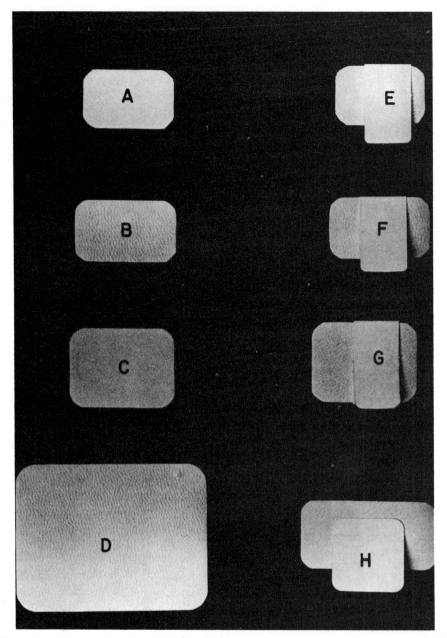

Figure 3-15. Types of intraoral film. (A) No. 0 children's periapical film, size ⅞″ x 1⅜″. (B) No. 1 periapical film, narrow-anterior, size ¹⁵⁄₁₆″ x 1⁹⁄₁₆″ (C) No. 2 regular periapical film, size 1¼″ x 1⅝″. (D) Occlusal film, size 2¼″ x 3″. (E) No. 0 bitewing film (under 6 years). (F) No. 1 bitewing film (6 to 9 years). (G) No. 2 bitewing film (adult). (H) No. 3 bitewing film (adult).

Kodak Company places a herringbone pattern in the lead foil backing that will appear in the radiographic image if the back of the packet is placed toward the tube during exposure.

All of the dental films manufactured at present are double-coated emulsion films. In order to identify the "tube side" of the film a "raised dot" is placed in the corner of the film. The raised portion of the dot is always toward the tube, and the depressed side of the dot is toward the tongue. A black dot on the printed label-side of the film packet locates the position of the "raised dot" on the x-ray film.

The older, slower films were coated with a single emulsion on one side of the film base (similar to photographic film). The emulsion side of the film (dull to reflected light) was always toward the tube and the non-emulsion side (shiny side) was always toward the tongue. When this film was developed and dried, it was read from the shiny or non-coated side, as if you were inside the patient's mouth looking out. This is why you still find some dentists today mounting and reading their films as if they were inside the patient's mouth looking out.

There are three types of intraoral dental film. They are as follows:

1. Periapical film
2. Bitewing film
3. Occlusal film

(1) *Periapical Film:* As the name suggests, the objective of the periapical film is to show the apex of the tooth and surrounding bone, but it should show the entire crown also. There are three sizes of periapical film: the #0 or child film, the #1 (narrow) adult anterior film, and the #2 (standard) adult film.

(2) *Bitewing Film:* The bitewing packet has a wing, or tab, on the side which the patient bites on. The posterior bitewing film shows the crowns of the maxillary and mandibular posterior teeth and their interproximal alveolar crests. The adult #3 posterior bitewing film is longer and narrower than the #2 standard periapical film. A tab attached to the No. 2 periapical film converts it to a bitewing film. In 9- to 12-year-old children a #2 standard film on each side of the arch is sufficient, but two #2 standard films on each side of the arch are usually necessary for adults. A bitewing film can be made for 5- to 9-year-old children by placing a tab on a No. 1 film, and one for children under 5 years of age by placing a tab on a #0 periapical film packet.

(3) *Occlusal Film:* The occlusal film is considerably larger than the periapical film and is so named because the patient bites upon the entire film. The objective of the occlusal film is to show large segments of the maxillary and mandibular arches and the floor of the mouth.

The sizes of these films are illustrated in Figure 3-15.

Radiographic Density

Density refers to the degree or gradation of "blackness" on a radiographic film. After the exposed film is processed, the film is viewed by placing it in front of an illuminator. It is this variation in the quantity of transmitted light through the film that identifies the image seen by the eyes. The heavier the deposit of the layer of black silver masses, the greater the quantity of light absorbed (and not transmitted), and the darker the area appears. Remember the darker areas on the film are regions of the anatomical part of the body that freely let the x-rays pass through to expose the film are called radiolucencies. A high degree of radiographic density gives a *dark* film; a *light* film has a thin or low degree of radiographic density.

Mathematically, film density is defined as the common logarithm* of the ratio of the intensity of the light beam of the illuminator as it strikes the radiograph (I) as compared to the amount of light transmitted through the radiograph (T). (I will always equal to 100%.)

$$\text{Density} = \log_{10} \frac{I}{T}$$

To illustrate: When the silver allows 1/10th of the illuminator or incident light through the radiograph, the ratio is 100/10 or 10/1 which is equal to 10. The common logarithm of 10 is 1, and therefore, the density of the film is equal to 1. Again, if the silver allows only 1/100 of the light to pass through the radiograph, the ratio is equal to 100/1 or 100. The common logarithm of 100 is 2. The exponent, 2, is the logarithm of 100 to the base 10.

The dental radiograph obviously contains a great many different densities in the various areas that comprise the image. These densities range from 0.4 in the relatively clear radiopaque areas (metallic restorations) to 3.0 in the blackest radiolucent areas. That is, the silver content allows approximately 1/2 of the light to pass through the radiopaque areas (density of 0.4), and only 1/100 of the light to pass through the blackest radiolucent areas (density of 3.0). The densities on the radiograph may be read directly by a photometer especially designed for measuring film densities. This device is called a *densitometer*.

Most illuminators are not intense enough to view a film having a density greater than 2.

Radiographic Contrast

Whereas radiographic density refers to the amount of light transmitted through a film, radiographic contrast is the difference between the amount of light transmitted by two or more areas of the film.

Mathematically, radiographic contrast can be expressed as:

$$\text{Contrast} = D_1 - D_2$$

where D_1 and D_2 are densities of two extreme black and white areas. The greater the difference between two radiographic densities on a film, the greater the radiographic contrast.

There are two general types of contrast. In short-scale contrast, the range of image densities is short, and the density differences between adjacent areas are great. In long-scale contrast the range of densities is wide, and the density dif-

---

* The power of a number is the product obtained when it is multiplied by itself a given number of times. Thus, $10^3 = 10 \times 10 \times 10 = 1,000$. The figure 3 is the *exponent*. The exponent used in raising 10 to a given power is called the *common logarithm* of the value. For example, the relation $1,000 = 10^3$ then will result in the statement "the common logarithm of 1,000 is 3." In symbols, this is usually written as $\log_{10} 1,000 = 3$. ($10^1 = 10$; $10^2 = 100$; $10^3 = 1,000$; $10^4 = 10,000$; $10^5 = 100,000$.)

ference between neighboring areas is small.

Radiographic contrast depends primarily on subject contrast and film contrast. Subject contrast represents the differences in absorption of an object to the x-ray beam. This absorption depends upon the atomic structure of the tissue and the wavelength of the x-ray—which results in the production of a number of different silver deposits on the radiograph. Each silver deposit has a certain degree of translucency or density when the radiograph is viewed on an x-ray illuminator. On the radiograph you will see variations in the degrees of density. Some areas will appear black, others gray, and others white. The black, the gray, and the white areas "contrast" with each other. You will be able to see a difference in the density of the various areas. Greater subject contrast exists between x-ray images recorded of amalgam restorations and dentin than with enamel and dentin.

Film contrast depends on the type of film and developer used. Certain film types are manufactured with more inherent contrast characteristics. The no-screen films have higher radiographic contrast than screen-type films.

Certain developing solutions produce greater radiographic contrast than the regular developing solutions. These are usually developing solutions that contain a more active alkaline (such as sodium hydroxide).

Exposure

The term "exposure" in radiography has many definitions.

In its strictly radiological sense, "exposure" denotes the amount of electric charge (positive or negative) per unit mass of air, produced when photons pass through an area. Exposure is such an important quantity that a unit in which exposure may be measured has been defined. This unit is called the roentgen and it is based on the ionization generated by radiation in air.

The roentgen (R) is defined as *that quantity of x or gamma radiation such that the associated corpuscular emission per 0.001293 gm of air produces, in air, ions carrying one electrostatic unit of electricty of either sign* (See Figure 3-16). What does it mean?

1. It is a unit of quantity, and, therefore, a unit of exposure. Exposure rate is measured in R per second (or per minute).

2. It applies to x- and gamma radiation and to no other type of ionizing radiation.

3. "Associated Corpuscular Emission" refers to the secondary electrons produced generally by a photoelectric or Compton interactions when photons are absorbed in a known volume of air. The measurement of the roentgen, therefore, must also include the ionizations caused by these secondary electrons ejected when photons are absorbed.

4. 0.001293 gm of air is the mass of 1 cc (unit volume) of dry air at $0°C$ and 760 mm Hg barometric pressure. This means the roentgen must be independent of atmospheric conditions.

5. The roentgen is a measure of air, and of no other absorbing medium.

6. An *electrostatic unit* is a quantity of electrical charge, which, if placed in a vacuum bulb one centimeter from another charge of the same type and just

as strong, will repel it with a force of *one dyne*.

A *dyne* is the amount of force or shove which can accelerate a mass of one gram one centimeter per second.

To form *1 esu* per 0.001293 gram of air, the radiation must produce 1.61×10^{12} ion pairs when absorbed in one gram of air.

In the International System of units (SI):

1 roentgen = 2.58×10^{-4} coulombs/ kilogram of air
(1 coulomb = 3.00×10^9 esu of charge)

Simply, the roentgen (R) is the unit of exposure measuring the amount of photon-produced air ionizations formed in 1 cc of air at standard conditions.

Radiographic exposure is also defined as the quantity of radiation received by a particular area of the film producing a given density on the processed film.

Radiographic exposure may be expressed in ergs/cm² or roentgens/cm². (1 erg is a unit of energy which can exert a force of one dyne through a distance of one centimeter.)

The response of a film to exposure is usually expressed graphically by plotting the density against the common logarithm of the *relative* exposure. (The study of quantitative relationships of exposure and density is called sensitometry). The resultant curve is called the film "characteristic curve" or the H and D curve (derived from Hurter and Driffield who first used these curves in 1890).

Since a standard unit for expressing radiographic exposure has not been devised as yet, exposures are given in relative values. The logarithm of exposure is used rather than quantity in order to compress the scale and make it easier to evaluate (See Figure 3-17).

When the slope of the characteristic

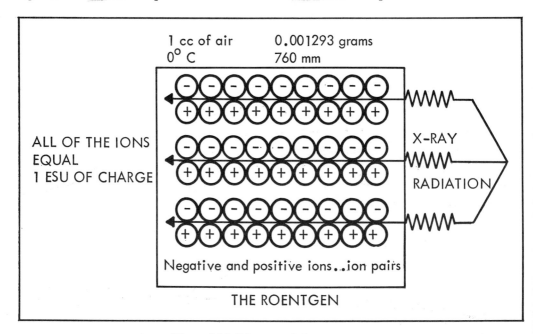

Figure 3-16. Diagram of the roentgen.

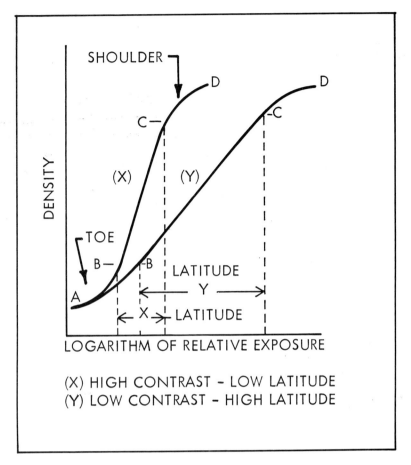

Figure 3-17. Characteristic curves for two different films. (Courtesy of William L. Bloom, John L. Hollenbach and James A. Morgan.)

curve is steepest, the film contrast is greatest.

Exposure for all practical purposes may be defined indirectly by the technical factor "mAs." This is the product of milliamperes (quantity) and the *time* during which the x-rays are produced. The higher the mAs, the greater the intensity of the beam, and subsequently, the more photons of energy that strike the sensitive emulsions of the radiograph.

Rule: The milliamperage required for a given exposure is *inversely proportional* to the exposure time. That is, the higher the milliamperage, the shorter the exposure time. The rule is expressed mathematically as:

$$\frac{mA_o}{mA_n} = \frac{T_n}{T_o}$$

("o" subscript refers to old and "n" subscript refers to new.)

Latitude

On the characteristic curve, film latitude is the difference between log exposure and a useful range of densities (See Figure 3-17). If the predetermined useful range of densities is 0.25 to 2.0, then a film with the greater latitude will have a greater range of exposures with this density range than a film with lower latitude. The film latitude varies with the reciprocal of film contrast. In other words, the greater the film latitude, the lower the film contrast.

Exposure latitude is the range of exposures of an x-ray film permissible for a good diagnostic result. The greater the exposure "error" that can be tolerated, the greater is the latitude of the radiographic exposure technic. Exposure latitude improves when the kVp is increased, and the film contrast decreases.

Film Sensitivity

The efficiency with which a film responds to x-ray exposure is known as *film sensitivity* or—more commonly— "speed." X-ray films that require very little exposure to x-radiation to produce a radiograph are said to be very sensitive, or very fast, or to possess high speed. Then exposure time and film speed vary inversely.

A high speed film requires a lower mAs factor to produce comparable densities on a film than a slower speed film. On the characteristic curve, a more sensitive film will be positioned farther to the left because it requires less exposure for a given density (See Figure 3-17).

Intraoral film speeds have been standardized on an alphabetical basis according to a speed range recorded in "reciprocal roentgens" (See Figure 3-18).

X-ray films are compared by determining their relative sensitivity. This is actually measured by determining the amount of x-radiation necessary to produce a certain density (or "blackness")

in the emulsion which has been processed in a rigidly controlled manner. For example, if Film E requires half as much x-radiation as Film F to produce the same blackness in the emulsion, Film E is said to be *twice as fast* as Film F.

The speed of the film is dependent upon the sensitivity of the emulsion and is governed by the manufacturer. This is accomplished in several ways:

1. Special x-ray film emulsion dyes which sensitize the silver bromide crystals to become more radiosensitive.
2. Film "ripening" process—the emulsion granules are maintained more constant in size and rendered more sensitive by bringing the silver emulsion up to a temperature of approximately 100°C and kept there for a few minutes.
3. Covering the cellulose acetate base on both sides will increase the speed of the film.
4. The thicker the emulsion and the larger the silver bromide grain size, the faster the speed of the film.

At the present time, manufacturers of dental film record the film speed on the outside of the packet in an alphabetical classification. For instance, (B) for the medium fast films which are the so-called radiatized films; (C) for the extra-fast films; and (D) for the ultra- and lightning-fast films. There is a two-fold increase in film speed between groups. This means that a dentist using film in one speed classification may use film in the next high speed classification by simply reducing the previous time by one-half.

The film emulsion is sensitive to a number of conditions. Some of these con-

SPEED GROUP

FILM BRAND

(A.S.A. PH 6.1 – 1961)   (reciprocal roentgens)

Periapical film			
None	A	slowest	1.5 – 3.0
DuPont "D" Kodak Radia–Tized IFI BH 1 Minimax Intermediate Rinn MF	B		3.0 – 6.0
IFI SBH 1 Minimax Extra Fast Rinn EF	C		6.0 – 12.0
DuPont "LF" IFi UBH–1 Kodak Ultra–Speed Rinn Super Minimax Triplex	D		12.0 – 24.0
None	E		24.0 – 48.0
None	F	fastest	48.0 – 96.0
Occlusal film Kodak Ultra–Speed Rinn Super	D		12.0 – 24.0

Source: Adapted from Guide to Dental Materials and Devices, Fourth Edition, 1968, American Dental Association.

Figure 3-18. Dental film speed—group ratings.

ditions are heat, light, x-rays, fumes, bending, and pressure. The high-speed emulsions are even more sensitive to these conditions.

All unexposed films show a certain amount of density after processing. This is called the *base density* of the film. It is a constant factor and is caused by the absorption of a small quantity of light during the manufacture of the film base. An average value for the base density of a film would be 0.07.

Fog is defined as the density of the film due to the development of unexposed silver bromide grains. A film may also become fogged by the accidental exposure of the film to radiant energy in the form of x-rays or light. Fogging will give the radiograph a hazy appearance.

If you want to determine whether your films are fogged or not, compare the density difference between an unexposed film that has been fully processed with one that has only been fixed, washed, and dried. A fog density in excess of .20 is objectionable. Fogging of a film interferes with contrast by increasing the density.

Fogging of films can be caused by several conditions:

1. *Age of Film:* Age fog is the result of using outdated film. All films have an expiration date because fog increases with time.

2. *High Temperature and High Humidity Storage:* High temperatures and humidity increases the production of fog. Ideal storage conditions are temperatures of 50° to 70°F and 40 to 60 percent relative humidity.

3. *Excessive Time and/or Temperature Development:* Processing solutions are chemicals that when applied to the invisible latent image of the exposed x-ray film produce a visible and permanent radiographic image. Radiographic density increases with the time of development and with the temperature of the developing solutions. For optimum results, the time and temperature method of development as recommended by the manufacturer is important. Excessive developing time will *increase* the density of the radiograph, while excessive fixing time will *decrease* the density.

4. *Inadequate Protection of Stored Films from X-Rays:* Do not store film adjacent to the x-ray machine in unprotected containers.

5. *Darkroom Safelight too Bright:* Allow 4 watts of light for each foot of distance from working bench when using the Wratten 6B filter or equivalent. A direct safelight should be a minimum of four feet above the working surface.

7. *Wrong Filter in Safelight:* The Kodak *Morlite*® filter is a special type of film that is designed for use with a special type of film only. Screen-type films should only be used with Wratten 6B filters and *not* with Morlite filters.

8. *Too Long Exposure to Safelight:* Fogging of your films will take place if you leave unwrapped films under the safelight for periods of time that are excessive for your safelight conditions.

9. *Light Leaks in the Darkroom:* As mentioned previously, the high speed films are very sensitive to light as well as x-rays.

Other Exposure Factors

In determining an exposure technic, there are several other variables which must be taken into consideration. These are (1) filtration, (2) collimation, (3) size and age of patient, (4) anatomic region, (5) use of grids, (6) source-film distance, (7) kilovoltage and (8) processing.

Filters

As previously mentioned, filters are thin pieces of aluminum, which are placed in the x-ray beam to absorb the unnecessary low photon energies. This will increase the penetrability of the x-ray beam. However, added filtration also absorbs some of the useful higher photon energies of the beam at the same time, which reduces the total quantity of the primary beam. This tends to reduce radiographic contrast and density. In order to compensate for this reduction the mAs must be increased.

Collimation

This is restricting or limiting the primary beam of radiation by use of a collimator or diaphragm. The collimator is usually composed of a sheet of lead in which an aperture has been cut of a size to permit x-ray coverage of a desired film area. It is located between the x-ray tube and the cone. Decreasing the size of the aperture decreases the production of scatter radiation which is produced when the primary radiation strikes the soft tissues of the patient. Scatter radiation increases the overall density of the radiograph and tends to decrease the contrast. Therefore, if the collimation is increased too much, the mAs may have to be increased.

Size and Age of Patient

The size of a patient varies greatly and exposure time for any patient, regardless of age, should be adjusted according to the patient's size. For the larger than average patient, increase the mAs by 50 percent. For the smaller than average patient, decrease the mAs by 25

percent or more. There are also some modifications to be made according to the patient's age. For patients over 50 years of age, increase the mAs by 25 percent; and for patients under 10 years of age, decrease mAs by 50 percent. In edentulous patients and patients between the ages of 10 and 15, the mAs should be decreased by 25 percent.

Anatomic Region Being Recorded

Several starting exposure technics for intraoral radiography exist. They all use the mandibular molar region as the baseline. The average exposure times for the various anatomic regions are given as percentages of the recommended exposure times for the mandibular molar region.

An exposure variation is recommended for the different areas of the oral cavity in order to compensate for the differences in the quantity of the hard and soft structures encountered. Greater amounts of exposure is required to penetrate areas which have thicker amounts of tissue.

In the table below, two different fixed kV technics are given where the mAs is the exposure factor of change.

RECOMMENDED AVERAGE EXPOSURES
GIVEN AS PERCENTAGES OF INCREASE OR
DECREASE OF AVERAGE MANDIBULAR
MOLAR EXPOSURE TIME

Anatomic Area	Exposure Percentage (Fixed kV Technic)	
Maxillary molar	+50	+33
Maxillary premolar	0	0
Maxillary cuspid	0	0
Maxillary incisor	0	+16
Mandibular molar	0	0
Mandibular premolar	−25	−16
Mandibular cuspid	−25	−33
Mandibular incisor	−25	−50
Posterior bitewings	0	0

Although fixed voltage technics are used almost universally in dental radiography, it is possible to use a variable kilovoltage technic. In this technic, the kilovoltage is varied according to the difference in the anatomic region and the mAs is fixed. The variable kilovoltage technic will tend to produce a complete radiographic survey that is without density variations between the different anatomic regions.

A TYPICAL VARIABLE kVp TECHNIC*

Type of Film: Eastman Kodak® Ultra-Speed
mAs: 10 mA at ¾ sec.
Source-Film Distance: 16″

	Male	Female
Maxilla		
Central-Lateral	78 kV	72 kV
Canines	80 kV	74 kV
Premolars	86 kV	80 kV
Molars	90 kV	84 kV
Mandible		
Central-Lateral	74 kV	68 kV
Canines	76 kV	70 kV
Premolars	78 kV	72 kV
Molars	81 kV	75 kV
Posterior Bitewings		
Premolars	65 kV	65 kV
	at 1¾ sec	at 1¾ sec
Molars	90 kV	90 kV

* According to Dr. Don Wagner of the University of Nebraska.

Use of Grids

A grid is composed of alternate strips of lead (approximately .005 inch thick), and non-opaque material used to absorb scatter radiation. When thicker body parts are radiographed, grids are placed between the patient and the film to absorb the emerging scatter radiation which tends to interfere with the definition of the radiograph. Although grids are used primarily in medical radiography, they have a place in dental radiography when the dentist is taking skull radiographs.

The ability of the grid to filter out the unwanted scatter radiation is measured by the grid ratio which is defined as the ratio of the height of the lead strips to the width of the nonopaque material. For instance, a grid with lead strips the height of 2.8 mm and a width of .35 mm for the nonopaque material will have a 2.8/.35 or 8:1 ratio.

A 16:1 grid will absorb twice as many scatter rays as an 8:1 grid. By absorbing the scatter radiation the radiographic contrast is improved. When grids are used, the mAs factor must be increased.

Grids may be either stationary or moving type. The stationary grid is light and portable and may be mounted on cassettes commonly used in skull radiography. The lead strips are recorded on the film as thin white lines. These white lines will first be perceptable if there are at least 80 white lines per inch. Some of the more expensive stationary grids have as many as 110 lines per inch.

These fine white lines on the radiograph can be removed completely by means of a moving grid. This principle of the moving grid was first introduced by Dr. Bucky in 1909. The grid is made to oscillate or move continuously in one direction. The grid motion is synchronized to start its movement just before the x-rays are set off.

Source-Film Distance

As mentioned previously, the exposure time varies directly as the square of the source-film distance. In other words, in

DECREASE IN EXPOSURE TIME	INCREASE IN KILOVOLTAGE		INCREASE IN EXPOSURE TIME	DECREASE IN KILOVOLTAGE	
	With Medium Speed Screens	Without Screens		With Medium Speed Screens	Without Screens
25%	7%	15%	25%	5%	10%
50%	20%	40%	50%	10%	18%
75%	50%	100%	75%	13%	25%
			100%	16%	30%

Figure 3-19. Approximate kilovoltage-time relationship. (Courtesy of Eastman Kodak Co.)

order to produce a given density at a different distance, it is necessary to vary the exposure directly as the square of the distance.

The formula for time-distance relations is expressed as follows:

$$T_n D_o^2 = T_o D_n^2$$
$$T_n = T_o D_n^2 / D_o^2$$

(subscript n = new and o = original)

Kilovoltage

Although the exposure time varies inversely to the kilovoltage, no definite mathematical relationship exists between the two. See the table in Figure 3-19 for the approximate kilovoltage-time relationship. This is only an approximate guide since the actual relationship depends upon both kilovoltage and subject contrast.

Processing

The objective of any exposure technic should be to provide the minimum amount of radiation to a patient and still produce a radiograph which has maximum diagnostic quality. The film developing process can provide a valuable test in determining whether a film has been exposed to the proper amount of radiation. Develop an exposed sample film for 8 to 9 minutes at the recommended temperature, fix and dry. This is overdevelopment; however, it is practically impossible to overdevelop properly exposed or underexposed film. If the film is dark, the film has been overexposed. If the film has the proper density, expose another film and develop this film at the recommended 5 minutes at 70°, fix and dry. If this film has a low density (light), the film has been underexposed. However, if the film is of the optimal density, the film has been properly exposed.

REFERENCES

Ennis, Berry, and Phillips: *Dental Roentgenology*, 6th ed. Philadelphia, Lea and Febiger, 1967.

Etter, Lewis E.: *Glossary of Words and Phrases Used in Radiology, Nuclear Medicine and Ultrasound*, 2nd ed. Springfield, Charles C Thomas, 1970.

Fuchs, Arthur W.: *Principles of Radiographic Exposure and Processing*, 2nd ed. Springfield, Illinois, Charles C Thomas, 1969.

Fundamentals of Radiography, 10th ed. Rochester, New York, Eastman Kodak Co., 1960.

Goodwin, Paul N.; Quimby, Edith H.; and Morgan, Russell: *Physical Foundations of Radiology,* 4th ed. New York, Harper & Row, 1970.

Guide to Dental Materials and Devices, 4th ed. American Dental Association, 1968.

Hendee, William R.: *Medical Radiation Physics,* Chicago, Year Book Medical Publishers, 1970.

Herz, Richard H.: *The Photographic Action of Ionizing Radiation.* Somerset, N. J., John Wiley & Sons, 1969.

Jaundrell-Thompson, F. and Ashworth, W. J.: *X-Ray Physics and Equipment,* 2nd ed.

Philadelphia, F. A. Davis, 1970.

Johns, H. E., and Cunningham, J. R.: *The Physics of Radiology,* 3rd ed. Springfield, Ill., Charles C Thomas, 1969.

McCall, John O., and Wald, Samuel S.: *Clinical Dental Roentgenology,* 4th ed. Philadelphia, W. B. Saunders, 1957, pp. 17-20.

Seeman, Herman E.: *Physical and Photographic Principles of Medical Radiography.* New York, John Wiley & Sons, 1968.

Ter-Pogossian, Michel M.: *The Physical Aspects of Diagnostic Radiology.* New York, Harper & Row, 1967.

Wuehrmann, Arthur H.: *Radiation Protection and Dentistry.* St. Louis, C. V. Mosby, 1960.

X-Rays in Dentistry. Rochester, N. Y., Eastman Kodak Co., 1962.

CHAPTER 4

DIAGNOSTIC QUALITY OF DENTAL RADIOGRAPHS

THE DIAGNOSTIC quality of a dental radiograph is dependent upon four conditions:

1. *Proper Visual Characteristics of Radiograph*
   a. Density
   b. Contrast
2. *Minimal Geometric Characteristics of Radiograph*
   a. Radiographic image unsharpness
      1. Geometric unsharpness
      2. Motion unsharpness
      3. Screen unsharpness
   b. Magnification
   c. Distortion
3. *Anatomical Accuracy of Radiographic Images*
4. *Adequate Coverage of Anatomic Region of Interest*

A clear understanding of the effects and significance of each factor will aid the student in the routine production of radiographs of diagnostic quality.

Visual Characteristics

The diagnostic quality of the radiograph is directly influenced by two visual characteristics of the radiographic image called *density* and *contrast.*

Radiographic Density

As mentioned previously in Chapter 3, density refers to the amount of "blackness" on a radiographic film. Density on your film is determined by the number of silver bromide crystals in the film emulsion that are exposed to radiation.

In final analysis, the quantity of metallic silver deposited in the emulsion is determined primarily by the exposure technic and the processing procedure.

Exposure Factors that Control Density

Listed below are the three important exposure factors which control density of a radiograph. In dental radiography, the first factor mentioned (mAs) is generally the factor of choice.

1. *Milliampere-Seconds:* The density or blackness of the radiograph varies directly and proportionately as the milliamperage (tube current) and the exposure time. Therefore, exposure time and milliamperage are interchangeable and considered as a *single* factor (mAs). For instance, the density of a radiographic image produced by a direct exposure of 2 seconds at 10 milliamperes is identical to the density of the image produced by an exposure time of 4 seconds at 5 milliamperes. The product of mA and exposure time is equal to 20 mAs in each instance. The higher the mAs the more x-rays that will strike the film and the greater the quantity of metallic silver deposited in the film emulsion. The quantity or (mAs) of the x-ray beam is usu-

ally measured by the use of a *roentgen meter.*

2. *Kilovoltage:* Kilovoltage is referred to as the "penetrating power" of the x-ray beam and influences density. The relationship between the exposure required and the kilovoltage is varied and is expressed by the formula:

$$E = mAs \times kV^n$$

Where E is the exposure intensity producing a certain density and is proportional to some power n of the kilovoltage. The nth power is a number lying between 2.0 and 4.5 which depends upon the:

1. Kilovoltage beam filtration.
2. Photo-chemical sensitivity of x-ray film.
3. Fluorescent intensity of intensifying screens (if used).
4. Thickness of region radiographed.

See Figure 3-19 on page 67 for a table giving the approximate exposure relationship for various changes in kilovoltage.

As the kilovoltage becomes greater, and the effective wavelengths of the x-ray beam become shorter, the penetration of the x-ray beam becomes greater. Therefore, a greater amount of x-radiation will strike the film emulsion, which in turn, will cause more metallic silver to be deposited in the emulsion. This will result in a higher radiographic density if all other factors remain constant.

3. *Source-Film Distance:* Since the intensity of an x-ray beam varies *inversely* as the square of the source film distance (inverse square law), the time of exposure necessary to maintain a constant density in a radiograph varies *directly* as the square of the focal-film distance. The smaller the distance between the focal spot and the film, the more x-rays that strike the film, and therefore, the *higher* the density. *Example:* Doubling the distance gives one-fourth the density—halving the distance gives four times the density. The relationship of the above three exposure factors that control radiographic density can be expressed in equation form:

$$\text{Radiographic Density} = \frac{kV^n \times mA \times \text{Seconds}}{D^2 \text{ (Source-Film Distance)}}$$

The density of the film is proportional to the exposure in milli-ampere-seconds and inversely to the distance squared. Also, density depends upon some power n of kilovoltage. As a rule of thumb, you may assume n equals (4) four and adjust accordingly to a lower number when a standard density is not achieved routinely by your technic.

Secondary factors affecting density:

1. *Patient Thickness:* Body parts which are thicker require more mAs or kVp in order to maintain a constant density.
2. *Development Conditions:* The ra-

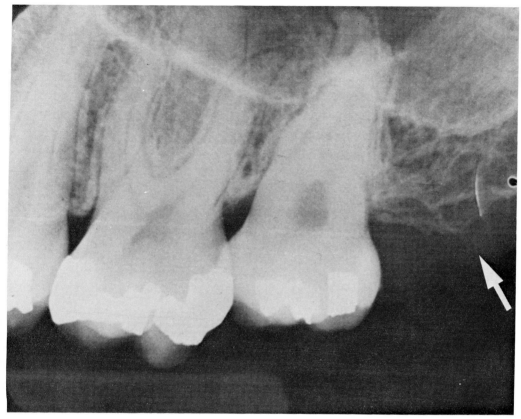

Figure 4-1. Radiograph of maxillary molar region. Notice thin shadow of soft tissue over bone in tuberosity area distal to maxillary 2nd molar.

diograph may be darker or lighter depending on whether the films are under- or overdeveloped. However, it is difficult to overdevelop a film which has been properly exposed.

3. *Type of Film:* High speed films require less mAs in order to cause a density change.

4. *Screens:* High-speed screens require less mAs in order to cause a density change in the radiograph.

5. *Grids:* The use of grids require more mAs in order to keep a constant density.

What Degree of Radiographic Density Is Most Desirable?

The desirable degree of radiographic density cannot be fixed as a permanent thing because one dentist may prefer a certain degree of density while another may prefer a greater or lesser density for the same region. The degree of radiographic density may be considered to be largely as a matter of individual preference. Of course, you do not want a film that is too dark or too light—you need the right amount of density to visualize the anatomic structures accurately.

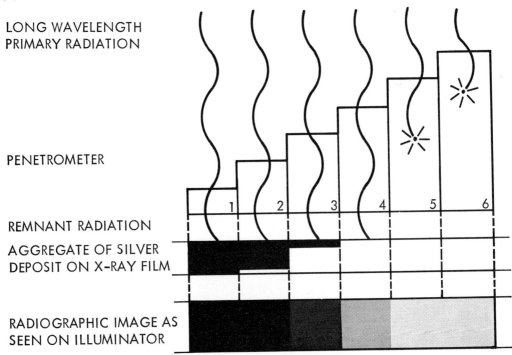

LONG WAVELENGTH
PRIMARY RADIATION

PENETROMETER

REMNANT RADIATION

AGGREGATE OF SILVER
DEPOSIT ON X-RAY FILM

RADIOGRAPHIC IMAGE AS
SEEN ON ILLUMINATOR

SHORT SCALE CONTRAST

Figure 4-2. Short scale contrast. (Courtesy of Mrs. Arthur W. Fuchs.)

In dental radiographs of correct density, the dentist should be able to see a faint outline of the soft tissues in edentulous spaces or distal to the third molar teeth when the radiographs are examined in the manner he habitually employs (See Figure 4-1).

Contrast

Contrast is the difference in densities visualized on radiographs. On the radiograph you will see variations in "blackness." Some areas will be black (radiolucent); other areas will be gray and other areas white (radiopaque). In the black areas a great many of the x-rays reached the film, while in the white areas, very few of the x-rays penetrated the object.

Contrast Is Primarily a Function of Kilovoltage

Contrast is affected primarily by kilovoltage; however, it can be affected by type of film, processing, and type of tissue (thickness and atomic number). The lower the kilovoltage, the higher will be the contrast. As the kilovoltage becomes higher, the contrast becomes less. The amount of kilovoltage that is applied will determine just how much "penetration" of the tissues is accomplished. If the kilovoltage is high (90 kVp), the wavelengths will be shorter, the penetration of the x-rays through the tissue will be greater, the density differences of adjacent areas are small, and the film will have *long-scale contrast*. If the kilovoltage is low

(65 kVp), the wavelengths will be longer, and the penetration will be less. The density differences between adjacent areas will be great, and the film will have *short-scale contrast.*

Long and short scale contrast can be illustrated by means of a *penetrometer.* The quality of an x-ray beam or its wavelength is usually measured by determining the rate of absorption in some material. A penetrometer is a radiographic testing device made of aluminum and built up in steps of varying thicknesses (See Figures 4-2 and 4-3). This shows an aluminum penetrometer or step-wedge being irradiated by x-rays;

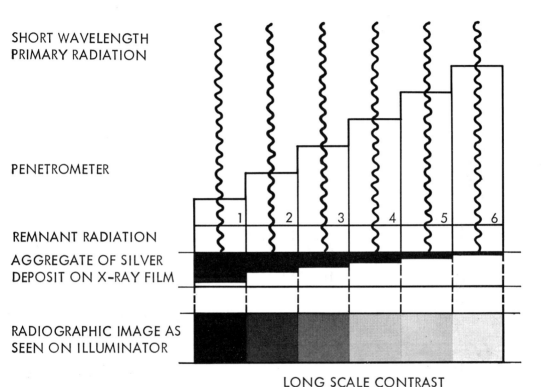

SHORT WAVELENGTH
PRIMARY RADIATION

PENETROMETER

REMNANT RADIATION

AGGREGATE OF SILVER
DEPOSIT ON X-RAY FILM

RADIOGRAPHIC IMAGE AS
SEEN ON ILLUMINATOR

LONG SCALE CONTRAST

Figure 4-3. Long scale contrast. (Courtesy of Mrs. Arthur W. Fuchs.)

DENSITY	CONTRAST	KVP	MA	SECONDS	MAS
Same	Less or Long-scale	90	15	.5	7.5
Same	Greater or Short-scale	65	10	2	20.0

Figure 4-4. Contrast-density relationship.

the exposed x-ray film in enlarged cross section is shown beneath the step-wedge or penetrometer; and the resulting radiographic image as it appears when viewed on the illuminator is depicted below the film cross section in both illustrations. The penetrometer demonstrates how long-scale contrast compares with short-scale contrast.

Relationship Between Contrast and Density

When the radiographic *contrast* is changed, the *radiographic density* of the film will be altered. However, when radiographic *density* is altered by itself, there will be no obvious change in the radiographic *contrast*. Why is this true?

A change in kilovoltage will produce a change in contrast. The higher the kilovoltage, the less will be the contrast. However, since kilovoltage is a controlling factor in radiographic density, an increase in kilovoltage will also increase the radiographic density. Therefore, when the kilovoltage is *increased,* the milliampere-seconds (a controlling factor in radiographic density) must be *decreased* in order to maintain the previous radiographic density. To illustrate this concept, examine the exposure table in Figure 4-4 for the maxillary molar region using ultraspeed film and a 16″ target-film distance.

Notice that the mAs using the 90-15 technic is 7.5, as compared with the 20 mAs for the 65-10 technic (Figure 4-4).

Film contrast cannot be varied by a change in milliamperage *unless* a variation in *voltage* is made to compensate for the milliamperage variation. The higher the mA, and the lower the voltage, the greater will be the contrast.

Radiographic density can be altered *without* changing the contrast. How is this accomplished? Milliampere-seconds is the *prime* factor in controlling radiographic density, but it is *not* a controlling factor in radiographic contrast. Therefore, a change in mAs will produce a change in radiographic density but not a noticeable change in contrast. *To illustrate:* Two radiographs of the same region can be made, one of greater density (higher mAs), and one of lesser density (lower mAs) with the kVp remaining constant in both radiographs. These two films will have differences in over-all *blackness* but the extreme blacks and whites of both films will remain the same.

Geometric Characteristics

The formation of an accurate radiographic image is dependent upon minimizing certain geometric characteristics which are present to a certain degree in every radiograph. There are three geometric characteristics and they are listed below:

1. Radiographic image unsharpness (diffusion of detail).
2. Magnification or enlargement of the radiographic image.
3. Distortion in shape of the radiographic image (unequal enlargement).

There will always be a certain amount of unsharpness, magnification, and shape distortion of the radiographic image for three reasons (See Figure 4-5):

1. X-rays originate from a definite area

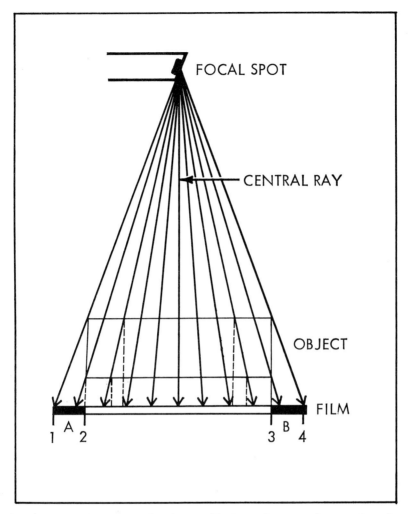

Figure 4-5. Diagram illustrating why there will always be some degree of unsharpness, magnification, and shape distortion in every radiograph. *Areas A & B penumbra* (areas of fuzziness of radiographic image). *Areas between 2 and 3:* actual size of image. *Areas between 1 and 4:* actual projected size of radiographic image.

rather than a point source. It is impossible to have a point source of x-rays because of the limited heating capacity of x-ray tubes. The source of radiation in modern dental x-ray machines varies from 0.8 mm to 1.5 mm square, depending upon the mA and kVp used.

2. X-rays travel in diverging straight lines as they radiate from their source of origin. This divergent quality of ionizing radiation is an important source of magnification.

3. The structures of the human jaws have depth as well as length and width. Therefore, in dental radiog-

raphy, a three-dimensional object is recorded upon the two-dimensional surface of a film. This results in unequal magnification of different parts of an object because of varying distances of these parts from the film. In dental radiography, the lingual cusps of the posterior teeth are magnified less than the buccal cusps because they are nearer the film.

In order to understand how these geometric characteristics can interfere with film image accuracy, let us first investi-

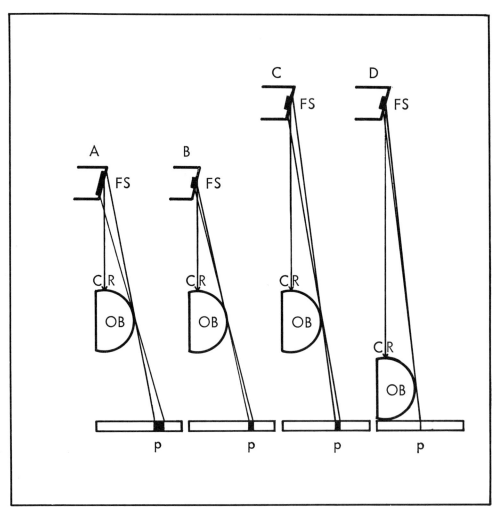

Figure 4-6. Diagrams illustrating how the accuracy of the radiographic image can be improved by decreasing the size of the penumbra (P). The penumbra effects image unsharpness and magnification. Notice the change in size of the penumbra (P) from A to B by decreasing the size of the *focal spot* of the anode. Notice the change in size of the penumbra (P) from B to C by increasing the distance between the *focal spot* and the *film*. Notice the change in size of the penumbra (P) from C to D by decreasing the distance between (OB) and the *film*. (Courtesy of Mrs. Arthur W. Fuchs.)

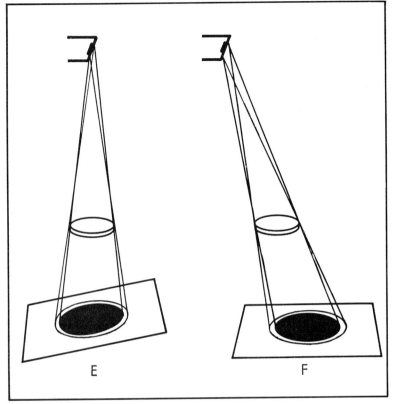

Figure 4-7. Diagrams illustrating the geometric effects of shape distortion of the radiographic image. If the object and the film are *not* parallel to each other, the shape of the image will be distorted as shown in *diagram E*. If the focal spot of the anode is not aligned perpendicularly to the object and the film, shape distortion will occur as seen in *diagram F*. (Courtesy of Eastman Kodak Co.)

gate how these same geometric characteristics are produced by light waves. After all, x-rays are no more than very short light waves which are invisible to the eye.

In order to demonstrate shadow formation by light, obtain a small light source (7½ watt bulb). Place your hand approximately an inch from the wall with the small light source positioned three feet from the wall. The shadow produced will be nearly the same size as your hand with its edges clear and well-defined. If you move your hand toward the light source, you will notice that the shadow of your hand will enlarge and its edges will become fuzzy and indistinct.

Next, substitute a large frosted bulb or a flashlight for the light source. You will notice this time that the hand shadow will have fuzzy edges even with your hand close to the wall. This fuzziness at the edges is caused by the large light source. The actual shadow is called the *umbra*, and the fuzzy shadow around the umbra is called the *penumbra* or the *area of unsharpness*. In order to minimize the unsharpness of your radiographic image, the penumbra must be reduced.

You can also distort your hand image by placing the light source in such a manner that the light waves strike your hand in an oblique direction rather than perpendicularly. This is called shape distortion.

In order to avoid confusion in comparing light waves and x-rays remember that light waves produce shadows by reflecting light from an opaque object. X-rays will penetrate this same object and will not produce a true shadow because details of the object will be visible in the processed film. Therefore, x-rays produce images rather than shadows.

Nevertheless, the same laws that apply to the shadow at the edge of the object (penumbra) apply to the details of the internal structures of the object. The five rules for accurate shadow casting by light waves are also applicable to x-rays in the formation of an accurate radiographic image.

Five Rules for Accurate Image Formation

1. The x-rays should proceed from as small a focal spot as conditions will allow.
2. The distance between the focal spot (source) and the object to be examined should always be as great as is practical.
3. The film should be as close as possible to the object being radiographed.
4. Generally speaking, the central ray should be as nearly perpendicular to the film as possible to record the adjacent structures in their true spatial relationships.
5. As far as is practical, the long axis of the object should be parallel to the film.

By following the above five rules, measures can be taken to minimize the inherent geometric characteristics found in every radiograph. The effects produced when these five rules are diagrammatically represented in Figures 4-6 and 4-7.

Factors That Influence Geometric Characteristics of the Radiographic Image

Radiographic Image Unsharpness

Radiographic image unsharpness is the fuzzy area surrounding the contour lines of the teeth and osseous tissues of the radiograph. Considering the relatively small size of the dental structures and tissues, it is very important that these areas of fuzziness or unsharpness be minimized in the dental radiograph. A dental radiograph must have maximum definition of detail, and the contour lines of the teeth and the osseous tissues must be clearly defined and distinct.

There are three types of radiographic image unsharpness (diffusion of detail by penumbra formation) found in the dental radiograph which all influence definition.

1. Geometric unsharpness
2. Motion unsharpness
3. Screen unsharpness

Geometric Unsharpness

Geometric unsharpness is the fuzzy outline of the radiographic image caused by the penumbra. The penumbra is produced by the size of the focal spot and is influenced by the source-object and the object-film distance.

1. The size of the effective focal spot of the x-ray tube
2. Focal spot-object distance, which is also known as source-object distance
3. Object-film distance

The smaller the size of the focal spot, the smaller the penumbra and consequently, the sharper the definition of the radiographic image (See Diagrams A & B of Figure 4-6). When the focal spot is relatively small (0.8 mm to 1.5 mm) the radiographic image is influenced very little by magnification.

The width of the zone of geometric unsharpness or penumbra can be illustrated by the following equation:

$$U_g = F \times \frac{d}{D}$$

U_g = Penumbra Size

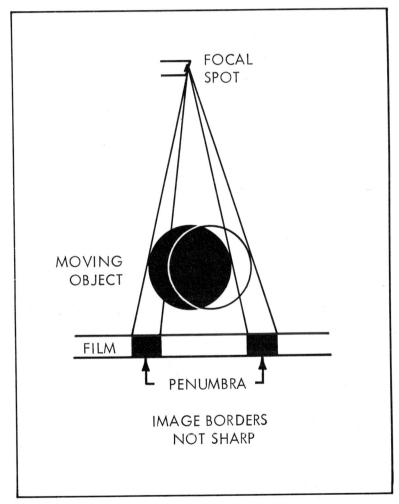

Figure 4-8. Diagram illustrating the influence of motion in producing image unsharpness. (Courtesy of Mrs. Arthur W. Fuchs.)

F = Focal Spot Size
d = Object-film distance in inches
D = Source-object distance in inches

In all situations, sharpness is improved when the source-object distance is increased (See Diagrams B & C of Figure 4-6).

The longer the object-film distance the greater the *unsharpness*. In the dental radiograph, the portion of the dental structure closest to the film will have the greatest sharpness. Therefore, the lingual cusp and the lingual root of a tooth will have more sharpness on the radiograph than the buccal cusp and the buccal root or roots, because they are closer to the film (See Diagrams C and D of Figure 4-6).

In summary then, geometric unsharpness can be minimized by reducing the width of the focal spot, reducing the object-film distance and increasing the source-object distance.

Motion Unsharpness

Motion by the patient, motion of the film, and/or motion of the tube, directly influences sharpness of the image definition. Even a slight motion of the film may cause motion unsharpness in the radiographic image. Any motion of the tube may cause vibration of the focal spot, which increases the size of the focal spot, thereby causing an increase in radiographic image unsharpness of the resulting images in the radiograph. The influence of patient movement on the definition of the radiographic image is illustrated in Figure 4-8.

The movement of the film without pa-

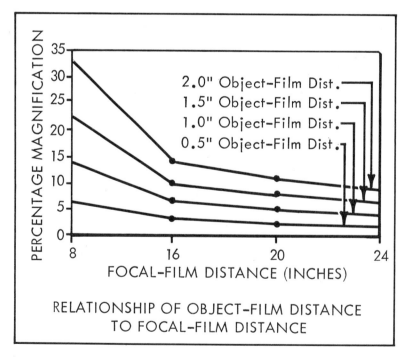

Figure 4-9. Relationship of the source-film distance to the object-film distance. (Courtesy of Dr. William Updegrave.)

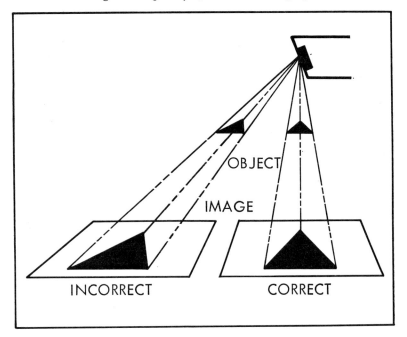

Figure 4-10. Shape distortion is produced by poor alignment.

tient movement during exposure will cause the greatest amount of motion unsharpness on the film.

Screen Unsharpness

Screen unsharpness is introduced to the radiograph when intensifying screens are used in extraoral radiography. The amount of unsharpness is dependent namely upon the thickness of the screen, the crystal particle size, and the film-screen contact.

Magnification

Magnification is the enlargement of the actual size of the object upon the projection of the radiographic image. The factors that influence magnification are the same factors that influence geometric unsharpness; however, the distance factors have more influence than the focal spot size.

Since the focal spot size is controlled by the manufacturer, the two distance factors are the only factors that can be controlled by the operator. It is possible to minimize magnification (enlargement) of the dental structures by increasing the source-film distance and reducing object-film distance to practical distances.

MAGNIFICATION FORMULAS. The *percent of magnification* of an object at any source-film distance (SFD) and the object-film distance (OFD) can be readily determined by the following formula:

$$\frac{SFD}{SFD\text{-}OFD} - \times 1.0\ (1 \times 100\%) = \text{Percent of Magnification}$$

Example: Determine the percent magnification of an object situated 1 inch from the film (OFD) when employing an SFD of 16 inches.

$$\frac{16}{16-1} - 1.00\ (1 \times 100\%) = .066 \text{ or } 6.6\%$$

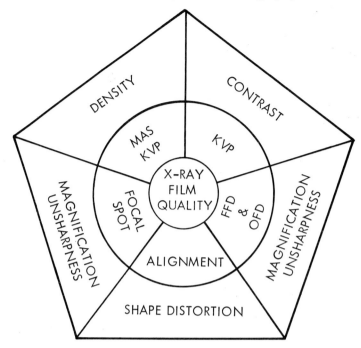

Figure 4-11. Summary of controlling factors of density, contrast, geometric unsharpness, magnification and distortion.

The graph in Figure 4-9 depicts the effect of source-film, object-film relationship on percentage of image enlargement or magnification.

THE RULE FOR MAGNIFICATION. The rule for magnification can be stated as a proportion:

The actual size of the object (tooth) is proportional to the size of the projected radiographic image of the object (tooth) as the source-object distance is to the source-film distance.

$$\frac{S_1 \text{ (Size of the Object)}}{S_2 \text{ (Size of the Image)}} = \frac{\text{Source-Object Distance}}{\text{Source-Film Distance}}$$

The source-object distance is measured from the source to an imaginary line at one half of the thickness of the object (tooth) to be radiographed.

Shape Distortion

Shape distortion of the radiographic image is a variation from the true shape of the anatomical structure radiographed. It results from an improper alignment of the object, the film, and the projected radiation. Shape distortion can be minimized by placing the film parallel to the major planes of the object and directing the central ray perpendicular to the major planes of the object and the film (See Figure 4-10).

If all other exposure factors remain constant, the factors listed in the table in Figure 4-11 will influence the x-ray image characteristics of density, contrast, geometric unsharpness, magnification and shape distortion in various ways.

Anatomic Accuracy

Anatomic accuracy occurs when the

anatomical structures are reproduced on the film in the exact relationship as they normally appear. A radiograph with anatomic accuracy will have a minimum of superimposition of images of adjacent structures. Anatomic accuracy is accomplished when the long axis of the teeth are parallel to the film and the radiation beam is perpendicular to both.

A radiograph is said to have anatomic accuracy when:

1. The labial and lingual cemento-enamel junctions of the anterior teeth are superimposed.
2. The buccal and lingual cusps of the posterior teeth (especially the molars) are superimposed.
3. The contacts of the teeth are opened in at least one of the projections of a given area.
4. The buccal portion of the alveolar crest is superimposed over the lingual portion of the alveolar crest.
5. There is no superimposition of the zygoma over the roots of the maxillary molar teeth.

Radiographic Coverage

It is important that the area of interest is well covered in the radiograph. In the periapical radiograph, an adequate amount of bone surrounding the apices of the teeth should be revealed on the radiograph.

Supplemental films taken at right angles to each other may be mandatory at times in order to localize the area of interest. Adequate coverage of area of interest depends upon several factors:

1. Proper alignment of film and the radiation beam to area of interest.
2. Proper selection of film types.
3. Proper selection of film projection technics.

Summary

Therefore, the diagnostic quality of your film is dependent upon the proper utilization of several factors. The functions of these factors is given below:

1. *Focal spot size* influences unsharpness and magnification of radiographic image.
2. *Source-film and object-film distances* influences density, unsharpness and magnification of radiographic image.
3. *Alignment of film and beam of radiation to object* influences anatomic accuracy, distortion and coverage of radiograph.
4. *Kilovoltage*
   a. regulates degree of penetration of tissues.
   b. influences scatter radiation fog.
   c. regulates contrast scale.
   d. determines exposure latitude.
   e. influences density of radiograph.
5. *Milliampere—Seconds (mAs)*
   a. regulates density of radiograph.

REFERENCES

Beck, James: *Syllabus of Dental Radiology.* University of Minnesota School of Dentistry, 1970.

Bloom, William J.; Hollenbach, John L.; and Morgan, James A.: *Medical Radiographic Technic*, 3rd ed. Springfield, Ill., Charles C Thomas, 1969.

Cheris, David, and Cheris, Barbara: *Basic Physics and Principles of Diagnostic Radiology.* Chicago, Year Book Medical Publishers, 1966.

Curby, W. A., and Wuehrmann, A. H.: Utilization of constant exposure factors for intraoral roentgenographic studies. *J Dent Res,* 32:790-795, December, 1953.

Ennis, LeRoy; Berry, Harrison; and Phillips, James E.: *Dent Roentgenol*, 6th ed. Lea & Febiger, 1967.

Files, G. W.: The relation, radiographically, of kilovolts peak to time of exposure. *Radiology*, 7:255, 1926.

Fitzgerald, G. M.: An investigation in adumbration, or the factors that control geometric unsharpness. *J Am Dent Assoc*, 34:5, 1947.

Fitzgerald, G. M.: Dental roentgenographic IV. The voltage factor. *J Am Dent Assoc*, 41:19-28, July, 1950.

Fitzgerald, G. M.: *Ginn's Review of Dentistry*. St. Louis, C. V. Mosby, 1949.

Fitzgerald, Gordon: Dental roentgenography I: An investigation in adumbration, or the factors that control geometric unsharpness. *J Am Dent Assoc*, 34:1-20, January, 1947.

Fitzgerald, Gordon: Roentgenologic rebuttal. *Oral Surg*, 13:1218, October, 1960.

Franklin, J. B.: The effect of aluminum filter disks in roentgenocephalometry. *Angle Orthodont*, 32:252, October, 1962.

Fuchs, Arthur: *Principles of Radiographic Exposure and Processing*, 2nd ed. Springfield, Ill., Charles C Thomas, 1971.

Hendee, William R.: *Medical Radiation Physics*. Chicago, Year Book Medical Publishers, 1970.

Jaundrell-Thompson, J., and Ashworth, W. J.: *X-Ray Physics and Equipment*, 2nd ed. Philadelphia, F. A. Davis, 1970.

Jacobi, Charles A., and Paris, Don Q.: *Textbook of Radiology Technology*, St. Louis, C. V. Mosby Co., 5th Ed., 1972.

Johns, Harold, and Cunningham, John: *The Physics of Radiology*, 3rd ed. Springfield, Ill., Charles C Thomas, 1969.

Langland, O. E., and Sippy, F. H.: A study of radiographic longitudinal distortion of anterior teeth using the paralleling technique. *Oral Surg*, 22:737-749, December, 1966.

Mattson, O.: Practical photographic problems in radiography with special reference to high voltage technic. *Acta Radiol, Supp 20*, 1955.

McCormack, Donald: Dental roentgenology: A technical procedure for furthering the advancement toward anatomical accuracy. *J Calif State Dent Assoc*, May-June, 1937.

McCormack, F. W.: A plea for standardized technique for oral radiography. *J Dent Res*, 2, 1920.

Muncheryan, H. M.: *Modern Physics of Roentgenology*. Los Angeles, Wetzel, 1940.

Radiology Specialist. Washington, D. C., Department of the Air Force, March, 1958.

Richards, Albert G.: Technical factors that control radiographic density. *Dent Clin North Am*, 371-377, July, 1961.

Seeman, Herman E.: *Physical and Photographic Principles of Medical Radiography*. New York, John Wiley & Sons, 1968.

Selman, Joseph: *The Fundamentals of X-Ray and Radium Physics*, 3rd ed. Springfield, Ill., Charles C Thomas, 1966.

Sweet, A. Porter: Dental seminar: radiographic density. *Dent Radiol Photogr*, No. 4, 1949.

Sweet, A. Porter: Peripheral geometry. *Dent Radiol Photogr*, 25, 1952.

Ter-Pogossian, Michel M.: *The Physical Aspects of Diagnostic Radiology*. New York, Hoeber Medical, 1967.

The Fundamentals of Radiography, 10th ed. Rochester, N. Y., Eastman Kodak Co., 1960.

TM-8-280, Military Roentgenology, Washington, D. C., U. S. Government Printing Office, 1944.

Updegrave, William: Simplifying and improving intraoral dental roentgenography. *Oral Surg*, 12:704-716, June, 1959.

Updegrave, William: High or low kilovoltage. *Dent Radiol Photogr*, No. 4, 1960.

Updegrave, W. J.: Higher fidelity in intraoral roentgenography. *J Am Dent Assoc*, 62:3, 1961.

Waggener, Donald T.: The Right-Angle Technique Using the Extension Cone. *Dent Clinics North Am*, 783-788, November, 1960.

Wuehrmann, Arthur: The long cone technic. *Prac Dent Monogr*, 3-30, July, 1957.

Wuehrmann, Arthur, and Manson-Hing, Lincoln: *Dental Radiology*. St. Louis, C. V. Mosby, 1965.

Wuehrmann, Arthur, and Monacelli, C. J.: Selection of optimum kilovoltage for dental radiography. *Radiology*, 57:240-246, August, 1951.

Wuehrmann, Arthur, and Curby, W. A.: Radiopacity of oral structures as a basis for selecting optimum kilovoltage for intraoral roentgenograms. *J Dent Res*, 31:27-32, February, 1952.

X-Ray Generation and Radiographic Principles in Dentistry. Milwaukee, X-Ray Department, General Electric Co.

CHAPTER 5

RADIATION HAZARDS AND PREVENTION

Biologic Effects of Ionizing Radiations

ALL IONIZING RADIATION is potentially harmful if excessive. X-rays, gamma rays, and cosmic rays are known as ionizing radiations since they ionize the substance which they strike.

Radiation striking a cell, or a chemical unit causes primarily ionization, and to a lesser extent excitation. This, in turn, effects chemical changes in the molecules of the cells. The cell may ultimately be damaged by these chemical changes or chain reactions.

Ionization is the separation of an atom into positive and negative ions by the influence of ionizing radiation. There are two major modes by which ionization is produced in dental radiography. They are by (1) photoelectric absorption and (2) Compton Scattering. These modes of ionization were described previously in Chapter 3.

Two main theories have been put forward to explain the damage to the cell caused by ionization and excitation:

The Target or Direct Action Theory

In the simplest form, it states that the cell contains a critical site or "target," and a single ionizing event or "hit" within this target will inactivate the cell; all hits outside the critical site will have no effect. Although this theory has very little support at present time, it remains a convenient means of discussing certain aspects of radiation damage to cells.

The Poison-Chemical or Indirect Action Theory

In contrast to the "target" theory, which assumes that the radiation attacks a discrete portion of the cell, the poison theory states that the radiation is absorbed somewhere within the cell which in turn causes chemical reactions to result which form toxic substances within the cell. These toxic compounds affect the vital substances of the cell secondarily. This is the reason for also calling the Poison Theory, the Indirect Theory.

Fundamentally, the harmful consequences of ionizing radiations to a living organism are due to the energy absorbed by the cells and tissues which form the organism. This absorbed energy (or dose) produces chemical decomposition of the molecules present in the living cells. (Molecules are formed when atoms are linked together by their electrons). The amount of the tissue decomposition appears to be related to the amount of ionization or number of ion pairs produced by ionizing radiations in the cells or tissues.

Measurement of Radiation Quantity

The ideal basis for the measurement of radiation quantity would be measurement of the ion pairs (or ionizations) taking place within the medium of interest.

The roentgen has long been the unit for measuring (1) the radiation as it emerges from the x-ray machine and (2) the energy absorbed by the unit. However, the roentgen is not the ideal unit for measuring radiation quantity because:

1. The definition of the roentgen makes it impossible to measure adequately above 3 MeV.
2. The roentgen is defined for electromagnetic radiation and not for other types of radiation such as electrons, protons and neutrons. These particles can also produce biologic chemical effects when absorbed.
3. Since ionization is an indirect measurement of radiation quantity, the roentgen is an indirect measurement unit.

Therefore, in 1956 a new unit of dose, the rad, was established by the International Commission on Radiological Units and Measurements (ICRU). At this meeting, the commission established the concept of *exposure*, which was to be measured in roentgens, and the *dose* to be measured in rads (a new unit). The word "dose" strictly connotes the deposition of energy per unit mass of the absorber.

The Rad

The rad is defined as an energy absorption of 100 ergs per gram of any material.

$$1 \text{ Rad} = 100 \text{ ergs/gm} = 0.01 \text{ joules/kg}$$

The rad is a somewhat larger unit than a roentgen since the roentgen is equal to 0.869 ergs of energy absorbed per gram of air or 93 ergs of energy absorbed per gram of soft tissue. The rad, however, is more nearly equivalent to the roentgen in mixed body tissue (hard and soft), and it is thus applicable to human exposure. Usually, it can be said that one roentgen of exposure will pro-

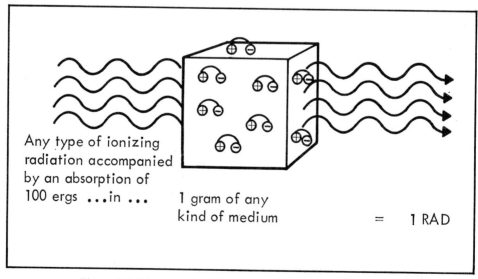

Any type of ionizing radiation accompanied by an absorption of 100 ergs ...in ... 1 gram of any kind of medium = 1 RAD

Figure 5-1. Diagram of a RAD. (Courtesy of Dr. I. Meschan.)

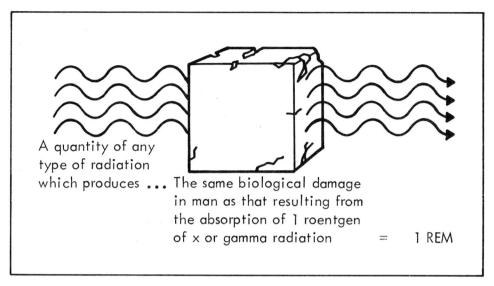

A quantity of any type of radiation which produces ... The same biological damage in man as that resulting from the absorption of 1 roentgen of x or gamma radiation = 1 REM

Figure 5-2. Diagram of a REM. (Courtesy of Dr. I. Meschan.)

duce about 1 rad of absorbed dose in mixed body tissue (1 erg equals the work done in moving a body 1 cm against a force of 1 dyne) (See Figure 5-1).

The Rem

A dose of one type of ionizing radiation may differ in its efficiency to elicit a chemical or biological effect in a medium than the same dose of a different type of radiation.

The relative biological effectiveness (RBE) expresses the effectiveness with which a particular ionizing radiation produces a certain chemical or biological effect.

The rad is a convenient unit for expressing energy absorption, but it does not take into account the biological effect of the particular radiation absorbed.

Therefore, a new unit of dose called the rem (roentgen equivalent man) was introduced taking into consideration the RBE. It was defined as:

$$\text{Dose (rems)} = \text{Dose (rads)} \times \text{RBE}$$

SOME RBE VALUES

Radiation	RBE
X-rays, gamma rays, electrons and beta particles	1.0
Fast neutrons and protons up to 10 Mv	10.0
Naturally occurring alpha particles	10.0

At present, the use of the RBE is restricted to the field of radiobiology and other terms have been introduced for use in the radiation protection field. These new terms are the quality factor (QF) and the distribution factor (DF). They take into consideration the different biological effects of various types of particulate radiation and the modification of the biological effect by the nonuniform distribution of internally taken isotopes. A more detailed account of these factors can be found in any radiation physics textbook.

Thus, the rem is a unit of biological

dose. In general, for x- and gamma radiation, the biological dose in rems is numerically equal to the dose in rads and roughly equal to the exposure dose in roentgens (See Figure 5-2). With the level of radiation energy used in dentistry, the following generalization can be made:

$$1 R = 1 Rad = 1 Rem$$

Somatic and Germinal Cells

Radiation affects two types of cells in the body. They are the somatic and germinal cells. The somatic cells constitute all the cells of the body except the germ cells of the reproductive organs. The germ cells of the reproductive organs are the ova of the female and the spermatozoa of the male. The changes brought about by radiation in the germinal cells cannot be detected in the exposed person, but the changes may be passed on to their offspring.

Factors Which Determine Biological Effects

Total Amount of Radiant Energy Absorbed

Generally, the more radiation that is absorbed by a tissue, the more damage that can be expected.

In measuring somatic changes from radiation, the effect usually cannot be detected until a minimum or threshold is exceeded. Of course, changes can occur if subthreshold doses are repeated. Genetic changes appear to have no thresholds; in other words, any given dosage will produce an effect of some kind.

There are exceptions to these accepted theories. Some studies have shown that leukemia and cancer production (somatic changes) have no threshold, and others have shown that certain genetic changes require a minimum dosage.

Rate of Absorption

The effects of radiation will be less if the total dose is divided rather than given in a single exposure. Exposures to radiation may be classified on the basis of the rate of absorption.

An acute exposure is a short intense exposure of ionizing radiation while chronic (protracted) exposures are continued exposures of lower intensity administered over a long period of time.

For instance, if a single acute skin dose of 600 rads administered within one hour to a local part produces erythema (redness in the skin), then it may take two doses of 425 rads each administered 24 hours apart to produce the same effect.

Body Part Exposed

The hazard of the radiation is increased when a larger part of the whole body is exposed at once. Local areas can receive larger doses of radiation without risk, whereas, if the same doses were given to the whole body it would be lethal to the patient.

For instance, if a single dose of 700 rads were given to a finger of a person, the finger would experience erythema and some injury with recovery; however, if the same dose (700 rads) was given to the whole body, the patient would die from acute radiation injury.

Species and Individual Differences

There is a wide variation in the response of individual species to whole body radiation. For instance, for animals exposed to 200 kV radiation the median lethal dose (MLD) will vary in the following manner: man, 450 rads; mice, 500 rads; and rabbits, 875 rads. There also may be considerable differences between individuals within a species. They may vary as much as 50 percent according to to their median lethal doses.

Variability of Radiosensitivity of Cells and Tissue

The response of the cell is governed by various factors which include:

1. *Mitotic Activity:* The cells that are more actively dividing are generally more sensitive to radiation.
2. The cells and tissues which are less differentiated or non-specialized are more sensitive to radiation.
3. Cells with an increased cellular metabolism tend to be more sensitive to radiation.

These factors explain the radiosensitivity of tumors, germinative tissues, the embryo, and rapidly growing tissues of younger animals.

Therefore, the tissues and cells of the body can be divided into two broad groups, the radiosensitive and the radioresistant. This division seems to parallel the rate of mitosis seen in various tissues.

1. *Radiosensitive group* (starting with the most sensitive tissue)
   a. germinal cells of ovary
   b. seminiferous epithelium of testis
   c. lymphocytes
   d. blood forming tissues
   e. intestinal epithelium
   f. skin
2. *Radioresistant group* (listed in decreasing order of sensitivity)
   a. most glandular tissues
   b. muscle tissue
   c. nerve tissue

Latent Period

Tissues do not always react immediately to a dose of x-radiation. There is a time lapse before any effects are seen; this is referred to as the latent period. The latent period merely represents the time interval until one is able to detect damage. There is a vast time range in the latent period. Those effects which appear within a matter of minutes, days, or weeks are called acute effects, and those which appear years, decades, and sometimes generations later are called long-term effects. In most cases, the larger the dose, the earlier is the appearance of injury. Where the doses are small and continued over a period of time, the latent period for some of the effects may be very long (25 years or more).

Following the exposure to radiation there is a certain amount of healing of damaged cells. The healing process can be one of replacement of the damaged tissue, or by recuperation of the injured cells. However, there is some residual damage occurring to some cells.

The radiation injury is carried within the nuclei of the cells and is passed on to its daughter cells. This is how the pathologic lesion can show up years later.

Accumulative Effect of X-Radiation

Of course, no radiation remains within the tissue after exposure. Some of the cells will recover by healing, while others will carry a residual biological effect. These biological effects will add up every time an individual receives a radiation dose. This is why x-radiation is said to be accumulative.

Of course, the amount of residual injury left within the tissue depends upon the dose delivered. The greatest amount

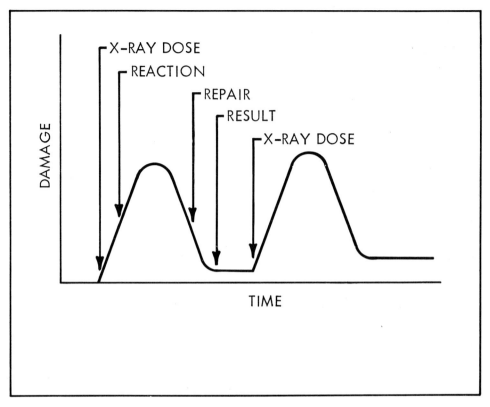

Figure 5-3. Diagrammatic representation of the accumulative effect of x-radiation. (Courtesy of Dr. Lincoln Manson-Hing.)

of healing of the damaged cells will occur within the first 24 hours. The residual biological effect within the cells which do not heal is called the accumulative effect of x-radiation (See Figure 5-3).

How Do Various Radiation Exposures Affect Human Beings?

The radiation hazard to human beings are of different types:

Large Amounts of Radiation to the Whole Body (Acute Exposure)

The possibility of this type of exposure in diagnostic radiography is very remote. It is seen in victims of atomic weapons and in individuals exposed accidentally to nuclear energy. When large doses are delivered to the whole body in a short period of time, the following effects may be seen:

Acute Dose	Probable Effect
0-25 Rads	No obvious injury
25-50 Rads	Possible blood changes but no serious injury
50-100 Rads	Blood cells changes, some injury, no disability
100-200 Rads	Injury, possible disability
200-400 Rads	Injury and disability certain, death possible

400 Rads   Fatal to 50%
600 rads or more Fatal

***Large Amounts of Radiation to
Limited Portions of the Body
(Acute and Chronic)***

Large measured doses are given to small parts of the body in order to treat serious illnesses such as cancer. The benefits of the radiation outweigh the hazards of the radiation in these cases. In the treatment of cancer, as much as 2,000 to 6,000 rads is delivered to a small area with reversible acute reactions and moderate chronic atrophic changes. There is always a possibility of latent

	TYPICAL VALUES IN MREMS	
	Whole Body mrem/year	Gonads mrem/year
I. Natural Background		
Cosmic Rays	38-75	
Terestrial Gamma	20-215	
Total	58-215	

The *average* annual whole body and genetically significant dose for the U.S. population is between 102 and *120* mrem/year.

II. Medical and Dental Radiation		
Medical	72	20
radiopharmaceuticals	1	0.26
Dental		0.15
Total	73	20.4
III. Miscellaneous Sources		
Nuclear power plants	1.0	1.0
Nuclear Testing (fallout)	4.0	4.0
T.V. & Consumer products	2.6	2.6
Total	7.6	7.6
Total Exposure All Sources:	138.6-295.6	

Source: Effects on populations of exposure to low levels of ionizing radiation, National Academy of Sciences, Washington, D.C., 1972.

IV. Doses associated with Dental Radiographic Procedures
   Dose per film—200 mrads
   Highest reported dose to any given region per CMRS—1500 mrads (maxillary central incisor)
   Genetically significant dose—no lead apron—0.5 mrads per CMRS
   Genetically significant dose—with lead apron—0.01-0.03 mrads per CMRS
   Average occupational exposure for:
      Medical and Dental personnel—200 mrem/year
      M.P.D. occupational workers—5 rem/year
      M.P.D. non-occupationally exposed individuals—0.5 rem/year (1/10th of occupational)
   Note: M.P.D. specifically excludes background and medical exposures

Figure 5-4. Sources of Population Exposure to Ionizing Radiation.

effects such as cancer, aseptic bone necrosis, and radiation cataracts showing up years later.

Small Amounts of Radiation to the Whole Body (Chronic Exposure)

There are two types of chronic whole body radiation: (1) background radiation and (2) radiation received from occupational exposure.

Background radiation comes from material sources and chronically exposes the entire world population each day (See Figure 5-4). It arises from three sources:

1. Cosmic rays
2. External radiation from radioactive materials in the environment
3. Internal radiation exposure from naturally occurring radioisotopes deposited in body by ingestion or inhalation

Background radiation contributes to an average yearly whole body dose of approximately 0.15 rem (or 150 mrem).

The dose rate from cosmic rays varies considerably at higher altitudes because of atmospheric absorption. In Denver, a person receives three times as much radiation from cosmic rays as a person living at sea level (50 mrems). Also, a jet airline pilot receives approximately 300 mrem per year from cosmic radiation. This is about six times the dose at sea level.

Dentists, dental auxiliaries, radiologists and x-ray technologists are exposed daily to small amounts of radiation to the whole body. This is a chronic type of exposure and is measured by the use of film badges. Maximum permissible limits for radiation exposure to the radiation workers have been determined by the National Committee on Radiation Protection.

Small Amounts of Radiation to Limited Portions of the Body (Acute and Chronic)

The patient is exposed to this type of radiation in diagnostic radiography. Biological effects (somatic or germinal) to patients are not likely to be critical with the small doses given in dentistry, but may be with repeated exposures, or where large and sensitive tissues are irradiated. The chief hazard to this type of radiation in dental practice is to the dentist who holds film in patients' mouths.

The Concept of Radiation Protection Guides

Since the use of ionizing radiation involves a certain risk to the patient, it must be balanced against the advantages gained by the use of the radiation.

Guidelines for the use of ionizing radiation were developed through the years because it became apparent to the early radiation workers that excessive exposure to this new form of energy was biologically undesirable. As our knowledge of the hazards of radiation increased, these limits have been revised downwards several times.

The International Commission on Radiological Protection (ICRP) states that the permissible dose for an individual is that dose, accumulated over a long period of time resulting from a single exposure, which, in light of present knowledge, carries a negligible probability of severe somatic or genetic injuries.

These radiation protection guides (maximum permissible doses) are directed to radiation workers and the general public. A radiation worker is an individual who participates in x-ray procedures, and therefore will be exposed to a certain amount of radiation as a part of his job.

For radiation workers, the maximum permissible accumulative dose rate to gonads, the blood-forming organs, and the lens of the eyes at any age over 18 is governed by the formula:

$$D = 5 \ (N—18)$$

where D is the tissue dose in rems and N is the age in years.

The maximum permissible dose to one who is occupationally exposed to radiation is 5 rem/year, or 0.1 rem/week.

The general public is allowed about 1/10th the amount of radiation exposure to the gonads, blood-forming organs and lens of the eyes as the occupationally exposed workers.

Radiation used for medical and dental diagnostic purposes is not counted toward the permissible amounts allowed the radiation worker and general public.

Needless to say, the dentist should try to use good clinical judgement in obtaining the maximum amount of diagnostic information from the least amount of radiation exposure to the patient that is practical.

General Effects of Radiation

Skin Reactions

Threshold doses for skin are relatively unknown. Skin reactions to radiation are determined by the injury to:

1. Blood vessels
2. Connective tissue
3. Epithelial cells

Erythema (or redness) to the skin will occur from high intensity radiation given for a short period (one hour) in the 400 to 2,000 rad ranges. In doses lower than this no erythema will occur. In the high dose ranges above 3,000 to 4,000 rads, the skin becomes thin, covered with dilated blood vessels and ulcerated. Cancer may develop from these acute doses; however, it is rare.

Cancer occurs (although not frequently) from a smaller dose repeated over months or years to a body part. This is the type of radiation effect seen in dentists who have held films in the mouths of their patients for years. The first clinical indication of any damage produced by x-rays administered in this manner is the appearance of chronic dermatitis.

The visible manifestations of x-ray damage to the hands or skin from low dosage radiation over a period of years can be divided into early and late symptoms.

The early signs:

1. Increased susceptibility to chapping and intolerance to surgical "scrub-up."
2. Blunting and leveling of the finger ridges.
3. Brittleness and ridging of the fingernails.

The late signs:

1. Loosening of the hairs and epilation.
2. Dryness and atrophy of the skin.
3. Progressive pigmentation, telangiectases, and keratoses.
4. Ulcerations, indolent in type (not painful).
5. Possibility of malignant change in tissue.

Using the better film technics, dentists can limit the exposure to the patient's jaws to 2 to 6 R per complete radiographic survey of 14 to 20 films. This is far below the threshold dose which is calculated as being between 400 to 2,000 rads.

Hematopoietic Injury (Lymphopenia, Leukopenia, Anemia, Leukemia, and Loss of Specific Immune Response)

Moderate whole body irradiation, such as 25 R, will produce transient changes in the blood count. Although the blood forming cells may be radiosensitive, they also have great recovery powers.

The usual picture of blood injury to radiation is leukopenia which in some cases may go to leukemia. It is very doubtful whether a single case of adult leukemia has ever occurred from acute doses of less than 200 rads to the bone marrow (Court-Brown and Doll, 1957).

Of the various neoplasms produced by whole-body radiation, the risk of leukemia is the greatest.

In the study of Japanese persons exposed to the atomic energy at Hiroshima and Nagasaki, the leukemia incidence increased after a latent period of ten years after exposure. The incidence has declined since then (Miller, 1969).

There is some evidence that low energy dosages directly to the fetus may result in childhood leukemia (MacMahon, 1962 and Stewart, 1968). However, this evidence is limited and inconclusive.

In some manner, not readily understood as yet, ionizing radiation can induce cancerous change (carcinogenesis) in man. Various epidemiological studies indicate relationship between radiation to various parts of the body and human cancer.

Cancer of the Skin

This was common during the early use of x-rays. Many of the early radiologists had multiple amputations for cancer of the arms and hands. Dr. C. Edmund Kells, one of the early pioneers in dental radiology, had an arm amputated because of skin cancer induced by continued exposures to radiation. There are only a few skin cancers seen today because the occupational exposure to the skin has been reduced to practically zero by the use of modern protective devices and procedures.

Bone Cancers

There is the tragic story of the radium-dial painters. They would moisten their brushes on their lips which were loaded with radioactive material before painting the dials. The radium entered the body through the mouth, and bone cancers appeared after a latent period of 15 years.

Lung Cancer

Austrian uranium miners were found to have a high percentage of lung cancer. The latent period was approximately 17 years and it was thought that the miners were exposed to radium gas in high concentration over a long period of time.

Thyroid Cancers

In previous years it was a practice to treat various disorders of neck, such as enlargement of the thymus gland and infected tonsils, with 300 rads of radiation or more. Years later a number of thyroid cancers resulted from such practices (Hempelman, 1960 and Hamford, et al., 1962).

It is interesting to note that less than 1 percent of the radiation delivered to the patient during a complete dental radiographic survey reaches the thyroid gland. This amount can be reduced to an infinite amount to the thyroid by using lead shields, and lead-lined cones.

Also, there have been no recorded cases of facial or thyroid cancers from the use of dental radiographic procedures.

X-Ray Therapy

There has been some recorded cases of cancer developing as a result of x-ray therapy of neoplasms of the body. The latent period varies from four to twenty-two years and the original dose is usually more than 3,000 rads (Cahan *et al.*, 1948).

In the treatment of diseases of the major salivary glands by x-ray therapy, doses of 2,500 to 3,000 R have been delivered over a period of one to two weeks. This is sufficient to dry the salivary glands (Wainwright, 1965), which has an indirect effect on caries production. It has not been established yet as to whether an increased caries rate in patients receiving massive doses of radiation for cancer of the jaws is due to physical changes of the tissues of the teeth or from a decreased salivary flow. It is probably due to both. Osteoradionecrosis of the jaws may occur from massive therapeutic doses of radiation delivered to the oral cavity for cancerous lesions. The usual procedure is to extract the teeth in the radiation beam or by the use of sound preventive measures on the remaining teeth.

Reduction of Life Span

Extensive data on mice has established that the average life span is diminished following a brief whole body radiation exposure or small amounts of radiation given over a long period of time. It has been found that the chief features of this syndrome is that it brings about an acceleration of the natural aging process resulting in a shortened life span (Curtis, 1961).

The results of these studies on animals are difficult to transfer to man. Life shortening has not been demonstrated in man following small doses of radiation.

It has been suggested that for every whole body exposure of 1R, the life span of an individual will be shortened by one day (Failla and McClement, 1957).

It was shown in a recent survey that dentists live on an average of 1.4 years longer than the rest of the white male population (Richards, 1968). This survey indicates that dentists have not suffered a shortening of life span from the occupational exposure to radiation.

Sterility (Temporary or Permanent)

A decrease in fertility in animals has been demonstrated from the exposure to ionizing radiation. Changes in the sperm count in the dog can be noticed if 0.5 R is given for long periods of time. However, it takes as much as 4.4 R per day exposure to female mice over a long period of time to produce sterility.

For humans, it takes as much as 600 R given in less than a week for women near menopause and nearly 2,000 R in a week directly to the reproductive organs to produce cessation of ovary activity. It is thought that it would require larger doses to produce sterility in the male. Doses of this amount to the whole body would be fatal.

Effects on Eyes

A "cataract" is a vision-impairing

opacity of the normally transparent lens of the eyes. It may cause blindness. Cataract formation is thought to be a "threshold" phenomenon in that it requires large doses of at least 600 R. The latent period is relatively long and varies inversely with the dose.

Genetic Changes

Offspring of man and animals arises from a single cell formed by the fusion of two germ cells, the ovum of the female and the sperm cell of the male. The germ cells (gametes) contain genes in the chromosome of their nuclei which determine what the offspring will be like.

A mutation is a change in the gene of a germ cell which will in turn change the inheritance of an offspring produced by this cell. Mutations occur in all living organisms; however, at a low rate. The cause of these natural mutations is unknown. Of course, genetic mutations have existed ever since the beginning of time.

Genetic mutations may be defective or they may be desirable. In the past, by the process of natural selectivity the defective mutations in a species tended to "die out" and the desirable mutations increased in number. However, modern civilization interferes with natural selectivity, and therefore, undesirable genetic mutations tend to be preserved.

At present, genetic defects in man may be the cause for about one out of every ten persons to fail to reproduce or die before maturity (McKusick, 1969). However, further study may modify these figures.

Ionizing radiation and chemicals are mutagenetic agents.

The most relevant information for determining the possible genetic damage induced by radiation in man comes from the extensive experimentation with the effects of radiation on the spermatozonia and oocytes in mice (Russell, 1969).

Scientists assume that there is no threshold dose for genetic effects, or no amount so low it wouldn't affect some genes sometime. They also suspect that one hit on a gene from radiation could act to mutate that gene.

The rate at which radiation is given was found to be highly important. For instance, a dose of 600 roentgens given in a short time will produce many more mutations than that same dosage given over weeks or months at a time.

The genetic harm from radiation is cumulative. This means that the genetic damage produced by radiation builds up, and it depends upon the total amount of gonadal exposures received by a person from their own conception to the conception of their last child (National Academy of Sciences, 1956).

It is not known whether what happens to mice genes from radiation can also happen to human genes. However, it is reasonable to believe that genetic effects in man follow the same general pattern.

The amount of radiation which will double (doubling dose) the natural mutation rate is not known. It has been estimated to be within the range of 30 to 80 R to the gonads per thirty years of life (National Academy of Sciences, 1958).

The maximum permissible dose from birth to age thirty to the general population from man-made radiation to the reproductive cells above natural background should be limited to 10 R (Taylor, 1957).

It has been estimated that a dental machine, operated at 65 kVp and 10 mA at an 8-inch source-film distance will deliver approximately one roentgen per second. Using fast film, the average exposure for each film is approximately 0.3 seconds. For a 14-film complete survey, then, the exposure to the face would be about 4.2 R. Research has shown that the male gonadal dose is about 1/10,000th the facial dose or 0.42 mR in this particular case (Richards, 1968). The average background exposure to an individual's gonads is estimated to be about 0.3 mR per day or 110 mR annually.

It is evident by this data, that the gonadal exposure for a dental complete survey is approximately the same amount that a person receives normally to his gonads from the natural background each day. This is a very small amount. A dentist may also use a lead apron draped over the gonadal area of a patient and reduce the exposure to zero.

Embryological and Developmental Effects

Considerable effects on growth and development can be shown in animals and man receiving radiation levels substantially greater than those expected from occupational exposure. For instance, continued whole body radiation to rats at a rate of 24 rads per week will produce growth inhibition. Slight retardation to growth and maturation were noticed in children exposed to atomic bomb radiation in Japan and Marshall Islands (Miller, 1968, 1969).

Effects of exposure during pregnancy on the embryo varies with dose and with age of the embryo. The fetus is more sensitive to radiation during its earliest stages of development (the first three months).

It has been shown that 25 R to the mouse embryo during the first half of the fetal life will produce obvious damage (Russell, 1952). A pregnant woman may have a miscarriage or stillbirth after 1,000 rads to the pelvis region; however, there are cases on record of pregnant women receiving doses of this level for treatment of cancer and still giving birth to normal children.

Routine radiological procedures (pelvimetry) of the fetus in the pregnant woman has been largely discontinued. It is now used only when it is indicated.

In one study conducted at Harvard School of Public Health of women irradiated during pregnancy, it was found that there was an increase in cancer (primarily leukemia and cancer of the nervous system) in the children born of these mothers, regardless of successful deliveries, color or sex. This data was collected from studies of 547,401 infants discharged from thirty United States hospitals from 1947 to January 1, 1959 (MacMahon, 1962).

A similar study produced opposite results. At a hospital in Chicago in 1948, pelvimetry was a routine procedure. After this year, pelvimetry was discontinued. A comparison was made between 1,008 infants exposed to radiation and 1,008 infants born after 1948 at this hospital. After a period of 15 years, 2,774 of these children were examined once again. No significant increase of leukemia, eye abnormalities or hemangiomas were noticed in the irradiated children (Griem et al., 1967).

It has not been proven at the present time whether the low intrauterine dose delivered during dental x-ray exposure can cause any increase in the number of malignancies or malformations among the offspring. However, in view of the importance of protecting the unborn child and in spite of the relatively low dose delivered to the fetus during most dental x-ray examinations, it would seem prudent to place additional shielding, such as a leaded apron, over the abdominal region of pregnant or potentially pregnant women during dental radiographic procedures.

Radiation Hazard Control

Although the amount of radiation exposure in the dental office is very small, the dentist should recognize that radiation exposure involves some hazard. The dentist has a professional responsibility to use x-rays in his dental practice; however, it is important for him to control the x-radiation in his office by all the practical means available in order to prevent any biological damage to himself, his workers, and his patients.

Limitations on Exposure to X-Radiation

LIMITS FOR DENTISTS AND DENTAL PERSONNEL. A permissible exposure is defined as the exposure to x-radiation that, in the light of present knowledge, is not expected to cause appreciable bodily injury to a person at any time during his lifetime (See Figure 5-5).

LIMITS FOR PATIENTS. The dental exposure of the patient to x-ray radiation shall be kept to the minimum level con-

Maximum Permissible Exposures[1] to Whole Body, Gonads, Blood Forming Organs, or Lens of Eye.

Average Weekly Exposure[2]	Maximum 13-week Exposure
0.1 R	3 R

Maximum Yearly Exposure	Maximum Accumulated Exposure[3]
5 R	5 (N − 18) R

1. Exposure of persons for dental or medical purposes is not counted against their maximum permissible exposure limits.

2. Used only for the purpose of designing radiation barriers.

3. N = Age in years and is greater than 18.
   The unit for exposure is the roentgen (R).

Figure 5-5. Limitations on exposure to x-radiations.

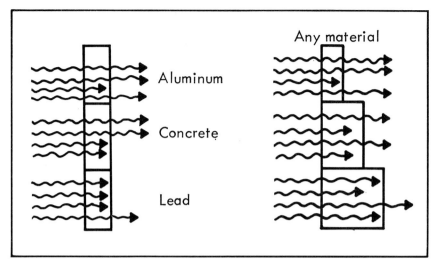

Figure 5-6. Shielding (relation of density and thickness of the shielding material).

sistent with diagnostic requirements. This limitation on exposure is determined in each case by the professional judgment of the dentist.

Sources of Radiation in the Dental Office

1. *Primary Radiation:* The direct radiation from the focal spot of the x-ray tube is called primary radiation. It passes through the aperture, collimator, and filter and emerges as the useful beam.

2. *Leakage Radiation:* All radiation coming from within the tube housing except the useful beam is called leakage radiation.

3. *Secondary Radiation:* Radiation emitted by any matter being irradiated with x-rays. Scattered radiation is a form of secondary radiation—it is radiation that, during passage through a substance, has been deviated in direction. It may also have been modified by an increase in wavelength. Secondary radiation originates mainly in the irradiated soft tis-

sues of the patient's face, the pointed plastic cone, and the filter.

Radiation Shielding

Any material interposed in an x-ray beam will absorb some of the radiation and thus reduce its intensity. The thicker the material and the greater its density, the more radiation it absorbs (See Figure 5-6). Good shielding can greatly reduce the occupational exposure of working personnel and radiation to areas surrounding the dental office.

Excellent results can be obtained by rigorous attention to proper shielding design of x-ray rooms and control booths and diligent use of protective aprons. A shielding design depends upon the radiation workload of the dental office.

The workload is expressed in milliampere seconds (mAs) per week. It is the product of the amount of current (mA) used per week multiplied by the amount of exposure time expressed in seconds. The workload is also related to the source-film distance, the tube voltage and film speed (Richards, 1968).

In the NCRP Report Number 35, a simple method for determining the workload for an x-ray machine is described. When an x-ray film box is opened, remove the box top. On the box top, place the date and machine identification. Do this with each box used during a specific period of time. When you have accumulated a number of box tops (possibly several months), determine the total number of films used during this time period. The unit of exposure used for upper molars is multiplied by the mA utilized for the machine. This product is divided by the number of weeks of the test. This will give you your weekly workload expressed in milliampere seconds. This workload figure will help you determine your barrier requirements by the use of appropriate tables.

EXAMPLE: (From NCRP Report No. 35, page 12)

Number of box tops	8
Number of films in each box	150
Total number of films	1,200
mA setting	10 mA
Longest exposure time	1 second
Total mAs during test period	12,000
Duration of test	10 weeks
Average mAs per week (average workload)	1,200 mAs/ week

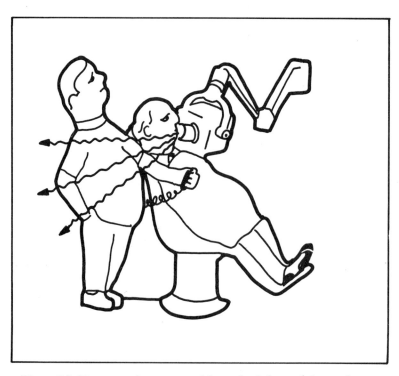

Figure 5-7. Never stand unprotected in path of the useful x-ray beam.

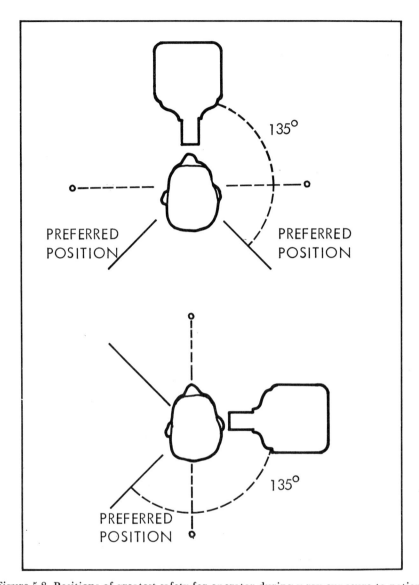

Figure 5-8. Positions of greatest safety for operator during x-ray exposure to patient.

Procedures for Protecting the Operator

Exposure of the operator of a dental x-ray machine to radiation can be minimized by the observance of the following operating procedures:

I. *Protection against exposure to primary radiation*

    A. The operator should stand at least six feet from patient and avoid the useful beam of primary radiation. When this is not possible, he should stand behind a protective barrier to radiation. Never stand unprotected in the path of the useful x-ray beam that passes from your x-ray tube aperture (See Figure 5-7). The primary beam can be avoided by standing behind the patient, if possible, and between 90° and 135° to the x-ray beam during x-ray exposure (See Figure 5-8).

B. In no case shall the film be held by the dentist or other dental personnel during exposure (See Figure 5-9).

C. Fluorescent mirrors shall not be used in dental examination (See Figure 5-10).

II. *Protection against exposure to leakage radiation*

A. Neither the tube housing nor the directing cone of the machine shall be hand-held during exposure (See Figure 5-11).

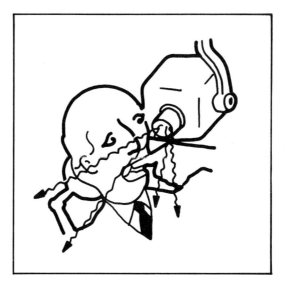

Figure 5-9. Never hold the film during exposures.

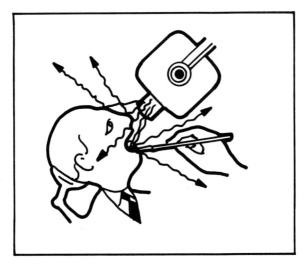

Figure 5-10. Never use an intraoral fluoroscopic mirror.

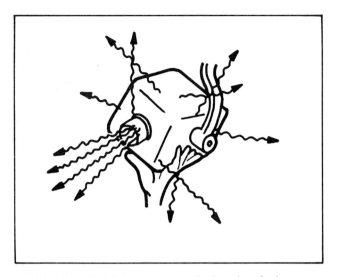

Figure 5-11. Never hold the cone or tube housing during exposure.

B. The x-ray machine should be tested for leakage radiation from the tube head. This can be accomplished by use of a sur-pac, which is a film device used for surveying dental x-ray machines. It may be obtained at no cost from a State Health Department. The sur-pac helps a health physicist determine the size and symmetry of primary beam, the x-ray output of the machine, the total filtration, and the presence of leakage radiation in a forward direction. Certain x-ray machines have a faulty ring which inadequately seals the tube head, which permits anterior leakage of radiation.

III. *Protection against exposure to secondary radiation*
The three sources of secondary radiation are the filter, the pointed plastic cone and the irradiated soft tissues of the patient's face. Secondary radiation can be minimized in the following manner:

A. The patients exposure, and indirectly the operator's exposure, should be reduced by using *high-speed films.* When one attempts to use high-speed films with older x-ray machines, the original mechanical timers may prove inadequate. There are several ways of adapting an old machine with a mechanical timer to the use of fast films. Mechanical timers are very inaccurate below "one-second" times.

1. Replace the mechanical timer with an electronic or synchronous motor timer.

2. Replace the short cone (8-inch TFD) with an open-ended cone to produce a target-film distance of 16 inches. This will increase the exposure time by four times. This procedure does not increase the

radiation exposure to the patient or the film.

3. Reduction of beam intensity by adding filtration. The image quality suffers somewhat with this procedure.

4. Reduction of the milliamperage, which would require a higher exposure time in seconds to achieve the same density.

B. The operator shall stand away from the patient's head during exposures. Safety increases with distance. A longer cord on the timer will permit the operator greater freedom of movement. He should be at least six feet away from the patient—if he cannot he should stand behind a lead protective barrier (See Figure 5-12). However, the safety requirements are determined by the workload of the machine. In the case of small offices, the dentist should step out of the room and position himself behind a wall.

C. Use of diaphragms or metal collimators to restrict the useful beam to a diameter of 2¾ inches when measured at the end of the directing cone.

D. Use of open-ended, lead-lined cones in place of the pointed, plastic cone. The pointed, plastic cones are sources of scatter radiation to the whole body as well as the gonads (Richards, 1962). This unnecessary scatter radiation can be reduced by use of an open-ended, lead-lined cone.

E. The operator should stand in a position where he cannot see the three major sources of secondary radiation (filter, cone, and patient's irradiated face). This will minimize the effects of secondary radiation produced by the exposure.

1. While exposing the region of the central incisors, the operator should stand at a 90-135° angle to the path of the central ray of the useful beam. This position is approximately behind the left or the right ear of the patient (Richards, 1960).

2. While exposing the other regions, the operator should stand behind the patient's head at an angle of 90-135° to the path of the central ray of the x-ray beam (See Figure 5-8).

IV. *Ancient dental x-ray machines with exposed overhead wires shall be replaced with modern shockproof equipment.*

V. *Film Badge Service.* The amount of x-radiation that reaches the body of the dentist or of the auxiliary dental personnel can be measured economically with a film badge. The use of the dental x-ray film and a paper clip will not accurately accomplish this determination. Film badges can be obtained on a weekly, biweekly, or monthly basis from numerous reliable film badge service companies in the country. (See appendix for film badge service listings.) At the laboratory, the film in the badge is

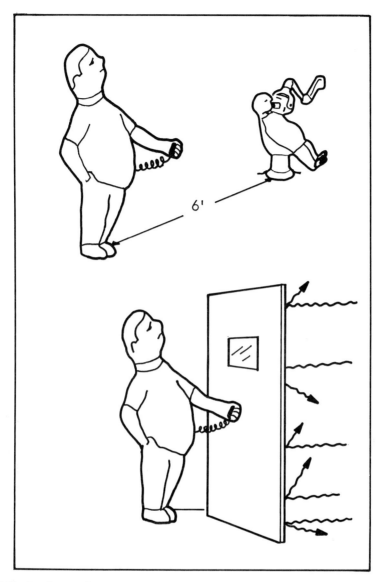

Figure 5-12. During each exposure stand at least 6 feet or more from the patient or behind a protective barrier.

carefully processed and its exposure evaluated. The amount of radiation recorded by the film badge is measure of the x-ray exposure of the wearer. He is notified by mail of the amount of his exposure. Film badges should be worn on the abdomen or hips.

Procedures for Protecting the Patient

Exposure of the head and body of the patient to x-ray radiation can be minimized by the observance of the following procedures:

I. The patient's exposure can be reduced by use of *high-speed films.*

The single most important factor in reducing radiation exposure to the dental patient is the use of high-speed film.

Without impairing the diagnostic quality of the film, high-speed films can reduce the radiation exposure to the patient as much as 85 percent.

Each film packet contains a lead film backing. This lead backing serves two purposes: (1) prevents fogging of film from backscattering of radiation and (2) absorbs much of the radiation which would otherwise expose tissues behind the film unnecessarily.

Some inexpensive film packets will contain inferior or thin lead backings. Therefore, it is recommended that only films of best quality with the highest speed be purchased.

II. *Collimators* shall be used to restrict the useful beam to an area no larger than 2.75 inches in diameter when measured at the end of the directing cone. The lead-lined open-ended cone should be used to reduce scatter radiation.

III. *Filtration* of the x-ray beam is used to remove the soft x-rays which expose the patient to unnecessary radiation.

Some filtration of the beam occurs when the x-rays pass through the glass window of the tube, the oil surrounding the tube, and portal which the rays emerge. This is inherent filtration and is measured in aluminum equivalents of filtration.

Usually it is necessary to add commercially pure aluminum discs to the useful beam in order to filter the beam according to recommended standards. The total filtration of the beam is the sum of the added and the inherent filtration.

The added filtration should be placed as near to the window of the tube housing as possible. Total filtration should not be less than that shown below:

Below 50 kVp　0.5 mm aluminum
50-70 kVp　　1.5 mm aluminum
Above 70 kVp　2.5 mm aluminum

IV. All films shall be *processed* according to the directions supplied by the manufacturers. In all instances use full development, such as 5 minutes at 68°F, or a time-temperature table based on these figures:

Development Temp	Time Min	
60°-62°F	9	
64°-66°F	7	
68°-70°F	5	Recommended
72°-76°F	4	
78°-80°F	3	

The exposure time can be reduced when the film is given full development. For instance, if the time of development (68°-70°F) is increased from three to five minutes, the radiation exposure may be decreased by 25 percent without interfering with the quality of the film image.

Only the best darkroom procedures should be employed. Radiographs ruined in the darkroom require repeated exposures to the patient.

V. *The film and the x-ray beam should be aligned correctly with the area of interest.* Retakes result-

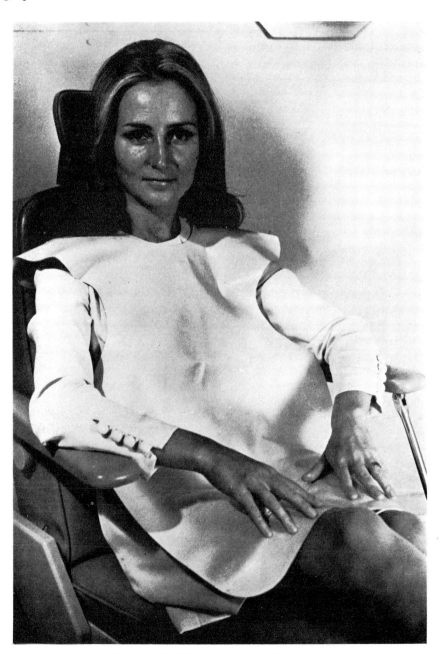

Figure 5-13. The use of the leaded apron.

ing from improper projection technics will expose the patient to unnecessary amounts of radiation.

VI. *Film holders should be used when taking dental radiographs.*

Film holders eliminate the necessity for the patient to hold the films in his mouth with his fingers. These devices not only remove the patient's hand from the x-ray beam, they also promote consistency and quality in the results.

VII. *The total radiation exposure given a patient must be justified by the amount of diagnostic information received.*

The welfare of the patient is the deciding factor. Dental films should be taken only when the information obtained will substantially aid in the diagnosis and prevention of disease. The periodic routine use of x-rays without a rational basis for their use should be avoided whenever possible.

VIII. *Have periodic radiation protection surveys made of your x-ray procedures.*

The dental sur-pac procedure, sponsored by the federal government, is a simple and rapid technic for the dentist to conduct. This procedure will check the size and symmetry of the beam of radiation, the approximate roentgen output, the total filtration, and any leakage in the direction of the face (Miller, 1963).

IX. *Film view box or illuminator should have a variable intensity source.* Many times this will eliminate the necessity of retaking a radiograph if the density is too light or dark.

X. *Leaded protective aprons* are suggested as a prudent measure to use with children, pregnant women or women in the childbearing age (Richards, 1963). Usually when the preceding recommendations

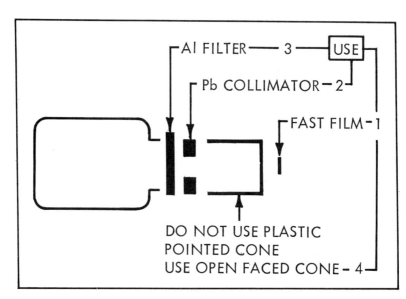

Figure 5-14. The three important methods of reducing radiation exposure to the patient: (1) fast film, (2) lead collimator and (3) aluminum filter.

have been followed, it is unnecessary to use the lead apron. When proper dental radiographic procedures are used, the gonadal exposure will not exceed the daily exposure from background radiation which is 0.3 mRems/day to 0.9 mRems/day. A clinical technic using 65 kVp-10 mA, short cone, 2.75 collimation, 2.25 mm of filtration, 14 ultra-speed films for a total exposure of 5.9 seconds was measured as exposing the gonads to .45 mRems to the gonads (Richards, 1958).

Whenever possible, direct the useful beam away from the gonads, thymus and thyroid regions of the patient. This can be done by tilting the patient's head or by using film holders which do not depend on uprighted head positions.

The leaded apron, when used, should have a protective equivalent of ¼ mm of lead. It will practically eliminate all the somatic and genetic exposure to the patient from leakage, scatter and secondary radiation (See Figure 5-13).

It should be remembered, though, that the leaded apron should not be a substitute for the use of ultra-speed film, full development, lead collimator and the aluminum filter. These are the primary methods in reducing the radiation exposure to the patient (See Figure 5-14). The lead apron is only a secondary measure.

Measurement of X-Ray Machine Output

The radiation output of the machine should be known under the conditions of kilovoltage, filter, and distance used. The output of dental x-ray machines is ordinarily expressed in terms of roentgens/second. The output will vary between the dental machines of different manufacturers and even between machines of the same model produced by the same manufacturer. It has been reported that a machine operating at a total filtration equivalent of 2.25 mm aluminum and 10 milliamperes of current, the output at 8 inches from the target was found to be *0.85 r per second* at 65 kilovolts peak and *1.68 r per second* at 90 kilovolts peak. Under these circumstances, if 0.85 r per second is delivered at a distance of 8 inches from the source at 65 kVp and 10 mA, .21 r would be delivered at 16 inches (Wuehrmann, 1960).

By the use of the sur-pac method, an estimation of the roentgen output of your machine can be determined for you.

Is Radiation Safe?

Nothing is perfectly safe, but—dental x-ray examinations can be made with very small amounts of radiation if the preceding recommendations are followed. The neglect of any one factor may very well nullify the advantages of attending to all the others. When modern techniques are used, there should be no cause for alarm regarding genetic damage or any other type of damage from dental x-ray exposure.

Dental x-ray films are essential to accurate diagnosis. Any amount of x-radiation needed to produce diagnostic films preliminary to dental treatment and supplementary films in course of treatment is safe, provided that the dentist has done everything possible to reduce such radiation to a minimum. To be sure, all radiation is harmful, and at least to some extent accumulative. But the ratio of harm to benefit leaves no doubt about the advisability of the continued use of x-radiation. This philosophy also applies to pregnant women and young children —if radiation is indicated, it should be used.

It is possible to produce a complete radiographic examination with no greater hazard to the patient's gonads than does his daily exposure to background radiation. If a lead apron is used, no radiation will reach the gonads at all.

Radiographic technics in dentistry should always be employed to achieve the greatest diagnostic information with the minimum dose to the patient, dental personnel and the public.

REFERENCES

Background material for development of radiation protection standard. Federal Radiation Council, FRC, Staff Report, No. 1, May, 1960.

Barr, J. H.: Radiation protection in dentistry for patients, operators, and office personnel. *J Am Dent Assoc,* 60:615, May, 1960.

Basic Radiation Protection Criteria, NCRP No. 39. NCRP Publication, Washington, D. C., January 15, 1971.

Basic Safety Standards for Radiation Protection. International Atomic Energy Agency (IAEA) Safety Series No. 9, 1967.

Blatz, H. (Ed.): *Radiation Hygiene Handbook.* New York, McGraw-Hill, 1959.

Buchholz, Robert E.: A Corpendium of Oral Roentgenology, USAF Hospital, Wright-Patterson Air Force Base, Ohio.

Budowsky, J. and others, *J Am Dent Assoc,* 52:55, May, 1956.

Cahan, W. G.; Woodard, H. Q.; Higenbothan, N. L.; Stewart, F. W.; and Coley, B. L.: Sarcomas arising in irradiated bone. *Cancer,* 1:3, 1948.

Chamberlain, R. H., and Nelsen, R. J.: A Practical Manual on the Medical and Dental Use of X-Rays with Control of Radiation Hazards. American College of Radiology.

Consumer Reports, The enormous benefits we owe to x-rays. September, 1961, pp. 493-501.

Court-Brown, W. N., and Doll, R.: Leukemia and aplastic anemia in patients irradiated for ankylosing spondylitis. *Medical Research Council Special Report, Series No. 295.* London, Her Majesty's Stationary Office, 1957.

Curtis, H. J.: Radiation-induced aging in mice. In Australian Conference on Radiobiology, 3rd, University of Sydney, 1960, London, Butterworth; 1961, pp. 114-122.

Dental Radiological Health Course Manual, Cincinnati, Ohio, Robert A. Taft Engineering Center, U. S. Department of Health, Education, and Welfare, Public Health Service, Bureau of States Service, Division of Radiological Health, January, 1961.

Ellinger, Friedrich: *Medical Radiation Biology.* Springfield, Ill., Charles C Thomas, 1957.

English: An analysis of the dangers of x-ray radiation. *Dent Rad Photo,* 25:1, 1952.

Ennis, LeRoy; Berry, Harrison; and Phillips, James A.: *Dental Roentgenology,* 6th ed. Lea & Febiger, 1967.

Failla, G., and McClement, P.: The shortening of life by chronic whole body irradiation. *Am J Roentgenol,* 78:946-954, 1957.

Fast Film Exposure and Processing in Dental Radiography. Public Health Service, Bureau of Radiological Health, Rockville, Maryland.

Franklin, J. B.: Radiation hazards in cephalometric roentgenography. *Angle Orthodontist,* 23:222-228, October, 1953.

Goodwin, Paul N.; Quimby, Edith H.; and Morgan, Russell H.: *Physical Foundations of Radiology,* 4th ed. Harper & Row, 1970.

Green: X-radiation reduction with 90-KVP technics. *Dent Rad Photo,* 2:36, 1958.

Griem, M. L.; Meir, P.; and Dobben, G. D.: Analysis of the morbidity and mortality of children irradiated in fetal life. *Radiology,* 88:347-349, 1967.

Hamford, J. M.; Quimby, E. H.: and Franz, V. K.: Cancer arising many years after radiation therapy. *JAMA,* 181:140, 1962.

Hempelman, L. H.: Epidemiological studies of leukemia in persons exposed to ionizing radiation. *Cancer Res,* 20:18, 1960.

Hendee, William R.: *Medical Radiation Physics.* Chicago, Year Book Medical Publishers, 1970.

Johns, Harold E., and Cunningham, John R.: *The Physics of Radiology,* 3rd ed. Springfield, Ill., Charles C Thomas, 1969.

Little, John B.: Cellular effects of ionizing radiation. *N Engl J Med,* 275:929-945, October 27, 1966.

MacMahan, B.: Prenatal x-ray exposure and childhood cancer. *J Natl Cancer Inst,* 28: 1173-1191, No. 5, May, 1962.

MacMahon, B., and Newill, V. A.: Birth characteristics of children dying of malignant neoplasms. *J Natl Cancer Inst,* 28:231-244, No. 1, January, 1962.

Manson-Hing, Lincoln: The fundamental biologic effects of x-rays in dentistry. *Oral Surg,* May, 1959, p. 562.

McKusick, V. A.: *Human Genetics.* New York, Prentice-Hall, 1969.

Medical X-ray and Gamma Ray Protection for Energies up to 10 MeV, Equipment Design and Use. NCRP, Report No. 33, NCRP Publications, February 1, 1968.

Medwedeff, Fred M.; Knox, William H.; and Latimer, Paul: A new device to reduce patient irradiation and improve dental quality. *Oral Surg,* 15:1079-1088, September, 1962.

Medwedeff, Fred M., and Knox, William H.: Radiation reduction for children. *J Tenn State Dent Assoc,* 42: October, 1962.

Merrian, G. R., and Focht, E. A.: A clinical study of radiation cataracts and their relationship to dose. *Am J Roentgenol,* 127:759, 1957.

Miller, J. W.: Summary of state dental radiological health activities. *Radiol Health Data Rep,* 4:1, 1963.

Miller, R. W.: Delayed radiation effects in atomic bomb survivors. *Sciences,* 166:569, 1969.

Miller, R. W.: Effects of ionizing radiation from the atomic bomb on Japanese children. *Pediatrics,* 41:257, 1968.

Model legislation for users of ionizing radiation in the healing arts. *Public Health Service,* Bureau of Radiological Health, January, 1970.

National Academy of Sciences: The Biological Effects of Atomic Radiation: Summary Reports, and a Report to the Public, 1958.

National Academy of Sciences: The Biological Effects of Atomic Radiation—A Report to the Public, 1956, p. 3.

National Bureau of Standards: Permissible Dose from External Sources of Ionizing Radiation, Handbook 59. Washington, D. C., U. S. Government Printing Office, 1954.

National Bureau of Standards: Medical X-Ray Protection Up to Three Million Volts, Handbook 76. Washington, D. C., U. S. Government Printing Office, 1961.

National Council on Radiation Protection and Measurements Report No. 35, Dental X-Ray Protection. NCRP Publications, March 9, 1970.

Paul, I. R.: Is our x-ray machine a hazard? *Oral Surg,* 11:282-288, March, 1958.

Physical Survey Manual, Dental X-Ray. Public Health Service Publication No. 1559, April, 1967.

Precautions in the management of patients who have received therapeutic amounts of radionuclides. *NCRP Report No. 37.* NCRP Publications, Washington, D. C., October 1, 1970.

Preliminary report on radiographic holding, paralleling and shielding devices. *J Am Dent Assoc,* 77:4:884-887, October, 1968.

Radiation Control for Health and Safety Act of 1967, Hearings before Committee on Commerce, United States Senate, 90th Congress, August 28-30, 1967, Washington, D. C., U. S. Government Printing Office, 1968.

Radiation hygiene and practice in dentistry, I. *J Am Dent Assoc,* 74:1032-1033, April, 1967.

Radiation hygiene and practice in dentistry, II. *J Am Dent Assoc,* 75:1197-1198, November, 1967.

Radiation hygiene and practice in dentistry, III. *J Am Dent Assoc,* 76:115-116, January, 1968.

Radiation hygiene and practice in dentistry, IV. *J Am Dent Assoc,* 76:363-364, February, 1968.

Radiation hygiene and practice in dentistry, V, *J Am Dent Assoc,* 76:602-603, March, 1968.

Radiation protection in educational institutions, *NCRP Report No. 32.* Washington, D. C., NCRP Publications, July, 1966.

Radiation Protection for Dentist and Patient. Washington, D. C., Government Printing Office, Superintendent of Documents, U. S. Department of Health, Education and Welfare, Public Health Service, Division of Radiological Health, 1962.

Report of Councils and Bureaus: State Radiation Protection Laws. *J Am Dent Assoc,* 60:126-218, 1960.

Richards, A. G.: Roentgen-ray doses in dental roentgenography. *J Am Dent Assoc,* 56:351, March, 1958.

Richards, A. G.: Roentgen ray radiation and the dental patients. *J Am Dent Assoc,* 54:476-487, 1957.

Richards, A. G.: Biologic effects of the x-ray used in dentistry. *Journal of the Michigan State Dental Association.* Vol. 40, July-August, 1958, pp. 188-191.

Richards, A. G.: Roentgen ray radiation and the dental patient. *J Am Dent Assoc,* 54:476-487, 1957.

Richards, A. G., et al.: The effective use of x-ray radiation in dentistry. *Oral Surg,* 16:294-304, March, 1963.

Richards, A. G., et al.: X-ray protection in the dental office. *J Am Dent Assoc,* 56:514, 1958; 57:31, 1959.

Richards, A. G.: New methods for reduction of gonadal radiation of patients. *J Am Dent Assoc,* 65:1-111, 1962.

Richards, A. G.: Dental x-ray equipment of the future. *Oral Surg,* February, 1960B, pp. 194-198.

Richards, A. G.: How hazardous is dental roentgenography? *Oral Surg,* 14:40-51, January, 1961.

Richards, A. G., et al.: X-ray protection in the dental office. *J Am Dent Assoc,* 56:514-519.

Richards, A. G.: Shielding requirements for installations. *J Am Dent Assoc,* 64:788-793, June, 1962.

Richards, A. G.: New conception dental x-ray machine. *J Am Dent Assoc,* 73:69-76, July, 1966.

Richards, Albert G.: Radiation protection via the pin hole camera. *Oral Surg,* 13:953-963, No. 8, August, 1960.

Richards, Albert G.: Radiation Control for Health Safety Act of 1967. Hearings Before Committee on Commerce, U. S. Senate, U. S. Government Printing Office, 1968.

Richards, Lloyd F., et al.: A study of radiation exposure in the private office. *Calif D A, Nevada D Soc,* 34:380-385. September-October, 1958.

Roney, Paul L., and Brown, Morton L.: Preliminary estimate of gonadal and genetic dose to the U. S. population from medical diagnostic roentgenololgy. *Population Exposure Studies,* National Center for Radiological Health, June 20, 1967.

Russell, L. B., and Russell, W. L.: Radiation hazards to embryo and fetus. *Radiology,* 58:369-377, No. 3, March, 1952.

Russell, W. L.: Factors affecting the radiation induction of mutations in the mouse, biological implication of the nuclear age. Proceedings of Symposium at Lawrence Radiation Laboratory, March, 1968, Atomic Energy Commission, Washington, 1969.

Sinclair: X-ray protection in dental radiography. *Dent Rad Photo,* 4:66, 1958.

Snavely, David R., et al.: Regulations, standards and guides pertaining to medical and dental radiation protection—an annotated bibliography. *Public Health Service,* U. S Government Printing Office, Washington, 1969.

Stewart, A., et al.: A survey of childhood malignancies. *Br Med J,* 1496, 1508, June, 1958.

Stewart, A., and Kneale, G. W.: Changes in the cancer risk associated with obstetric radiography. *Lancet,* 1:104, 1968.

Taylor, L. S.: Maximum permissible radiation exposure to man. *Radiation Res,* 6:573-576, 1957.

Trubman, Aaron: Radiation protection of dental personnel. *J Am Dent Assoc,* 65:751-754, No. 6, December, 1962.

Wainwright, W. W.: *Dental Radiology.* New York, McGraw-Hill, 1965.

Wainwright, William and Vallanyi: Radiation

hazards. *Prac Dent Monogr,* January, 1959, pp. 3-31.

Wuehrmann, Arthur H.: *Radiation Protection and Dentistry.* St. Louis, C. V. Mosby, 1960.

Wuehrmann, Arthur H., and Manson-Hing, Lincoln: *Dental Radiology,* 2nd ed. St. Louis, C. V. Mosby, 1968.

Yale, S. H., and Goodman, L. S.: Reduction of radiation output of the standard dental x-ray machine utilizing copper for external filtration. *J Am Dent Assoc,* 54:354, 1957.

Yale, Seymour: Radiation control in dental office. *Dent Clin North Am,* July, 1961, p. 355.

CHAPTER 6

INTRAORAL PROJECTION TECHNICS

minimize shape distortion of the radiographic image.

Through the years, two intraoral projection technics have been devised to minimize image distortion; each are based upon entirely different principles.

1. The bisecting principle
2. The paralleling principle

A N INTRAORAL projection technic prescribes the precise alignment of the x-ray beam, the long axes of the teeth, and the plane of the film in order to

THE BISECTING PRINCIPLE

The bisecting principle is based upon the geometric principle which states that two triangles are equal if they have two equal angles and a common side. It is called the "rule of isometry." (Isometry is defined as equality of measurement.) (See Figure 6-1.)

In 1904, Dr. Weston Price, an American dentist, first applied the rule of isometry to intraoral radiographic projection technic. When this rule is ap-

plied to dental radiography, it is used to determine the *correct vertical angulation* of the tube or cone. (Vertical angulation is the up and the down movement of the tube or cone.)

When the bisecting principle of isometry is applied to an intraoral radiographic technic the rule is this:

"The central ray must be directed through the apex of the tooth, perpendicular to a line bisecting the angle formed by the

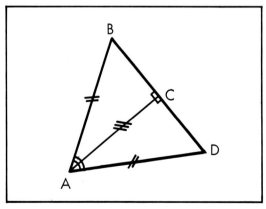

Figure 6-1. The *rule of isometry*—angle (a) is bisected by *line AC. Line AC* is perpendicular to *line BD. Angle DAC* is equal to *Angle CAB*, and *Angle ACD* is equal to *ACB*. Therefore, two angles are equal and they have a common side—it then can be said that *triangle DAC* is equal to *triangle CAB*. (Courtesy of Dr. LeRoy M. Ennis.)

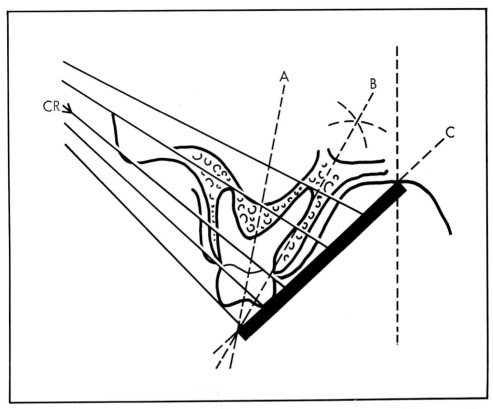

Figure 6-2. The rule of isometry applied to the intraoral radiographic technic commonly called the bisection-of-the-angle technic. Line A = long axis of the tooth, Line C = long axis of the film, Line B = the bisecting line, CR = path of the central ray directed perpendicular to line B.

mean plane of the long axis of the tooth and the mean plane of the film." (See Figure 6-2.)

This rule applies admirably to plane surfaces that have only length and width, but has certain shortcomings when applied to structures such as the teeth which have depth as well as width and length. Nevertheless, this procedure has served the profession well and does have certain advantages.

If the bisecting angle rule is neglected in the slightest manner, the resulting radiographic image will be distorted. Elongation of the length of the actual image of the tooth will result if the x-ray beam is directed perpendicular through the mean plane of the long axis of the tooth rather than through the bisecting line.

Foreshortening or shortening of the radiographic image will occur when the x-ray beam is directed perpendicular to the plane of the film, rather than the bisecting line (See Figure 6-3).

The bisecting technic is for the most part practiced with the short cone (8 inches SFD). If the short cone is used, it should have an open, flat face.

The long or extension cone may also

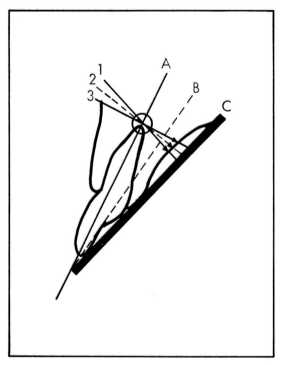

Figure 6-3. If the central ray is directed as photon (1) perpendicular to the film—the radiographic image will be *foreshortened;* if the *CR* is directed as photon (3) perpendicular to the tooth—the radiographic image will be elongated. (Courtesy of Dr. LeRoy M. Ennis.)

be used with the bisecting technic. Source-film distances of 20 and 18 inches have been used in the past, but the 16-inch source-film distance seems to be the most practical distance to use in most dental offices. The advantage of the extended source-film distance is that it minimizes geometric unsharpness and magnification of the radiographic image.

In order to determine the correct alignment of the central beam, the film and the teeth, using the bisecting technic, the following procedures must be considered:

1. Head Position
2. Film Placement
3. Vertical Angulation of the Tube
4. Horizontal Angulation of the Tube
5. The Point of Entry of the Central Beam

Head Position

When using the bisecting technics with the digital method of holding the films in the mouth, the head position is quite important. The rule for head position is as follows: *The occlusal plane of the teeth to be radiographed should be parallel to the floor; and the sagittal plane of the head should be perpendicular to the floor.*

The *maxillary orientation line* is an imaginary line drawn from the tragus of the ear (cartilagenous projection located just before the ear hole or external auditory meatus) and the ala of the nose (wing of the nose). This line should be parallel to the floor when radiographing the maxillary teeth (See Figure 6-4).

The *mandibular occlusal plane* changes when the mouth is opened. Therefore, tilt the patient's head slightly backwards so the occlusal plane of the mandible will

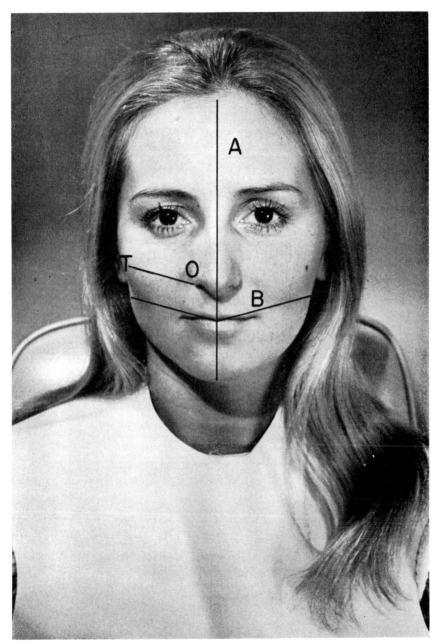

Figure 6-4. The head divided into four quarters by sagittal plane *A* and the occlusal plane *B*. The line *TO* is the tragal-ala line which is parallel to the occlusal plane B.

be parallel to the floor when the mouth is opened. Make sure that the patient does not open too wide as this will contract the muscles of the floor of the mouth and make it difficult to place the film. If the patient tenses the muscles of the floor of the mouth, have him relax these muscles by swallowing.

The *sagittal plane* of the skull divides the skull vertically in the *midline* into right and left halves. The sagittal plane of the skull should be *perpendicular* to the floor prior to placing films into mouth for the bisecting-digital technic (See Figure 6-4).

Film Placement

The rule for film placement in the bisecting-digital technic is this: The center of the film is positioned behind the center of the region to be radiographed.

The most popular complete periapical examination (often called the full-mouth survey) using the bisecting technic is the 14-film survey. The films are of the #2 or standard periapical film size. The following areas are covered:

One film in each of the 4 molar areas = 4 films

One film in each of the 4 premolar areas = 4 films

One film in each of the 4 canine areas = 4 films

One film in each of the 2 midline incisor areas = 2 films

TOTAL 14 films

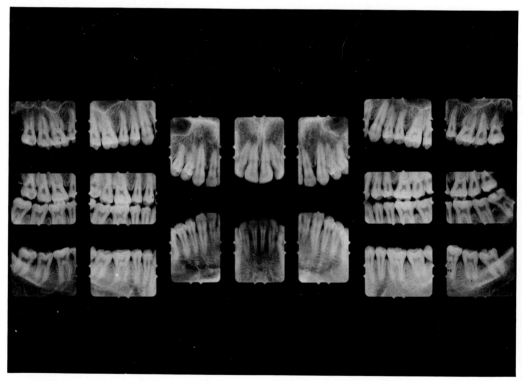

Figure 6-5. Typical complete radiographic survey taken by bisecting angle technic utilizing a short cone (8″ SFD).

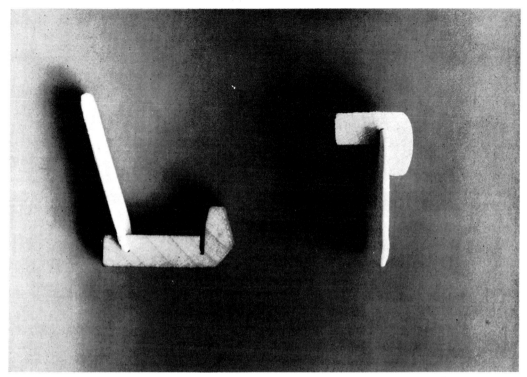

Figure 6-6. Wooden film holders. *Left:* Film holder used for mandibular posterior and anterior projections in paralleling technic. *Right:* Film holder used for mandibular posterior projections in bisecting and paralleling technics.

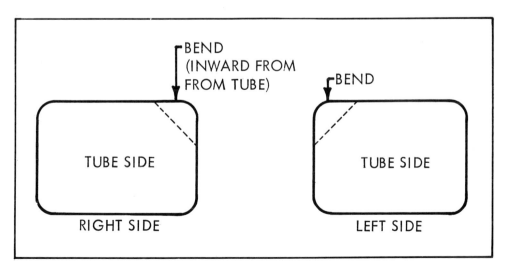

Figure 6-7. In the digital bisecting technic, bend the film for the maxillary premolar projection as shown above.

The number one narrow film is a much more desirable film than the number two regular for use in the anterior portion of the mouth. It may require one or two more projections; however, it prevents distortion from film bending, and it is much easier to place.

In positioning the films in the mouth for the molar and premolar projections, place the long axes of the film packets horizontally to the long axes of the teeth. The canine and incisor projections require the placement of long axes of the film packets vertically to the long axes of the teeth (See Figure 6-5).

When using the bisecting technic, the film packets may be held in the mouth by the patient's fingers (digital method) or by means of film holders. The digital method has been in use for the longest period of time, and is the most undesirable. It places the patient's hand in the primary beam of radiation.

The film is held in the mouth by the patient's thumb for the maxillary projections and by the patient's forefinger for the mandibular projections. In radiographing the right side of the mouth the patient's left hand is used, and vice versa. This is why it is always a good suggestion to have the patient wash his hands before this technic is used because he will be placing his hands into his mouth.

Always make sure that approximately ⅛ inch of the film appears below the occlusal plane of the teeth. If this is overlooked, partial images of crowns of the teeth will be seen on the finished radiograph.

Many times the film for the maxillary premolar teeth is intentionally bent sharply across the upper anterior corner which is placed in the region of the lingual surface of the opposite lateral incisor. The premolar projection must reveal the distal surface of the canine because this surface is usually not seen on the canine projection (See Figure 6-7).

In taking the maxillary canine projections with #2 regular film, it may be necessary to bend the film in the upper

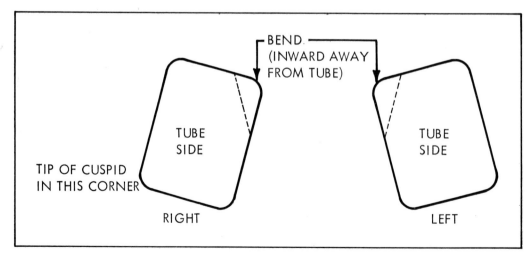

Figure 6-8. In the digital bisecting technic, bend the film for the maxillary canine projection as shown above.

anterior corner in order for the film to fit lingually to the opposite premolar region. The patient holds the film with his thumb on the bend to make sure that the film is not placed too far back in the mouth which will cause you to miss the lateral incisor in this projection (See Figure 6-8).

Two cotton rolls may be placed between the film and the teeth in the anterior projections to prevent distortion from film bending.

Vertical Angulation of the Tube or Cone

The *rule for vertical angulation* in the bisecting technic is this: Direct the central beam through the apices of the teeth in area to be examined, perpendicular to the line bisecting the angle formed by the planes of the long axes of the tooth and the plane of the film.

Due to variations in the arrangement, inclination and angulation of the teeth in the jaws, the angle formed by the plane of the film and the long axes of the teeth for any given area of the mouth varies from one patient to another.

In the normal maxillary arch, the roots of the teeth are inclined palatally from the vertical with the premolars having the most perpendicular roots. The maxillary incisors have the greatest inclination, and the maxillary first molars rarely tilt more than 15 degrees from the vertical. Also, the palatal depth is much higher in the posterior region of the maxilla than the incisor region, which has an effect on the angle formed by the film and the long axes of the teeth. Therefore, the vertical angulations in the maxilla are governed by the inclinations of the teeth from vertical and the palatal depth.

In the mandible the inclination of the teeth are not as pronounced from the vertical as in the maxillary arch. The roots of the anterior teeth slant inwards, the premolars are fairly vertical, and the roots of the molars slant outward slightly. The muscle attachments in the floor of the mouth modify the mandibular

FILM	MAXILLARY RANGE	MAXILLARY STARTING ANGLE	MANDIBULAR RANGE	MANDIBULAR STARTING ANGLE
Molar	$+25°$ to $30°$	$+30°$	$0°$	$0°$
Bicuspid	$+35°$ to $40°$	$+40°$	$-5°$ to $-10°$	$-10°$
Cuspid	$+45°$ to $50°$	$+50°$	$-15°$ to $-30°$	$-15°$
Incisor	$+55°$ to $65°$	$+55°$	$-15°$ to $-30°$	$-20°$
P. Bitewing		$+10°$		

Figure 6-9. Ranges of vertical angulation for short cone bisecting technic.

FILM	MAXILLA	MANDIBLE
Molar	+25°	+5° (Fixed Angle)[1]
Bicuspid	+35°	− 5°
Cuspid	+45°	− 10°
Incisors	+45°	− 15°
P. Bitewing	+10°	

Figure 6-10. Starting Angles (Adults) Long Cone (16″ TFD) Bisection of the Angle Technic. [1] The +5° vertical angulation is a fixed angle meaning that practically every mandibular molar shot is taken at +5° above the horizontal.

vertical angles more than the inclinations of the teeth.

The muscle attachments in the floor of the mouth are deep in the molar region, less deep in the premolar region and high in the incisor region. The angle formed by the long axes of the teeth and the film is much greater in the regions where the muscle attachments are high. Consequently, the vertical angulations of the tube will be greater in areas where the muscle attachments are high in the mandible. As you can see, it is very difficult to devise routine vertical angulations which will be accurate for any given region for every patient.

To aid the operator, certain ranges of vertical angulations have been devised into which the majority of the patients fall. These ranges are used only as a guide by the operator; the exact angle to be used for each region for each patient must be determined after the film has been placed in the mouth. The ranges of prescribed vertical angulations for both the long and the short cone bisec-tion of the angle technics are listed in Figures 6-9 and 6-10. Notice that the long cone vertical angulations are generally less than those listed for the short cone.

Horizontal Angulation

The *rule for horizontal angulation* is this: As the tube moves around the arch, the x-ray beam is directed perpendicular to the mean tangents of the facial surfaces of the teeth under examination. The flat face of the cone should be placed parallel to the horizontal plane of the film.

If there is an error in the horizontal angulation, overlapping of the radiographic images will result. The mean tangents of the facial surfaces of the teeth will vary from one region to another.

As you move around the dental arches the mean tangents of the facial surfaces of the teeth will not be the same. The mean tangents will generally be the same for the following groups of teeth: molars, premolars, canines, and incisors. Therefore, the horizontal angulation must be adjusted for each of these regional exposures. Since the dental arches vary so much as to size and shape from one person to another, no predetermined set of angles can be used (See Figure 6-11).

Point of Entry

The *rule for the point of entry* in the bisecting technic is this: The x-ray beam is directed through the center of the area to be radiographed.

The objective here is to completely cover the film with the cone of radiation. If this is not done, a "cone cut" or partial image will be seen in the finished radiograph.

If the x-ray beam is directed through the apices of the roots of the teeth, an adequate amount of periapical bone will be seen surrounding the apices of the roots of the teeth in the resulting radiograph. This is prerequisite in a periapical radiograph. Use the apices of the central teeth of the group as your guide for your point of entry.

In the maxillary arch, the points of entry can be established by the use of external landmarks oriented to the ala-tragal line (See Figure 6-12A).

In the mandible, the root apices can be established by estimating the points of entry from the lower border of the mandible. This is usually the width of the thumb ($1/4$ inch) (See Figure 6-12A).

Since the mouth is opened during the taking of the mandibular radiographs,

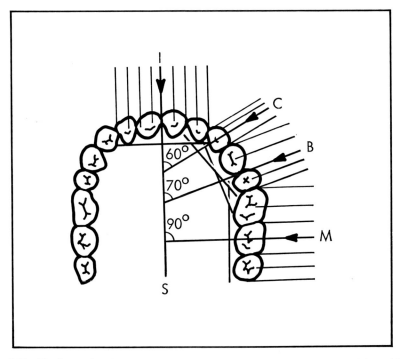

Figure 6-11. Horizontal tube movement around head (M—Molars, B—Bicuspids, C—Cuspids, I—Incisors).

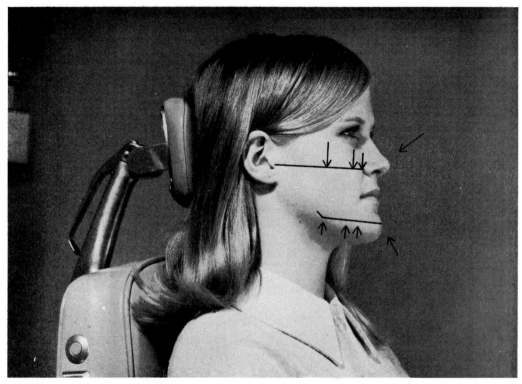

Figure 6-12A. Points of entry for bisecting technic.

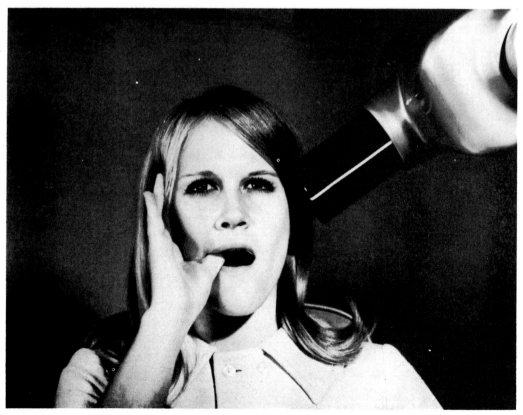

Figure 6-12B. Maxillary molar projection. (Digital bisecting short cone technic.)

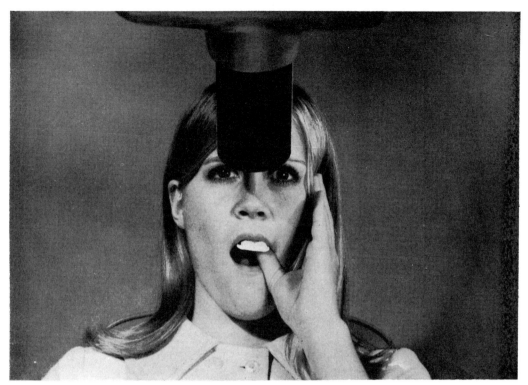

Figure 6-13. Maxillary midline projection. (Digital bisecting short cone technic.)

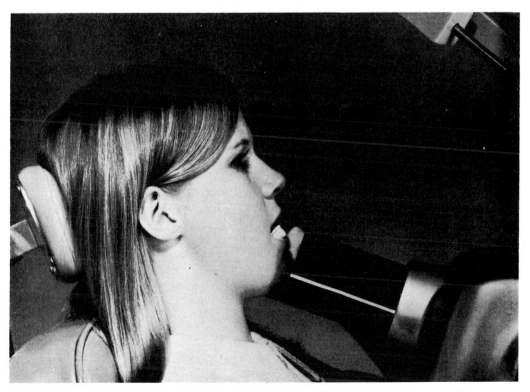

Figure 6-14. Mandibular midline projection. (Digital bisecting short cone technic.)

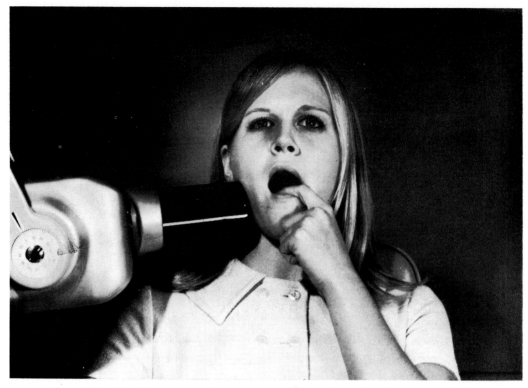

Figure 6-15. Mandibular premolar projection. (Digital bisecting short cone technic.)

the crowns of the teeth can be generally used as landmarks in determining the approximate locations of the apices of the mandibular teeth.

In placing films into the floor of the mouth, care must be taken not to injure these sensitive tissues. Never force films into place; glide them gently and firmly to place. Then guide the patient's index finger to the proper position to hold the film.

You may be required to crease the lower anterior border of the premolar film prior to placement. This is the most sensitive area in the floor of the mouth. The situation is complicated even more if a mandibular torus (boney projection) is present.

The bisecting-angle technic using the finger retention is illustrated in the following figures: Figure 6-12B—maxillary molar region, Figure 6-13—maxillary midline region, Figure 6-14—mandibular midline region, and Figure 6-15—mandibular premolar region.

Use of Film Holders with Bisecting Angle Technic

Recently, film holders have been designed to standardize the five variables in the bisecting technic, which are (1) vertical angulation, (2) horizontal angulation, (3) head positioning, (4) film positioning and (5) point of entry of the x-ray beam.

The Rinn® Bisecting Angle posterior

and anterior film instruments offer a practical method of eliminating some of the distracting features of the bisecting-angle technic using the finger-retention or digital method. These instruments are designed to automatically indicate the horizontal and vertical angulations, minimize distortion from film bending and eliminate cone cutting.

A set of Rinn anterior and posterior bisecting angle instruments consists of a periapical bite-block, an indicator rod, and a locator ring.

Periapical Bite-Block (See Figure 6-16)

The biteblock is designed to support and retain the film packet. The bite-block has a film backing, which is tilted at an average angle for the bisecting technic (See Figure 6-17). Also, the backing aids in the prevention of film distortion.

Indicator Rod

The indicator rod is used in aiding the operator in positioning the correct horizontal and vertical angulation of the x-ray cone.

Locator Ring

If desired, the locator ring can be placed on the indicator rod, and used to aid the operator in locating the correct alignment of the cone and the film. In addition, the locator ring prevents "cone cutting."

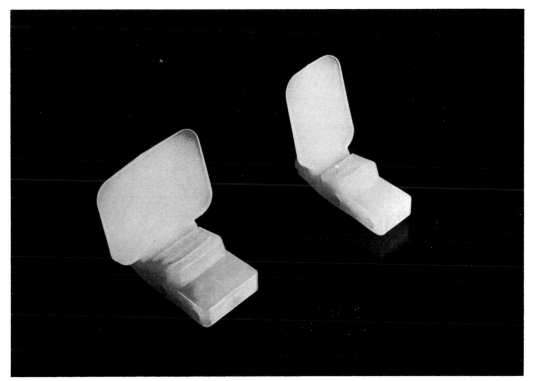

Figure 6-16. Rinn Bisecting Angle Bite Block. (*Left:* posterior bite block, *Right:* anterior bite block.)

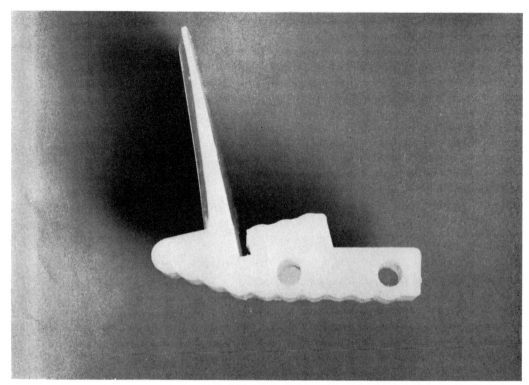

Figure 6-17. Side view of Rinn Bite-block showing off-set backing.

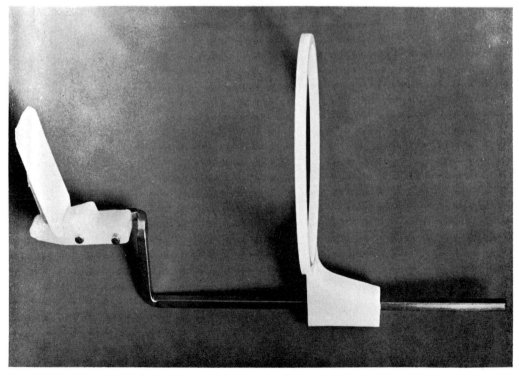

Figure 6-18. Assembled Rinn Anterior Bisecting Instrument.

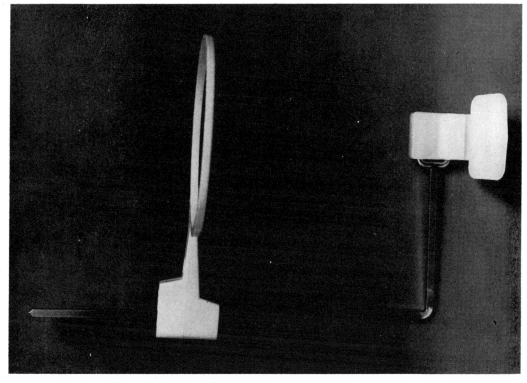

Figure 6-19. Assembled Rinn Posterior Bisecting Instrument.

By use of a film holder such as the Rinn bisecting instruments, vertical and horizontal film angles need not be memorized, and head positioning is not critical. Moreover, correct film placement and retention is accomplished with less strain on the patient (See Figures 6-18, 6-19).

The technic is described as follows:

Maxillary and Mandibular Anterior Regions (See Figures 6-20, 6-21, 6-22, 6-23):

1. With film vertically placed in anterior block, insert in mouth, center film with area of interest, and position as close to lingual surface of crowns as anatomy permits. Narrow (No. 1) films are recommended.

2. Instruct patient to close firmly on block to retain film in place. A cotton roll may be inserted between opposing teeth and block to increase stability.

3. Slide locator ring on rod to approximate skin surface and align cone with rod and ring on vertical and horizontal planes.

Mandibular and Maxillary Posterior Regions (See Figures 6-24, 6-25, 6-26, 6-27):

1. With film horizontally placed in posterior block, insert in mouth, positioning block on occlusal and centering film (#2 regular) on areas of interest as close to lingual surface as anatomy permits. (Relief of an-

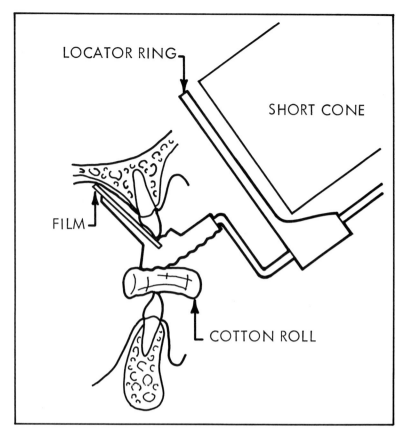

Figure 6-20. Diagram showing the correct positioning of Rinn bisecting film holder and cone for maxillary incisor region.

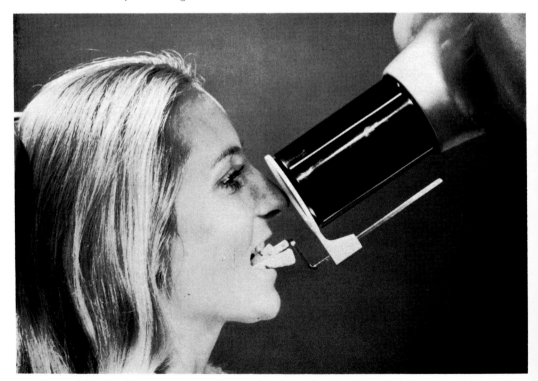

Figure 6-21. Maxillary anterior region. (Rinn Bisecting Instrument). Note use of cotton roll on opposing teeth to stabilize the film holder.

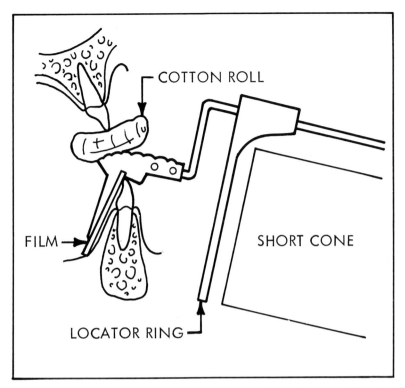

Figure 6-22. Diagram showing the correct positioning of Rinn Bisecting Film Holder and cone for mandibular anterior region.

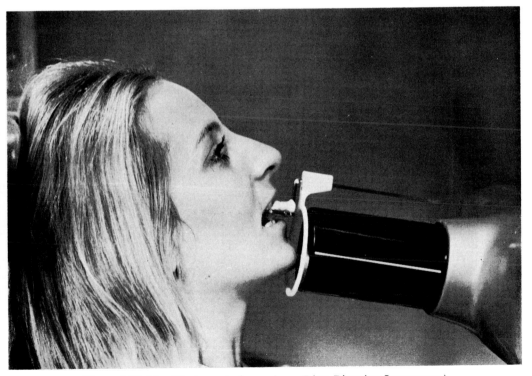

Figure 6-23. Mandibular anterior region. (Rinn Bisecting Instrument.)

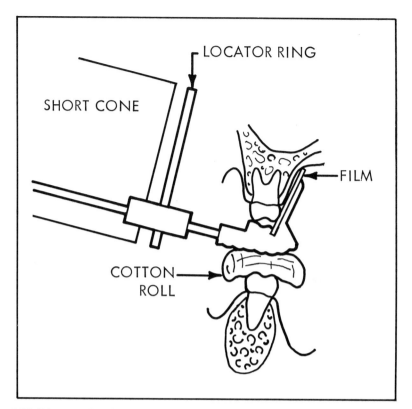

Figure 6-24. Diagram showing the correct positioning of Rinn Bisecting Film Holder and cone for maxillary posterior region.

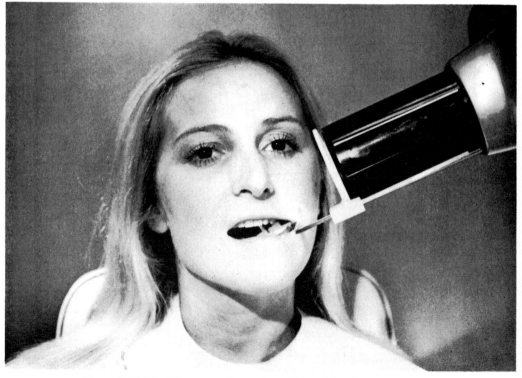

Figure 6-25. Maxillary posterior region. (Rinn Bisecting Instrument.)

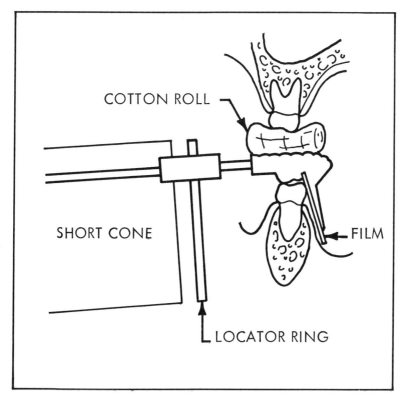

COTTON ROLL

SHORT CONE

FILM

LOCATOR RING

Figure 6-26. Diagram showing correct positioning of Rinn Bisecting Film Holder and cone for mandibular posterior region.

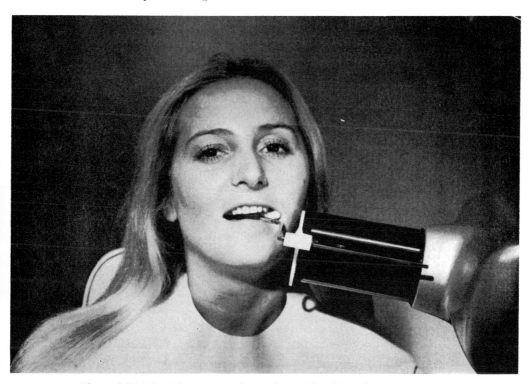

Figure 6-27. Mandibular posterior region. (Rinn Bisecting Instrument.)

terior superior corner of film facilitates positioning in premolar region.)

2. Instruct patient to close firmly on block to retain this film in place. A cotton roll may be inserted between opposing teeth and block to insure stability.

3. Slide locator ring on rod to approximate skin surface and align cone with rod and ring on vertical and horizontal planes.

PARALLELING OR RIGHT-ANGLE TECHNIC

The paralleling or right intraoral radiographic technic is based upon the paralleling principle. The paralleling principle in essence follows the five rules of accurate image formation (discussed in Chapter IV) in order to minimize the undesirable image characteristics of unsharpness, magnification, and shape distortion (See Figure 6-28).

Basically, the fundamental rules for the paralleling technic are these:

1. The films are placed in the mouth in a position which is parallel to the long axes of the teeth.

2. The central ray of the x-ray beam is directed perpendicular or at right angles to both the long axes of the teeth and the plane of the film.

In order to achieve parallelism be-

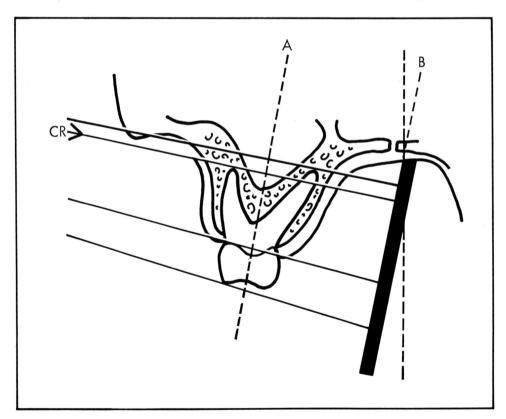

Figure 6-28. Diagram illustrating the relationship of the film and teeth in the paralleling (right angle) technic.

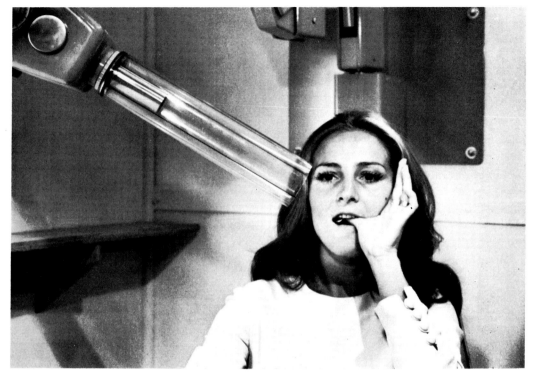

Figure 6-29. The long cone can be used with the bisecting technic.

tween the film and the long axes of the teeth, the object-film distance will have to be increased (especially in the maxillary arch). Of course, this goes against one of the five rules of accurate image formation which states: "The film must be as close to the object as possible." Therefore, to compensate for the undesirable image characteristics of geometric unsharpness and magnification caused by this procedure, the source-film distance is increased. This is probably why this technic has been referred to as the "long cone" technic in the past, but in reality this is a misnomer because the extension cone is not the basis of the technic; it is only a secondary feature of the technic. Remember that the extension cone can also be used with the bisecting technic (See Figure 6-29). Source-film

distances of 18 and 20 inches have been used in the past, but the source-film distance of 16 inches seems to be the most practical distance to be used in most dental offices.

Film Holders

As you may suspect, the most common problem experienced in the past with the paralleling technic has been the proper retention and placement of the film packet in the mouth. The film must be placed as nearly parallel to the long axes of the teeth as possible, maintaining a flat plane at all times, and retaining the film in position until it is properly exposed. Various film holders have been designed to overcome these problems associated with film retention and alignment.

There are four film holders that seem to be most popular. They are the (1) Rinn Snap-a-Ray®, (2) Fitzgerald Instruments, (3) Rinn XCP Instruments® and (4) Precision X-Ray Instruments.

The Rinn Snap-A-Ray Film Holder

This is a simple plastic film holder that can be used in both the anterior and posterior regions of the mouth. It does not have a film backing with it, thus the film may bend, and therefore, cause image distortion. However, it is a very useful film holder, in that it can be used in various areas of the mouth with patients who cannot tolerate a film backing (See Figure 6-30).

Figures 6-31 and 6-32 illustrate the cor-rect use of the Rinn Snap-A-Ray instrument in both the anterior and posterior regions of the mouth.

The Rinn Snap-A-Ray film holder is particularly useful for the following projections:

1. Mandibular premolars and molars. Since these teeth have almost perpendicular roots, the film can be positioned in close approximation to the teeth. However, the Snap-a-Ray does not have an alignment rod to aid the operator in obtaining the proper vertical and horizontal angulations.
2. Maxillary and mandibular impaction projections

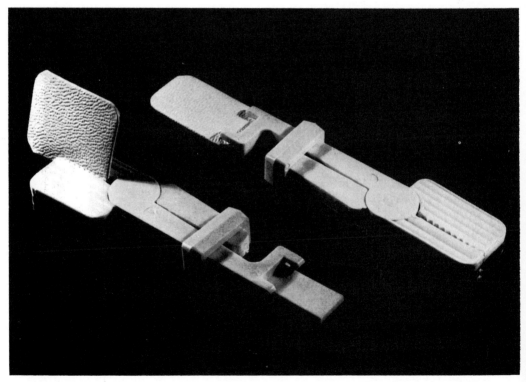

Figure 6-30. The Rinn Snap-a-Ray Film Holder. (*Left*—posterior projections; *Right*—anterior projections.)

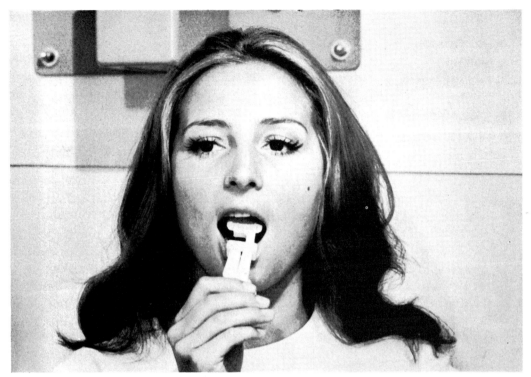

Figure 6-31. Use of Rinn Snap-a-Ray Instrument in anterior region.

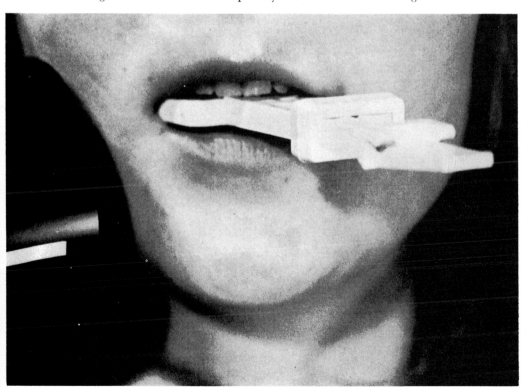

Figure 6-32. Use of Rinn Snap-a-Ray Instrument in posterior region.

3. Patients with a hypersensitive gag reflexes.
4. Children and edentulous projections
5. Endodontic projections

Fitzgerald Hemostat

This hemostat was specially designed by Dr. Gordon Fitzgerald of the University of California. The hemostat differs from the usual surgical hemostat in that the serrations on the beaks run lengthwise rather than across the beak. The hemostat comes complete with a rubber bite block and suitable metal film backings. (The instrument is sold by the Rocky Mountain Speciality Company, Denver, Colorado.) It is especially useful with patients who have a limited degree of mandibular openings (See Figure 6-33). The hemostat film holder with the metal backing and rubber bite block is used primarily in radiographing the maxillary posterior teeth (6-34).

The patient retains the forceps within the mouth by biting against the rubber bite-block with his maxillary and mandibular incisors.

After the patient bites on the rubber-bite block, rotate the film and film backing until it is parallel with the long axes of teeth being radiographed. The

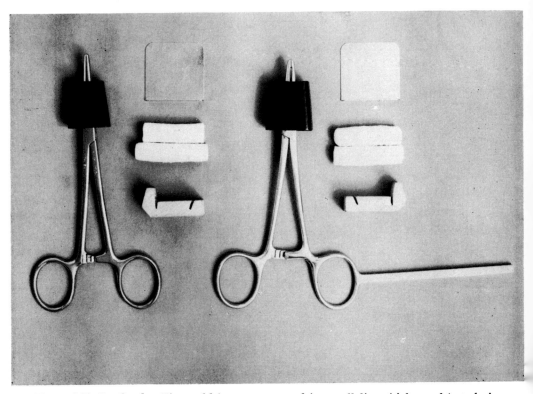

Figure 6-33. Dr. Gordon Fitzgerald instruments used in paralleling (right angle) technic. Note hemostat with rubber bite block, metal backing and specially designed wooden bite block for anterior region. (The hemostat on the right has an angulator to aid in positioning cone.)

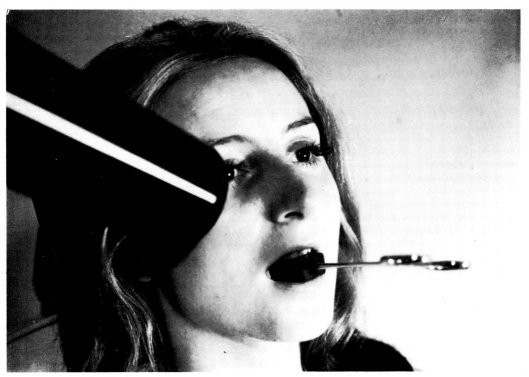

Figure 6-34. Use of Fitzgerald Hemostat in maxillary posterior region.

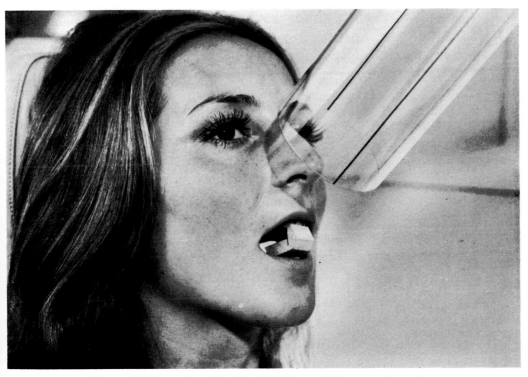

Figure 6-35. Use of wooden bite-block in maxillary anterior region.

film should be placed against the palate and, usually, parallel with the midline.

Direct the beam of radiation through the apices of the teeth at right angles to the teeth. The vertical angle is determined by position of hemostat handles. For the horizontal angle, direct the x-ray beam through the interproximal spaces of the teeth.

The wooden bite-blocks are used for the anterior teeth (maxillary and mandibular) and mandibular premolars. The patient retains the wooden bite-block in the mouth by his teeth. The use of the patient's hands is not necessary (See Figure 6-35).

In the maxillary anterior projections, the film is inserted into the slot in the small end of the wooden film block and the patient bites on the large end of the film block. With mandibular anteriors and premolars, insert the film in the slot in the large end of the bite-block and have the patient bite on the small end of the block. The digital method is used in the mandibular molar region.

In utilizing the Fitzgerald technic the sagittal plane of the head should be perpendicular to the floor. As in the bisecting-angle technic, the occlusal planes of the maxillary and mandibular teeth should be parallel with the floor when

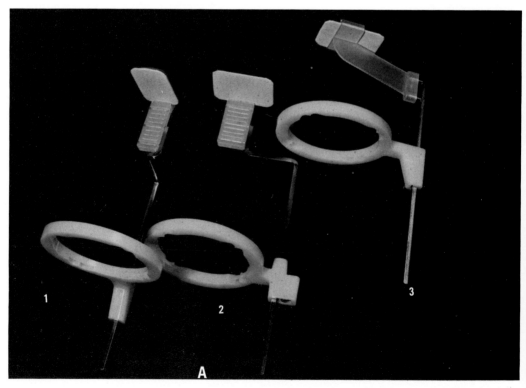

Figure 6-36A. Rinn X-C-P instruments to be used with the long rectangular P.I.D. (Cone) (1) anterior instrument, (2) posterior instrument, (3) bitewing instrument.

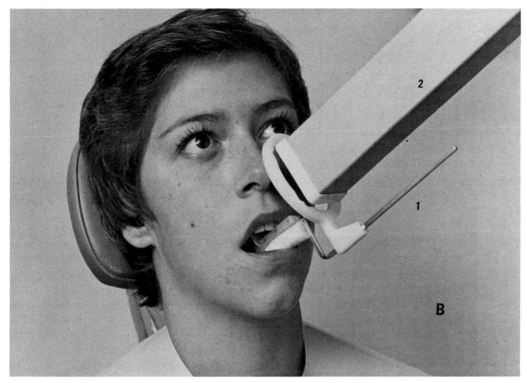

Figure 6-36B. Illustrates the use of the maxillary anterior instrument using (1) Rinn's Rectangular Film Placement Holder with the (2) rectangular beam limiting device.

radiographing maxillary and mandibular teeth respectively.

The Rinn XCP Instruments (Xtension-Cone-Paralleling.)

This is a set of two instruments, an anterior and a posterior instrument, which were designed by Dr. William J. Updegrave of the School of Dentistry, Temple University at Philadelphia. Each instrument consists of three parts:

1. *Anterior and posterior plastic bite-blocks.* These are designed to retain the film packet by means of tension created by a semiflexible plastic backing.

2. *Indicator rod.* These are made of stainless steel, and are used to align the x-ray cone with film. There is an anterior offset rod and a posterior right-angle rod designed to insert into the receptable holes of their respective bite-blocks.

3. *Locator ring.* They are made for sliding onto the rods to establish alignment of the cone with the film. This also prevents "cone cutting."

The Rinn XCP instruments have been modified to include a rectangular-shaped extension cone and a rectangular shaped locating ring (See Figure 6-36). To aid in the alignment of the cone with the locator ring, the cone can be rotated on its own axis. This modification will accomplish two things:

a. Reduce radiation exposure to the patient.

b. Simplifies cone and film alignment.

CLINICAL PROCEDURE FOR PARALLELING OR RIGHT ANGLE TECHNIC USING THE RINN XCP INSTRUMENTS.

1. Wash your hands and assemble the following:

  a. Twenty x-ray films (eight #1 films and twelve #2 regular films)

  b. Four bitewing tabs on four of the #2 films

  c. Two #2 cotton rolls

  d. Paper napkins to blot the films

  e. Rinn XCP Posterior and Anterior Instruments

  f. Rinn Snap-A-Ray Instrument.

2. Number the films with a crayon-type pencil. Do not use a lead pencil or a ball point pen as they will make a latent image on the sensitive film emulsion which will be seen when the radiographs are processed. The films are numbered for three reasons: (a) to prevent the omission of a film in your survey, (b) to facilitate the "wet reading" of a complete mouth survey and (c) to simplify the mounting procedure. (See Figure 6-37A for a typical adult paralleling survey and Figure 6-37B for the complete survey mount used at L.S.U.).

3. Seat patient in dental x-ray chair and adjust the chair so that the patient's maxillary occlusal plane is parallel to

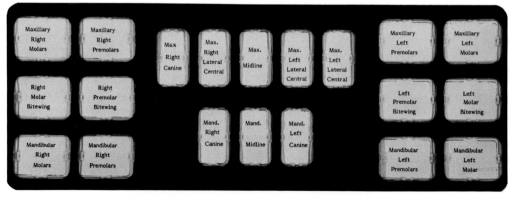

Figure 6-37A. Typical complete radiographic survey using the paralleling technic. (Note that the number one narrow film is used in anterior region.)

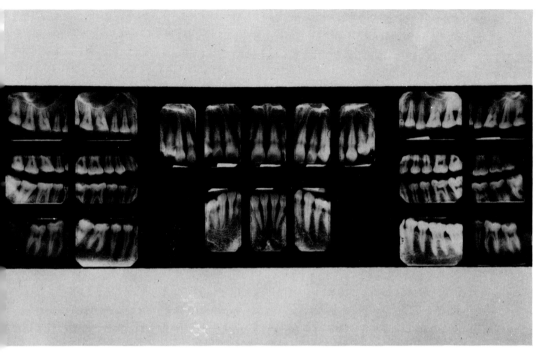

Figure 6-37B. Typical complete radiographic survey. (8 posterior films, 8 anterior films, and 4 posterior bitewings.)

the floor and the midsagittal plane is perpendicular to the floor. Also, the height of the chair should be adjusted to accommodate the operator's height. In general, the chair is lowered for the maxillary arch and raised for the mandibular arch projections. If a lead apron is used in your office, drape the patient's torso with an apron at this time.

4. Examine the patient's oral cavity for anatomical variations such as palatal height, tori, and arch size. Have patient remove his glasses, and introral appliances such as dentures and removable partial dentures. Give the patient the responsibility of keeping his own glasses and his own intraoral appliances for safekeeping. It is nice to have a waxed paper bag or a nap-

kin available for the patient to place his removable intraoral appliances.

5. Turn on the x-ray unit and adjust the milliamperes, kilovoltage and time of exposure before making any exposures. This should be done prior to placing any film in the patient's mouth.

6. Place the film into the XCP instrument biteblock in the following manner:

Posterior Instrument:

a. Place printed side of the #2 film-packet against backing support of bite-block and insert horizontally (sometimes the mandibular premolar film is placed vertically) into slot using a downward motion and at the same time placing slight pressure against the backing support to open slot (See Figure 6-38).

b. Holding the right angle portion of indicator rod anterior to the bite-block, and away from the film, insert the pin in the proper holes. (The three holes allow a choice for the desired lingual positioning of the film. Usually the most anterior holes are used in the maxillary projections and the posterior holes in the mandible.)

Anterior Instruments:

a. Place printed side of #1 film packet against backing support of the bite-block and insert vertically into slot using a downward motion and at the same time placing slight pressure against the backing support to open the slot.

b. Holding the off-set portion of the indicator rod away from the biting surface of the block, insert the pin in the proper holes (See Figure 6-39).

7. Place the black dot on the printed side of the film into the slot of the posterior and anterior biteblocks to prevent superimposition of this dot over the periapical end of the radiographic image of the tooth. The dot should always be placed toward the occlusal line. The black dot on the printed side of the film packet identifies the position of the raised, embossed dot on the radiographic film. The raised portion of the dot is always toward the cone of radiation, so therefore is the side of the film to

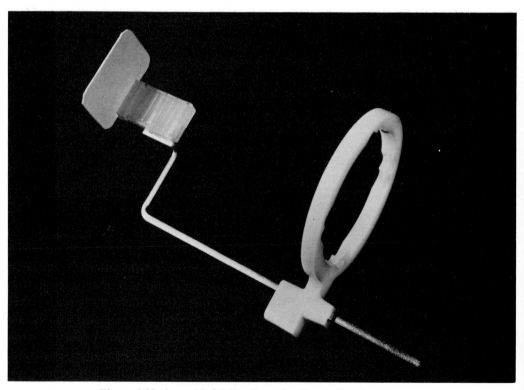

Figure 6-38. Assembled Rinn Posterior Paralleling Instrument.

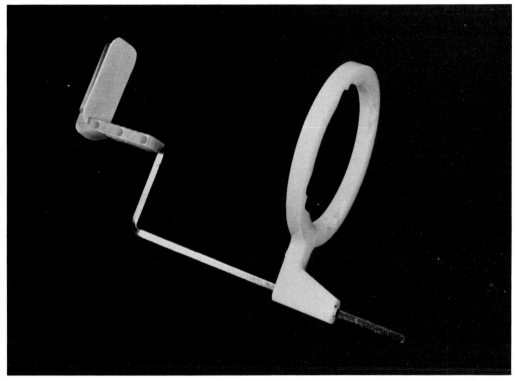

Figure 6-39. Assembled Rinn Anterior Paralleling Instrument.

ward the teeth. The dot, then, identifies the right or left side of the patient. The position of the raised dot is not important when using the bitewing film.

8. There are *six factors* to consider in alignment of the cone with the film in the paralleling technic utilizing the Rinn XCP instruments: There are three factors to consider in the placement of the film in the mouth and three factors to consider in the alignment of the cone:

Three factors to consider in the placement of film:

a. Place film so that it covers the prescribed teeth to be examined for each region of the oral cavity:

(Scope of examination for each region is listed below.)

Upper Molar Region: The radiograph should show all of the 3rd molar or tuberosity, 2nd molar and the 1st molar.

Upper Premolar Region: The radiograph should show all of the premolars, and the distal portion of the canine.

Upper Canine Region: The radiograph should show the canine centered upon the film.

Upper Central and Lateral Region: The radiograph should show all of the central and lateral incisors on the film (right and left side).

Upper Midline Region: The radiograph should show all of the cen-

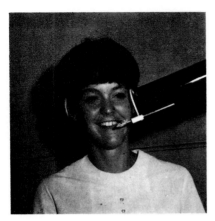

Figure 6-40. The maxillary posterior projection. Two-thirds of the cone shows above the alignment rod.)

tral incisors centered on the film.
Lower Molar Region: The radiograph should show all the mandibular molars on the film.
Lower Premolar Region: The radiograph should show all of the premolars and the distal of the canine.
Lower Canine Region: The radiograph should show all of the canine centered on the film.
Lower Midline Region: The radiograph should show all of the central incisors and the laterals on the film.
Molar Posterior Bite-Wing: The radiograph should show the interproximal regions of maxillary and mandibular molars.
Premolar Posterior Bite-Wing: The radiograph should show the interproximal regions of the maxillary and mandibular premolars and the distal surfaces of the maxillary and mandibular canines.
b. Position the film parallel to the long axes of the teeth being radio-

graphed and rest the bite-block on occlusal surface. (In most patients film will be located in midline of palate for maxillary posterior projections).
c. Position the film parallel to the lingual surfaces of the teeth to be examined. Instruct the patient to close teeth firmly on bite block to retain film in position. A cotton roll is placed routinely on the opposite side of the bite-block in all projections to increase comfort and stability.

The locator ring is used to produce positive alignment of the cone with the film. When the locator ring is not used, there are three factors to consider in positioning the cone:
a. Position cone so that cone is *vertically* parallel with the indicator or alignment rod. In the maxillary posterior arch projections, two thirds of the cone should extend *above* the alignment rod (See Figure 6-40). In the mandibular posterior arch projections two thirds

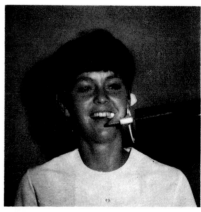

Figure 6-41. The mandibular posterior projection. (Two-thirds of the cone shows below the alignment rod.)

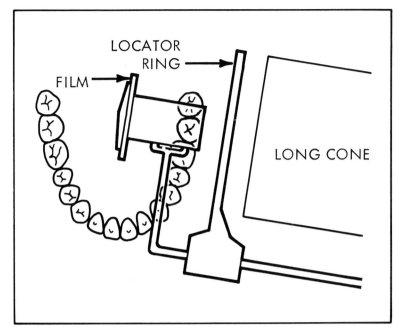

Figure 6-42. Diagram of cone positioned correctly for horizontal angulation for posterior projection. (Courtesy of Dr. William Updegrave.)

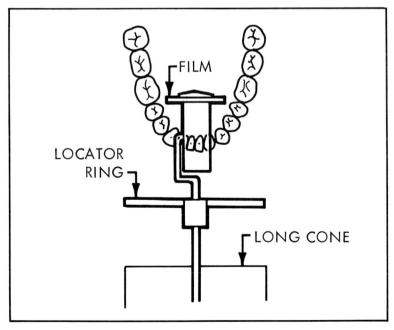

Figure 6-43. Diagram of cone positioned correctly for horizontal angulation for anterior projection. (Courtesy of Dr. William Updegrave.)

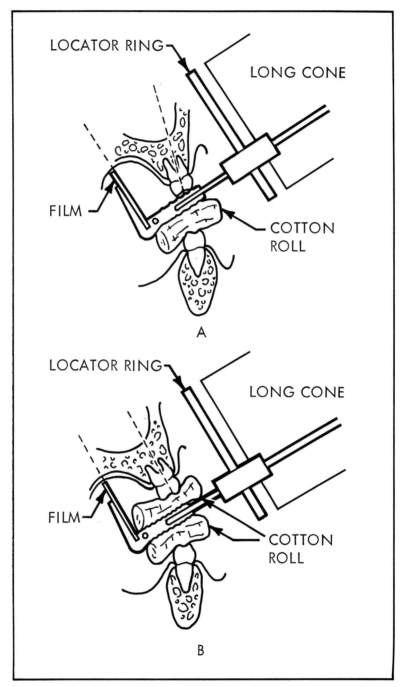

Figure 6-44. A.—Diagram of alignment of film and cone in patients with average-sized palatal vaults. B.—Diagram of alignment of teeth and cone in patients with shallow palatal vaults.

of the cone should extend below the indicator or alignment rod (See Figure 6-41). The correct cone alignment with the alignment rod should be done from the side of the cone, making sure that your eyes, the alignment rod, and the cone are in the same position while sighting. Vertical shape distortion and cone cutting will occur if this is not done properly.

b. Position the cone so that the cone is horizontally parallel to the alignment rod when viewed from behind the tube head. See Figure 6-42 for the posterior projections and Figure 6-43 for the anterior projections. Overlapping will occur if the horizontal angulation is incorrect.

c. Position the cone so that the cone of radiation completely covers the film. Sight along the anterior edge of the cone making sure that the cone covers the anterior border of

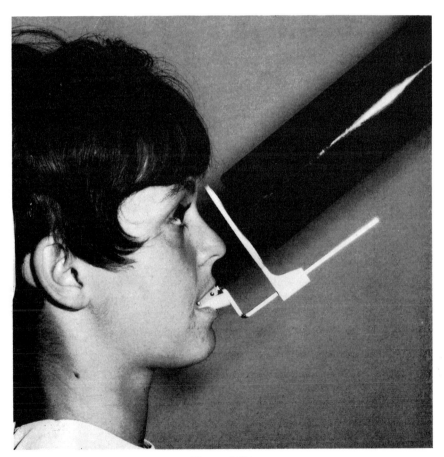

Figure 6-45A

Figure 6-45A & Figure 6-45B. Technic for positioning the film, and the cone in the maxillary anterior region using the Rinn XCP Instruments.

the biteblock and film. If this procedure is done incorrectly, "cone cutting" will occur.

ALIGNMENT SUGGESTIONS USING THE RINN XCP INSTRUMENTS.

Maxillary Posterior Region:

Low or Shallow Palates: When a patient has a low maxillary palate, it is difficult to achieve absolute parallelism between the film and the long axes of the teeth. First, the film must be placed as far lingually as the length of the biteblock and the anatomy will allow. A discrepancy in parallelism of 15° and below is usually tolerable. If the error in parallelism exceeds 15°, use two cotton rolls, one on each side of the biteblock. This will allow for more parallelism between the film and the teeth; however, the periapical coverage will be reduced. Usually, this procedure is acceptable in most instances, especially if the teeth have medium-sized or short roots (See Figure 6-44A and 6-44B).

Inadequate Periapical Coverage

If greater periapical coverage is desired, increase the vertical angulation of the cone by five to fifteen degrees greater than the instrument rod indicates.

Maxillary Anterior Region:

Position the film well posterior in the mouth parallel to the long axes of the anterior teeth being examined. Instruct patient to bite on block to retain it in position. Place cotton roll (#2) on underside of block to increase comfort and stability (See Figure 6-45).

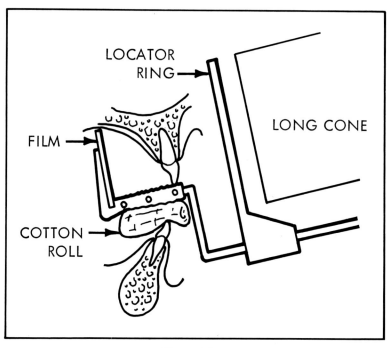

Figure 6-45B

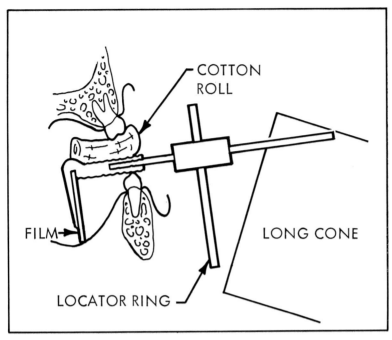

Figure 6-47. Diagram showing technic for using Rinn XCP instrument in the mandibular premolar region to alleviate the problem of inadequate coverage by using a negative cone angulation.

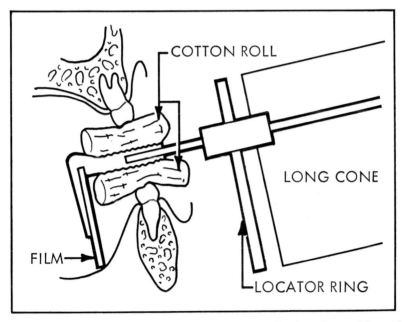

Figure 6-48. Diagram of the use of two cotton rolls to alleviate the problem of inadequate periapical coverage in the mandibular premolar region.

place yourself at least six feet behind patient and depress the timer switch button, holding it down until the exposure is completed.

10. Remove holder and film from patient's mouth, remove film from the film holder, blot film lightly to remove moisture and deposit film in proper receptacle. Proceed to next film and complete the periapical survey.

11. When all projections have been completed, remove exposed films from receptable, place in envelope and identify properly.

12. Dismiss patient.

Precision X-Ray Instruments

These instruments were developed by Dr. F. M. Medwedeff of Nashville, Tennessee. They are rectangular collimating film positioning instruments constructed of stainless steel. The adult periapical set consists of three instruments: (See Figure 6-49A and 6-49B.)

1. Anterior instrument for maxillary and mandibular placement.

2. Posterior instrument for right maxillary and left mandibular placement.

3. Posterior instrument for left maxilliary and right mandibular placement.

LOADING THE INSTRUMENT.

Load the film packet in the instrument with the printed side toward the backing support, and the dot toward the biteblock. After the film touches the

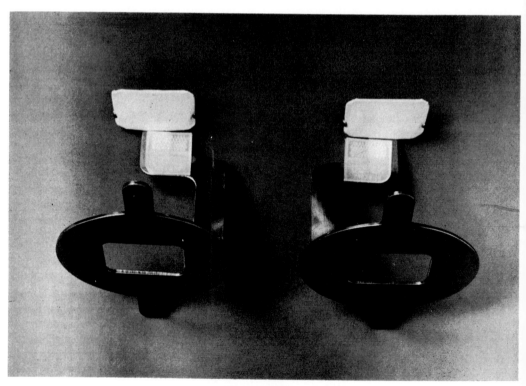

Figure 6-49A

Figure 6-49. Precision X-Ray Film Holders: A. posterior instruments.

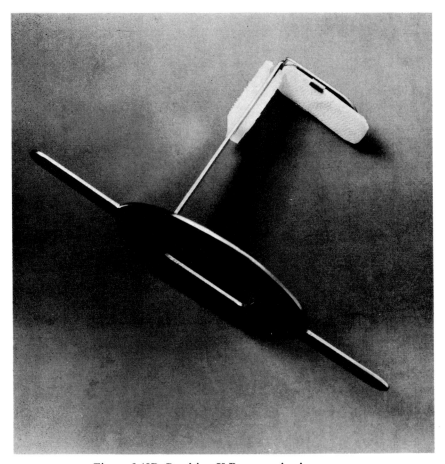

Figure 6-49B. Precision X-Ray anterior instrument.

support bar, move the biteblock tightly against the film.

POSITIONING THE INSTRUMENT.

1. Grasp the instrument with your finger through the rectangular opening.
2. Insert the anterior film into the oral cavity with the film horizontal. This will enable the film to pass into the mouth without requiring the patient to open widely.
3. Rotate the instrument into position so the film edge will contact the palate or the floor of the mouth. Make sure that the film is parallel to the teeth in both the vertical and hori-

zontal planes. Place the biteblock on the teeth to be examined.

4. Have the patient close down on the biteblock to hold it in position. The extended tab on the collimator may be used by the patient to further assist in the retention of the film holder.
5. If teeth are missing or malposed, a cotton roll placed in the biteblock will assist in the proper alignment.

CONE-FACE SHIELD ALIGNMENT.

The cone is aligned to the film by placing the open-faced cone in contact with the face shield of the film holder.

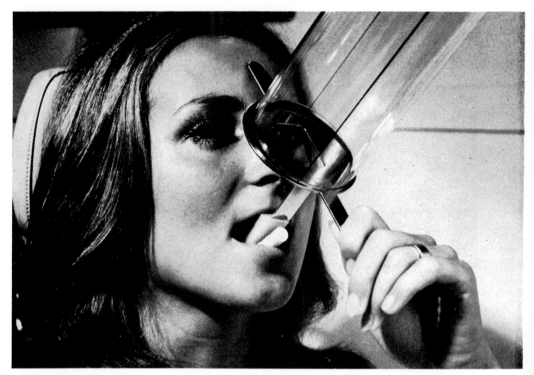

Figure 6-50. Demonstrates the use of Anterior Precision Instrument in maxillary anterior region.

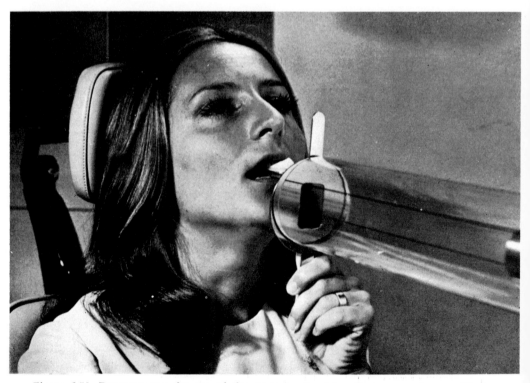

Figure 6-51. Demonstrates the use of the Anterior Precision Instrument in mandibular anterior region.

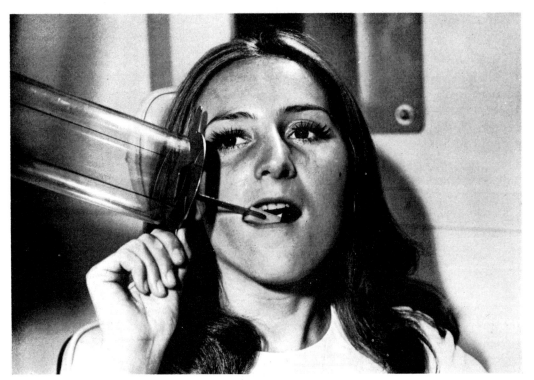

Figure 6-52. Demonstrates the use of the Posterior Precision Instrument in posterior maxillary region.

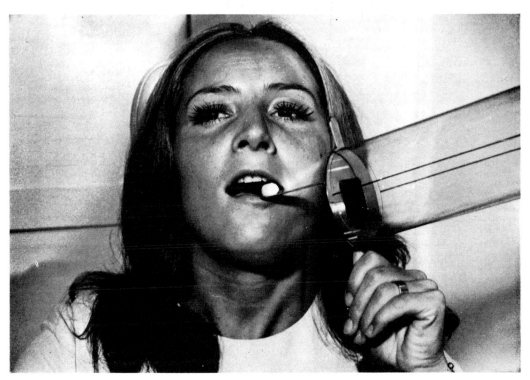

Figure 6-53. Demonstrates the use of the Posterior Precision Instrument in posterior mandibular region.

If the alignment of the face of the cone and the face shield of the film holder is in error by four degrees, or more, "cone cutting" may appear on the resultant radiograph. One suggestion is to bring the cone a few millimeters from the face shield, and then move the patient's head gently with both hands until the face of the cone touches the face shield. This will prevent "cone cutting" and provide stabilization of the patient's head. Figures 6-50 to 6-53 illustrate the use of the Precision X-Ray instruments in various regions of the jaws.

Posterior Bite-Wing Film Technic

In 1926, Dr. Howard Raper of Indiana University announced the bitewing technic for detecting interproximal caries. The posterior bitewing film reveals the crowns and adjacent tissue of the teeth of both jaws on one film.

A bitewing film has a wing or tab attached to the pebbled side of the film.

When the tab is placed on the occlusal surfaces of the mandibular posterior teeth, and the patient closes on the tab, the film will be held in a lingual position to the maxillary and mandibular crowns.

There are two sizes of adult bitewing films:

1. Adult or No. 3 Bite-Wing Film— this is a long, narrow film, designed to record the crowns of all the posterior teeth, both maxillary and mandibular. This type of bitewing film is not recommended because there is a slight amount of distortion in the film from conforming to a curved arch, and many times this film does not reveal all

of the interproximal surfaces of all the posterior teeth.
2. No. 2 or Standard Size Bite-Wing Film—A single No. 2 bite-wing is not long enough to record all posterior crowns in an adult mouth so in the adult, one No. 2 bite-wing film should be used in the molar region, and one No. 2 bite-wing film should be used in the premolar region.

Head Position

Regardless of the type of cone you may be using, the sagittal plane should be perpendicular to the floor, and the tragal-ala line should be parallel to the floor.

Film Placement and Retention

Step 1: Place the bitewing tab or wing on the occlusal surface of the mandibular molars or premolars with the lower edge of the film packet placed in the vestibule between the tongue and the teeth. The anterior edge of the premolar bitewing film should extend to the mesial surface of the mandibular canine and the molar bitewing film should be placed at the midline of the mandibular 2nd premolar.

To avoid overlapping of the contact points, the film should be positioned perpendicular to invisible lines drawn through the embrasures of the teeth.

To do this, in the molar bitewing projection, the anterior border of the film packet should be a greater distance from the lingual surfaces of the teeth than the posterior border.

If the person has a shallow vault, the film should be placed even a greater distance away from the lingual surfaces of the teeth. This will enable the person to close down on the bite-wing tab with less difficulty.

Step 2: Fold down half of the bite-wing tab over the buccal surface of the teeth. This should be done before the tab is placed on occlusal surfaces of the teeth. With the index finger of one hand, press against the lower lingual border of the film to keep it upright. Use the index finger of the other hand to press the tab against buccal surface of the mandibular teeth.

Step 3: Now remove the finger which is pressing against the back of the film, and instruct the patient to close slowly against the bite-wing tab in his normal bite. The patient will not close against your index finger because it is pressing against the buccal surfaces of the lower teeth. After the patient has closed against the bite-wing tab, remove your finger from the tab.

Vertical Angulation

Short Cone (8″ SFD)
   + 10° vertical angulation
Long Cone (16″ SFD)
   + 8° for molar region and
   + 6° for premolar region

If the palate is shallow, the upper border of the film will be forced lingually by the palate on closure. The vertical angle may have to be increased in this case to prevent shape distortion of the maxillary crowns.

Usually the maxillary premolars and molars tilt buccally (sometimes as much as 15 degrees from the vertical) while the mandibular premolars and molars

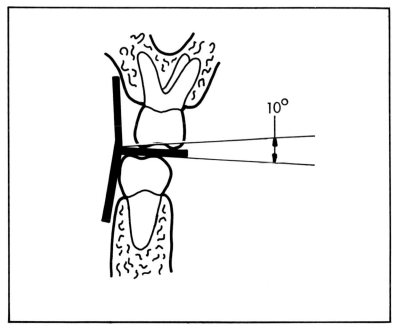

Figure 6-54. Diagram showing the position of the bitewing film in proper relationship to the crowns of the teeth. (Courtesy of Dr. LeRoy Ennis.)

slant very little from the vertical. Therefore, in order to compensate for this discrepancy, and prevent distortion of the
crowns, a compromise vertical angulation
is used for the bitewing projections (See
Figure 6-54).

Horizontal Angulation

Direct the central beam through the
interproximal embrasures of the crowns
of the teeth under examination. The flat
face of the cone should be horizontally
parallel to the film packet.

Point of Entry

Direct the central beam through the
occlusal plane of the teeth toward the
center of the film packet. In order to
prevent "cone cutting," gently pull back
the corner of the lips, and observe
whether the anterior periphery of the
cone is covering the anterior border of
the film. In the molar projection, attach
the tab flush with the anterior margin of
the film. This will serve as a landmark
for the anterior border of the film, when
the patient's teeth are closed together.
In the premolar projection, the anterior
margin of the film can be readily seen.

In order to prevent cone-cutting, use
the teeth as landmarks in the following
manner:

Molar #2 Bite-Wing Film: Align the

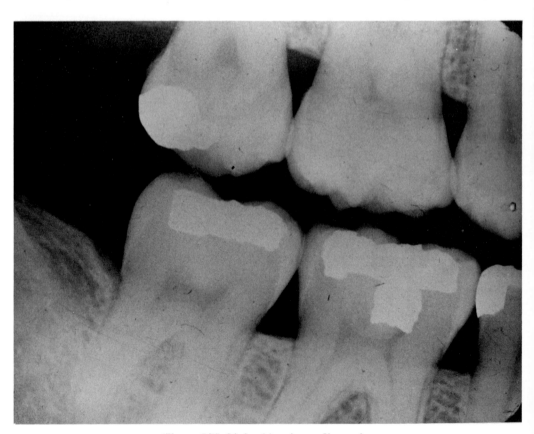

Figure 6-55. Molar bitewing radiograph.

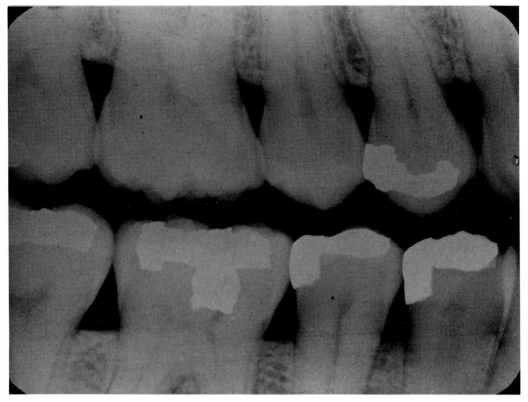

Figure 6-56. Premolar bitewing radiograph.

anterior margin of the cone with the interproximal space between the maxillary 1st premolar and the maxillary canine. Direct the central ray through the occlusal plane of maxillary and mandibular teeth (See Figure 6-55). *Premolar #2 Bite-Wing Film:* Align the anterior margin of the cone with the interproximal space between the maxillary lateral and central. Direct the central ray through the occlusal plane of the maxillary and mandibular teeth (See Figure 6-56).

Both the Rinn and Precision X-Ray companies have developed instruments to aid the operator in the correct alignment of the cone, the teeth and the film

during the bitewing projections. These instruments are available commercially.

The Practical Use of the Long Cone In the Dental Office

One of the reasons given by dentists in the past for not using the long or extension cone technic in their dental practices is that they do not have enough room. This is not a valid reason anymore, because with the use of appropriate film holders, the patient's head position can be adjusted to compensate for the lack of space in almost all dental operatories. If necessary, radiographs may be taken in the supine position. Also, the Pennwalt Corporation manu-

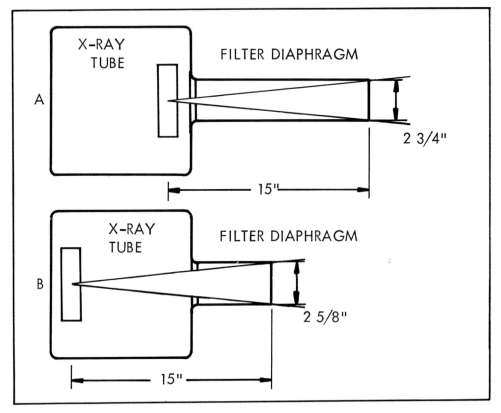

Figure 6-57. The Richards' built-in extended source-skin distance tube without the use of long external cone. (Courtesy of Prof. Albert Richards.)

factures an x-ray machine designed by Professor Albert Richards of University of Michigan which incorporates an extended source-film distance within the body of the x-ray tube housing. Therefore, this machine looks very similar to the conventional short cone machine; however it employs an extended source-film distance. This is accomplished by locating the x-ray tube in back of the x-ray head behind the transformers (See Figure 6-57).

REFERENCES

Appleman, Robert M.: The extended tube technique in intraoral roentgenology. *Am J Roentgenol* 62:881-889, No. 6, December, 1949.

Barr, J. H., and Grone, Paul: Palate contour as a limiting factor in intraoral x-ray technique. *Oral Surg,* 12:459, April, 1959.

Carr, Jack D., *et al.: Manual for Dental Radiology.* Indiana University, School of Dentistry, 1960.

Dempster, W. T.; Adams, W. J.; and Duddles, R. A.: Arrangement in the jaws of the roots of the teeth. *J Am Dent Assoc,* 67:689, December, 1963.

Ennis, LeRoy M.: The bisecting technique versus paralleling. *Dent Clin North Am,* 779-781, November, 1969.

Ennis, LeRoy M.; Berry, Harrison; and Phillips, James E.: *Dental Roentgenology,* 6th ed. Philadelphia, Lea & Febiger, 1967.

Fitzgerald, Gordon M.: Dental roentgenography I. *J Am Dent Assoc,* 34:1-20, No. 1, January, 1947.

Fitzgerald, Gordon M.: Dental roentgenography II. *J Am Dent Assoc,* 34:160-170, No. 3, February, 1947.

Fitzgerald, Gordon M.: Dental roentgenography III. *J Am Dent Assoc,* 38:293-303, No. 3, March, 1949.

Fitzgerald, Gordon M.: Dental roentgenography IV. *J Am Dent Assoc,* 41:19-28, No. 1, July, 1950.

Fitzgerald, Gordon M.: Roentgenographic rebuttal. *Oral Surg,* October, 1960.

Gilbert, R. R., and Hanan, Lewis: Duplication and quality control for intra-oral roentgenographic use in clinical periodontics. *Oral Surg,* 26:31, July, 1968.

Kaletsky, Theodore: A simple way to produce consistently accurate intraoral roentgenograms and a modification of the technic of dental roentgenography. *J Am Dent Assoc,* 26:390, March, 1939.

LeMaster, C. A.: A modification of technic for radiographing upper molars. *J Nat Dent Assoc,* 8:328, 1921.

MacMillan, H. W.: The structure and function of the alveolar process. *J Am Dent Assoc,* 11:1059, November, 1924.

McCall, John, and Wald, Samuel: *Clinical Dental Roentgenology,* 4th ed. Philadelphia, W. B. Saunders, 1957.

McCormack, Donald: Mechanical aids for obtaining accuracy in dental roentgenology. *J Am Dent Assoc,* 40:144-153, No. 2, February, 1950.

McCormack, Donald: Dental roentgenology: A technical procedure for furthering the advancement toward anatomical accuracy. *J Calif State Dent Assoc,* May-June, 1937, p. 89.

McCormack, Franklin: Plea for standardized technic. *J Dent Res,* 11:467, September, 1920.

Medwedeff, F. M., Knox, W. H., and Latimer P.: A new device to reduce patient irradiation and improve dental film quality. *Oral Surg,* 15:1079-1088, September, 1962.

Medwedeff, Fred M., and Ellan, Paul D.: A precision technic to minimize radiation. *Dent Surv,* 43:45, October, 1967.

Pature, B.: Roentgenographic evaluation of alveolar bone changes in periodontal disease. *Dent Clin North Am,* March, 1960.

Peterson, Shailer: *Clinical Dental Hygiene.* St. Louis, C. V. Mosby, 1959.

Price, Weston A.: The technique necessary for making good dental skiagraphs. *Dental Items of Interest,* 26:161-171, 1904.

Raper, H. R.: Uses of bitewing radiographs. *Dent Surv,* 30:763, June, 1954.

Raper, Howard: Advantages and disadvantages of three radiodontic technics. *Dental Surv,* 1404, November, 1955.

Raper, Howard: Critical analysis of three radiodontic technics—introduction. *Dent Surv,* 731, June, 1955.

Raper, Howard: Criticism of mathematical angulation technic. *Dent Surv,* 986, August, 1955.

Raper, Howard: Mathematical angulation technic. *Dent Surv,* 863, July, 1955.

Stafne, Edward C.: *Oral Roentgenographic Diagnosis,* 3rd ed. Philadelphia, Saunders, 1969.

Updegrave, W. J.: Radiographic examination. *Current Therapy in Dentistry,* Vol. II. St. Louis, C. V. Mosby, 1966.

Updegrave, William: Simplifying and improving intraoral dental roentgenography. *Oral Surg,* 12:704-716, June, 1959.

Updegrave, William J.: Dental radiography with the Rinn bisecting angle instruments. Elgin, Illinois, Rinn Corporation, 1967.

Updegrave, William J.: Paralleling extension cone technique in intraoral dental radiography. *Oral Surg,* 4:1250-1261, October, 1951.

Updegrave, William J.: Simplifying and improving intraoral dental roentgenography. *Oral Surg,* 12:704-716, June, 1959.

Updegrave, William J.: High and low kilovoltage. *Dent Rad Photogr,* 33:71, No. 4, 1960.

Updegrave, William J.: Higher fidelity in intraoral roentgenography. *J Am Dent Assoc,* 62:1-22, January, 1961.

Updegrave, William J.: New horizons in periapical radiography. Elgin, Illinois, Rinn Corporation, 1966.

Waggener, D. T.: The principles of the long cone technique. *J Neb Dent Soc,* 24:3, 1947.

Waggener, D. T.: Newer concepts in dental roentgenology. *J Can Dent Assoc,* 17:363-370, July, 1951.

Waggener, Donald T.: The right-angle technique using the extension cone. *Dent Clin North Am,* 783-788, November, 1960.

Waggener, Donald T.: *Oral Roentgenographic Technique.* University of Nebraska.

Waggener, Donald T.: The principles of the long tube technique. *J Neb Dent Soc,* 24:3, 1947.

Wainwright, W. W.: *Dental Radiology.* New York, McGraw-Hill, 1965.

Wege, W. W.: A technique for sequentially reproducing intraoral film. *Oral Surg,* 23:454-461, April, 1967.

Weissman, Donald D., and Longhurst, Gerald E.: *Manual of Rectangular Field Collimation for Intraoral Periapical Radio-graphs.* Los Angeles, University of California at Los Angeles, 1971.

Weissman, Donald D., and Longhurst, Gerald E.: Clinical evaluation of a rectangular field collimating device for periapical radiography. *J Am Dent Assoc,* 82:580-582, March, 1971.

Williams, Sam W.: The paralleling technique for intraoral roentgenology. *J Am Dent Assoc,* 43:419-433, No. 4, October, 1951.

Wuehrmann, Arthur: The long cone technic. *Prac Dent Monogr,* 3-30, July, 1957.

Wuehrmann, Arthur H.: What are the advantages of a long cone on a dental machine? *Oral Surg,* August, 1961.

Wuehrmann, Arthur H., and Manson-Hing, Lincoln R: *Dental Radiology,* 2nd ed. St. Louis, C. V. Mosby, 1968.

X-Rays in Dentistry. Eastman Kodak Company, Radiography Markets Division, Rochester, N. Y., 1969.

CHAPTER 7

CORRECT MANAGEMENT OF RADIOGRAPHIC PATIENTS

IN ORDER TO reduce radiographic retakes, the operator must know how to manage each patient individually. There are certain patient variations which should be considered before beginning your radiographic procedures.

Anatomical Variations

1. Maxillary and mandibular tori.
2. Maxillary palatal vault shape, size and depth.
3. Height of muscle attachments in floor of mouth.
4. Size of the tongue (tongue thrust).
5. Height of the patient. (A tall person will oftentimes have longer rooted teeth; the crowns of the teeth may give you some indication here.)
6. Size of the patient:
   a. A larger patient may require more exposure time in order to avoid low density films.
   b. A small patient may require less exposure time in order to avoid high density films.
   c. Edentulous patients will require less exposure time to avoid high density films.
7. Patients with "fat cheeks" (obese individuals). This will require more exposure time in order to avoid low density films.

8. People with ruddy, red complexions: These patients have more blood in these tissues and may require more exposure time in order to avoid low density films.
9. Thin patients: These people will usually require less exposure time to maintain the desired density.

Age of Patient

The recommended exposures are based on requirements for adults 20 to 50 years of age, average build, and with teeth present. For patients under 12 years of age, the exposure time may have to be decreased to maintain the desired film density. For patients over 50 years of age the exposure time may have to be increased to maintain the desired film density—the pulps of these teeth have reduced in size considerably. However, many of the elderly individuals have a condition called osteoporosis of the bone. In this condition, the cortex of the bone becomes thin and the trabeculae of the cancellous bone becomes reduced in number. Naturally, the exposure time should be reduced in a patient with this condition.

Apprehensive Patient

Usually apprehensive patients are highly nervous individuals who have hypersensitive mouths. They usually have a low pain threshold. Your first contact with these individuals should be a pleasant one, and you should be extremely careful in the placement of the films in the mouths of these patients.

It is imperative that you should employ a rapid and accurate radiographic technic.

Gagging Patient

Gagging is the involuntary effort to vomit. It is caused by the gag reflex, and is very annoying in intraoral radiography. Some patients have an extremely low threshold for the gag reflex.

The receptors for the gag reflex are located in the soft palate, the lateral posterior one-third of the tongue, and the region of the retromylohyoid space. The ninth or the glossopharyngeal cranial nerve governs the sensibility of these areas and also controls the reflex movement of swallowing, gagging and vomiting (See Figure 7-1).

The mechanism of the gagging reflex is set off by initial irritation to the soft

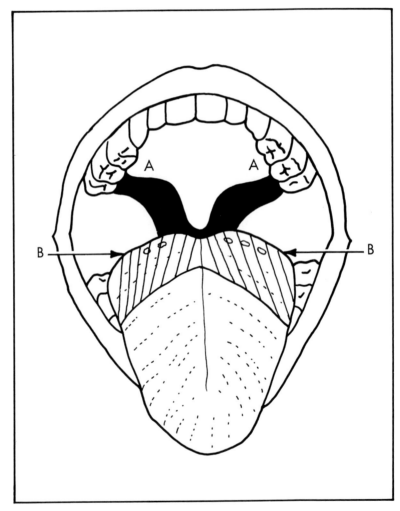

Figure 7-1. Areas of the oral pharynx and the posterior one-third of the tongue where the receptors for the gag reflex are located. These areas are innervated by the 9th or glossopharyngeal nerve—see areas (A) and (B).

palate or the posterior third of the tongue, and subsequently conveyed by afferent nerves to the gag center in the medulla oblongata. There is an outflow from this nerve center by way of efferent nerve fibers to the muscles envolved in gagging. The gag reflex proceeds by a series of reactions:

1. First, there is the cessation of respiration.
2. Followed by the contraction of the thoracicoabdominal and oropharyngeal muscles. (Sometimes food is regurgitated into the larynx, the oropharynx and the mouth.)

The two stimuli which commonly initiate the gag reflex are:

1. The psychic stimuli
2. The tactile stimuli

In order to eliminate or diminish the gag reflex we must diminish or eliminate these stimuli from the patient. How is this accomplished?

Reducing the Psychic Stimuli

People with the accentuated gag reflexes are usually highly nervous and highstrung individuals with very hypersensitive oral tissues. The following is a list of methods to aid in the management of these individuals:

1. Your first contact with these patients should be a pleasant one, and you should make every effort to give the person confidence in your ability to perform the service which you are about to render. Discuss his problem in a kindly and sympathetic manner, and try to gain the patient's confidence.
2. Do the anterior regions of the oral cavity first and the most sensitive maxil-

lary molar regions last. Maybe by then the patient's fears from psychic stimuli will be forgotten, and these sensitive areas in the oral cavity may be radiographed without incident.

3. Try to divert the patient's attention from the unpleasant prospect of gagging to some other interest or preoccupation:

   a. Tell the patient to think of something else.
   b. Have him bite hard on the biteblock; the pain may divert his attention.
   c. Instruct the patient in breathing exercises. These will keep his mind off of what he is doing, and besides, if the patient is breathing, he cannot gag. Remember that the first reaction in the gag reflex is the cessation of breathing. An excellent method is to tell the patient to breathe "rapid and shallow." The breathing should be audible to the operator. This should be demonstrated to the patient.

Reducing the Tactile Stimuli

Some people have accentuated gag reflexes because of hypersensitive pharyngeal areas. Patients suffering from chronic sinus trouble (the well known postnasal drip) are the worst gaggers. An accumulation of mucus and saliva into the nasal or oropharynx may initiate the gag reflex with these people.

Methods to alleviate the tactile stimuli are as follows:

1. The film should be placed positively and firmly in the mouth and retained in position without movement. Carry the film into the mouth parallel with the plane of occlusion, until you are in prop-

er position, then rotate the film to touch the palate. Film holders such as the Rinn Snap-a-Ray are very useful in the positive placement and retention of the film.

2. The exposure of the film should be done as quickly as possible by using a rapid radiographic technic. The timer is preset; the cone is placed for the approximate horizontal and vertical angulations; the film is placed into the mouth and then exposed as quickly as possible. Most people can stand the uncomfortable feeling for a few seconds. For example, for projections in the maxillary molar region:

a. Preset the timer.

b. Place film in Rinn Snap-a-Ray holder.

c. Place patient's head in correct position (mid-sagittal plane perpendicular to the floor and tragal-ala line parallel to the floor).

d. Adjust vertical angulation to +30 degrees and place center of cone over the point of entry (apices of maxillary 2nd molar). Adjust the horizontal angulation by paralleling the face of the flat-ended cone to the buccal surface of the maxillary molar crowns.

e. Place film quickly and firmly into position to cover maxillary molar region. Have patient close firmly on bite block.

f. Expose film.

3. If the before mentioned procedures do not work, you may use the following methods:

a. Some people give the patient a drink of ice water which is supposed to dull the sensory nerve endings.

b. Others have placed ordinary table salt on the tip of the tongue.

c. Others use a topical anesthetic which may be of the viscous or spray type. When using the spray type topical anesthetic, spray the anesthetic on the palate and the posterior third of the tongue and have the patient EXHALE WHILE YOU ARE DOING THIS. Wait a minute for the anesthesia to take effect. Benzocaine is the active ingredient of this topical anesthetic. The anesthesia lasts for approximately 20 minutes. You should be cautioned in the use of the spray topical anesthetic. Do not give it to any individuals who are allergic to benzocaine or have a tendency toward bronchial complications. If the topical spray is inhaled it could cause an aspiration pneumonitis, an inflammation of the air passages of the lungs which could be quite serious. You will soon discover, though, that the topical anesthetic procedure is used infrequently anyway.

Extreme Cases with Accentuated Gag Reflexes

There are some patients with accentuated gag reflexes. It is usually impossible to take an intraoral periapical radiograph on these individuals. This happens infrequently, but when it occurs, it is recommended that you use one of the following technics:

a. Right and left lateral jaw radiographs.

b. Maxillary topographical occlusal radiograph.

c. Mandibular incisor occlusal radiograph.

d. Attempt bite-wing films using a smaller sized film (size #1 or #0 films).

e. Panoramic radiograph.

REFERENCES

Dresen, O. M.: Control of the gagging patient. *Texas Dent J*, 65:332-333, 1947.

Ennis, LeRoy, and Berry, Harrison: *Dental Roentgenology*, 5th ed. Philadelphia, Lea and Febiger, 1959, pp. 104-105.

Hannah, Ruhamah, *et al.: Manual for Dental Radiology*. Indiana University School of Dentistry, 1960, pp. 19-20.

Landa, J. S.: *Practical Full Denture Prosthesis*. Dental Item of Interest Publishing Co., Brooklyn, N. Y., 1947, pp. 268-279.

Lozier, Matthew: Etiology and control of gagging reflex in the practice of intraoral roentgenography. *Oral Surg*, 2:766-769, 1949.

McCall, John, and Wald, Samuel: *Clinical Dental Roentgenology*, 4th ed. Philadelphia, W. B. Saunders, 1957, pp. 23-25.

Moss, Aaron A.: The confident dentist can eliminate gaging by waking hypnotic suggestion. *Dent Surv*, 26:198-199, 1950.

Richards, Albert: The control of gagging in dental radiography. *Dent Radiol Photogr*, No. 2, 1950.

Silha, Robert: Roentgenographic service for gagging patient. *Oral Surg*, January, 1962, p. 64.

Stephens, Douglas W.: Physiological and psychological approach to the problem of gagging. *Dent Surv*, 25:1795-1797, 1949.

Common Errors

1. Projection Errors

2. Exposure Errors

3. Processing Errors

CHAPTER 8

PROCESSING AND FILM MOUNTING PROCEDURES

E VEN THOUGH the finest x-ray equipment is used and the most exact-
ing radiographic technic is employed,
the radiograph may be of inferior quality if the processing of the exposed x-ray
film is carelessly executed.

Processing the film completes what the
exposure started. It produces a visible,
lasting image of the latent image created
by the x-rays. When the x-rays strike the
light-sensitive silver salts (silver bromide, AgBr) in the film emulsion, the
energy is stored in the form of a latent
image. The latent image becomes visible
after the film is immersed in certain
chemical solutions which change the exposed AgBr salts into particles of metallic silver. The term for the several operations that collectively produce the visible, permanent images is *processing*.

Processing consists of developing, rinsing, fixing, washing, and drying operations and they are all carried out in a
darkroom.

The Darkroom

It is very important that the darkroom
be designed to make film processing an
efficient, precise, and standardized procedure. Since the processing operations
are carried out in near-total darkness,
every piece of equipment must be in its
specific place. Figure 8-1 illustrates a
well-designed darkroom. For efficiency's
sake, the room should be large enough

to avoid crowded conditions and the
equipment should be arranged so as to
expedite the flow of work. The size of
an x-ray darkroom for a dental office can
be as small as 3 by 3 feet for an individual dentist; however, for a group practice installation a 4 by 6 foot darkroom
would be more adequate and convenient.

Processing rooms cannot be used as
storage rooms or for any other procedure
in the dental office that will contaminate
the films with dust or fumes. The darkroom must provide adequate bench
space and adequate facilities for proper
developing, fixing, washing and drying
of the films.

If development and drying are done
in the same room it is recommended
that some means of ventilation be provided to supply the room with fresh air
as well as exhausting the heated air from
the dryer. A room temperature of 70°F
is recommended. If humidity is a problem, especially in parts of the country
where the climate is hot and humid, air
conditioning is a must in these dental
offices. When the temperature of the
processing room exceeds 90°F, the x-ray
films may become sensitized by heat
alone.

There are certain minimum requirements which every darkroom should
have:
  1. Light-tight room
  2. Both safelight and white-light il-
     lumination
  3. Processing tanks
  4. Hot and cold running water

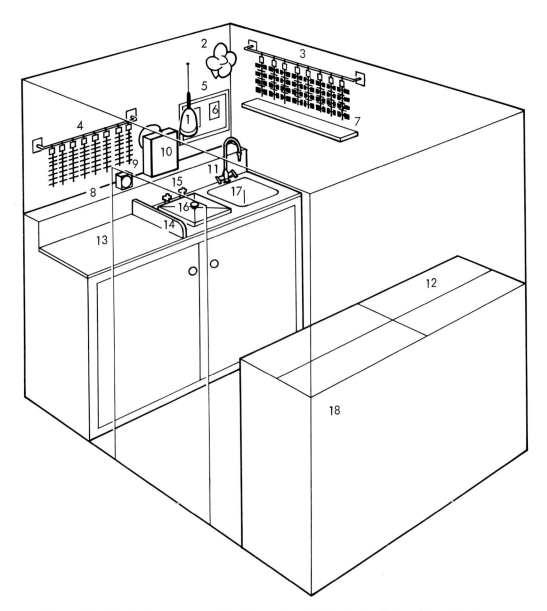

Figure 8-1. (1) Darkroom lamp (2) Electric fan (3) Rack for drying films (4) Storage rack for intraoral hangers (5) Bulletin board (6) Exposure and processing chart for dental x-ray films (7) Drip pan (8) Shelf (9) Timer (10) Utility safelight lamp (11) Gooseneck faucet (12) Loading area (13) Processing area (14) Splashboard (15) Hot and cold water valves (16) 8 x 10 dental processing tank (17) Utility sink (18) Supply cabinet for chemicals, cassettes, and other accessories. (Courtesy of Eastman Kodak Co.)

5. Accurate thermometer and interval timer
6. Fresh water tank for film washing
7. Drying racks or dryer
8. Adequate storage space

Light-tight Processing Room

The first requisite of a processing room is the exclusion of all external light. Dental film emulsions are extremely sensitive to visible light, and any light leaking around a door or window will fog and spoil the films. It is advantageous to have a lock on the darkroom door in order to eliminate the possibility of someone opening the door unexpectedly.

Light leaks in the darkroom may be tested in the following manner: Place unexposed films half covered with the black protective paper in various locations in the room where films are normally loaded and unloaded. Leave for 3 minutes in the dark and process in the usual manner. Any visible degree of fog in that portion of the film not covered by the black paper is indicative of light leaks.

Fluorescent lights should not be used as overhead lights in the darkroom because there is often a short afterglow that may fog the first few films opened after the light has been turned off. For the same reasoning, fluorescent illuminators in the darkroom are also contraindicated.

Processing Tanks

There are several ways in which a film may be developed; however, the standard *time-temperature* tank method is almost universally employed. This method is virtually foolproof and provides an excellent means for checking x-ray exposures. The manufacturer formulates an x-ray developer to give the most

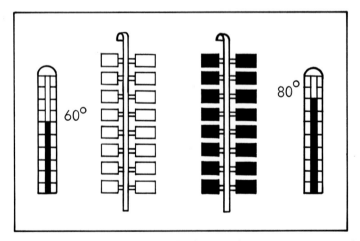

Figure 8-2. In the time-temperature method of processing, a temperature of 70°F at 5 minutes is recommended. Temperatures much below this will *not* allow chemical action to proceed at the required speed, and there is danger of underdevelopment. On the other hand, temperatures much above 70°F may cause some fogging on the film, or make the emulsion softer and more subject to change. You must remember that a properly exposed film cannot be overdeveloped in a reasonable amount of time (10 minutes).

desirable radiographic quality upon *full* development of the x-ray film within a limited temperature range. Hence it is understandable that variations from the optimum in temperature or developing time must be carefully compensated to maintain proper quality (See Figure 8-2).

Tank processing is the simplest and most efficient procedure for developing, rinsing, fixing, and washing films with accurate control. The all-important factor, temperature, can also be regulated and the processing time thereby standardized. The hub of the processing room obviously is the processing tank.

The processing tank contains two parts: The master tank and the insert tanks.

1. *Master Tank:* The master tank serves as a water jacket to hold the insert tanks and is usually large enough to provide space between the insert tanks for rinsing and washing of films when necessary.

2. *Insert Tanks:* The insert tanks are removable containers for the individual processing solutions (developer and fixer) and are spaced in the master tank.

There are many types and sizes of tanks available commercially. A practical one for the dental office consists of a master tank and two removable insert tanks of the one-gallon capacity.

Processing tanks are made of either enamel, earthenware, hard rubber, or stainless steel (AISI Type 316 stainless steel with 2-3% molybdenum). Never use reactive metals such as tin, copper, zinc, aluminum, or galvanized iron. Do not use tanks or other containers that have been soldered, because the reaction

of the solution with the solder metals causes chemical fog on the film. The removable inserts of the tank should be made of stainless steel in order to accommodate more rapidly to changes in temperature of the water in the master tank. Also, stainless steel is more easily cleaned.

To determine the capacity of a tank, measure the inside dimensions and reduce to gallons by using the following mathematical formula:

$$\frac{\text{Width} \times \text{Length} \times \text{Depth (solution level)}}{231 \text{ (\# of cubic inches in gal)}}$$

Cover the developer and fixer tanks when not in use to keep out dust and to reduce the rate of evaporation and oxidation. Many tanks are supplied with covers, but if one is needed, it can be made of water resistant, resin-bonded plywood.

CLEANING PROCESSING TANKS

The action between the mineral salts in the water and carbonate in the developing solutions produces a deposit on the inside walls of the developing tanks. A commercially prepared stainless steel tank cleaner can be used to remove these deposits. After using the tank cleaner, rinse the tank with fresh water and wipe out the tank with a clean cloth. Do not use abrasives such as "kitchen cleansers" in the tanks. These abrasives react unfavorably with the developing solution.

RUNNING HOT AND COLD WATER

X-ray processing solutions are most effective when used with a comparatively narrow range of temperatures. Below 60°F, some of the chemicals are definitely sluggish in action, which may cause underdevelopment and inadequate fixation. Above 75°F, they work too rapidly and may produce fogging of the film. A temperature of 70°F is recommended for three reasons:

1. The optimum quality of the radiograph is attained at this temperature. The contrast and density of the film are most satisfactory and fog is kept to an acceptable low level.
2. The processing time is practical.
3. With modern solution-tempering devices, a temperature of 70°F is usually conveniently maintained. The temperature of the water in the master tank is controlled by a thermostatic or manual mixing value in the water supply. This is the reason why hot and cold running water is essential. The temperature of the water in the master tank in turn controls the tempera-

ture of the processing solutions in the insert tanks.

Thermometers and Interval Timer

Proper control of the processing time is dependent upon the temperature of the solutions, and a good thermometer is an indispensable processing room accessory. There are two types: (1) a tank thermometer that is plainly marked with both Centigrade and Fahrenheit scales, and has a steel clip on the back formed into a hook to hang the thermometer in the tank, (2) another type is the floating, stirring rod type of thermometer. It is all glass and can also be used for stirring small quantities of processing solutions. An interval timer is also important in order to control time of development and fixation.

Correct Safelight

The processing room must be provided with both white and safelight illumination. White light is desirable when such work as cleaning the tanks and preparing the solutions is done. Reliable

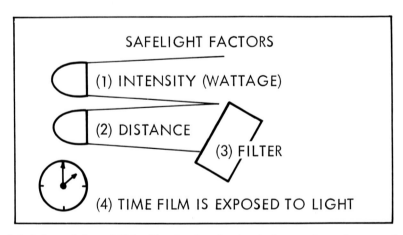

SAFELIGHT FACTORS

(1) INTENSITY (WATTAGE)

(2) DISTANCE

(3) FILTER

(4) TIME FILM IS EXPOSED TO LIGHT

Figure 8-3. Safety of the safelight illumination in the darkroom depends upon four factors: (1) wattage (2) distance (3) filter and (4) time exposed to the safelight.

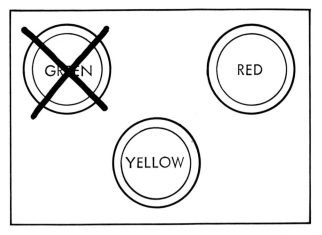

Figure 8-4. A green filter is not recommended for safelights. A red or yellow filter may be used. (Courtesy of Eastman Kodak Co.)

safelight lamps are an indispensable item, since their function is to provide adequate light of a quality that is safe for x-ray films during handling and processing. Remember that films are sensitive to light until after fixation.

Since excessive exposure of the film to safelight illumination will result in fog, three factors concerning safelight lamps must be carefully considered (See Figure 8-3). They are:

1. Type of filter
2. Intensity of illumination
   a. Wattage of bulb
   b. Distance of safelight lamp above the work area
3. Time film is exposed to the safelight

TYPE OF FILTER

Whatever the type of lamp, a correct filter that provides the proper color of light is essential. X-ray films have the

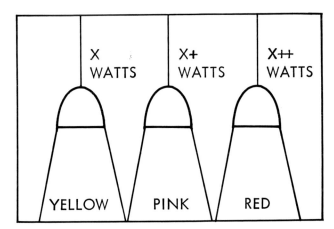

Figure 8-5. A larger bulb is needed in pink and red filters because the filters give off less light with the same wattage. (Courtesy of Eastman Kodak Co.)

highest sensitivity to the blue-green region of the spectrum. The x-ray film is less sensitive to light in the opposite region of the spectrum—the yellow and red region. It is obvious that a blue filter cannot be used; neither can a green filter as it is too close to the blue (See Figure 8-4). Therefore, safelights are safest when made with amber or red filters. Since yellow is closer to green than red in the spectrum, a person can see better under a yellow filter than a red filter. This is the basis of using film emulsions which are not sensitive to the yellow light, such as the Kodak Morlite® film. These film emulsions are especially designed for the yellow Morlite filters (See Figure 8-5). Screen films cannot be used with the Morlite filters.

Never use a red or ruby bulb as a safelight. While the light from such a bulb may look safe because it is dim, such illumination will surely fog x-ray film. In order to use the least amount of light for your safelight lamp, the *Wrat-* *ten® Series 6B filter* is the filter of choice. This filter transmits light predominantly in the yellow-red portion of the spectrum. A small amount of green is transmitted by the Wratten Series 6B filter (See Figure 8-6).

INTENSITY OF ILLUMINATION

The intensity of the illumination of the safelight is controlled by wattage of the bulb and distance of the safelight from the workbench.

With two lamps at the same distance, one having a 7½-watt bulb and the other a 10, the intensity of the 10-watt bulb will naturally be greater than that of the 7½. If two safelights are used, both of which are individually safe, the area of overlap of the beams at the working surface may not be safe (See Figure 8-7).

The recommended distance for safelight lamps is 4 feet above the working surface. If you are using the newer faster ultra-speed films you should use a 7½-

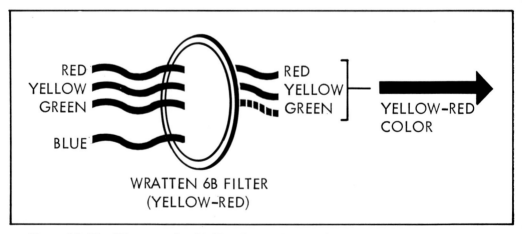

RED
YELLOW
GREEN

BLUE

WRATTEN 6B FILTER
(YELLOW-RED)

RED
YELLOW
GREEN

YELLOW-RED
COLOR

Figure 8-6. The Wratten series 6B filter is especially designed for use with screen films. It transmits light predominantly in the yellow-red portion of the spectrum, and filters out all the blue light that could fog the x-ray film. (Courtesy of Eastman Kodak Co.)

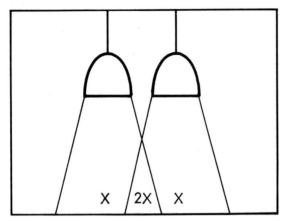

Figure 8-7. When the beams of two safelamps overlap, there is as much as 2X the light in the area of the overlap. (Courtesy of Eastman Kodak Co.)

watt bulb at this distance. Never shorten this distance unless compensation is made by using a bulb of lower wattage. Remember the inverse square law applies to light illumination: the intensity of light varies inversely as the square of the distance. In brief, if we have x intensity at 4 feet, we will have 4x intensity at 2 feet, and ¼x intensity at 8 feet (See Figure 8-8).

Therefore, the intensity of safelight illumination on the film varies with distance and also with the wattage of the bulb (See Figure 8-9). For instance, the intensity is the same when a 15-watt bulb is used at 6 feet, a 10-watt bulb at 5 feet, and a 7½-watt bulb at 4 feet. The correct intensity can be obtained by adjusting either the distance or the bulb wattage or both.

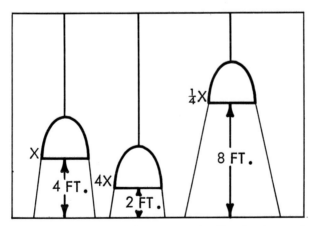

Figure 8-8. The inverse square law applies to safelight illumination as it does for x-radiation. The light intensity is 4 times greater at ½ the distance, and ¼ as much at twice the distance. (Courtesy of Eastman Kodak Co.)

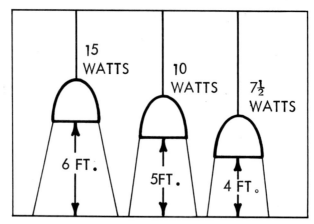

Figure 8-9. Intensity of illumination varies with safelight-to-film distance and wattage of the bulb. (Courtesy of Eastman Kodak Co.)

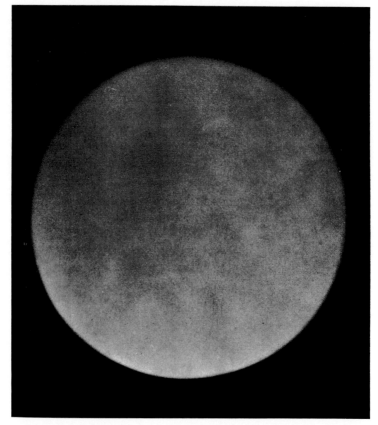

Figure 8-10. A simple method for checking the safelight illumination is to place coins on unexposed films and expose them to your safelight for various periods of time. Develop the films under normal conditions and determine the time limits of your safelight. If you can see the outline of the coin, your safelight is unsafe. This is an illustration of an unsafe safelight.

THE TIME THE FILM IS EXPOSED
TO SAFELIGHT

It must be made crystal clear that there is no such thing as an absolutely *safe* safelight. The Wratten Series 6B filter is the best that can be used, but the film will be fogged if it is exposed too long to light even with this filter. Because x-ray films exposed with intensifying screens are considerably more sensitive to safelight illumination than dental films are, extra precautions are necessary to avoid the danger of fogging them. How long can film be exposed to safelight illumination before fog becomes apparent? The answer to this question must be determined in the processing room under safelight conditions.

SAFETY OF ILLUMINATION TEST

A simple method of checking the safety of illumination of the safelight is as follows: (See Figure 8-10.)

Remove six dental x-ray films from their packets and lay them on the working surface of the bench beneath the safelight lamp. Place a small coin on each film. Expose each film to the safelight illumination for the following sequence of exposure times—1, 1½, 2, 2½, 3 and 3½ minutes—for the six films used. Develop the films in the usual manner. After the films have been cleared in the fixing bath, examine each film before an illuminator. If you can see the outline of the coin on the film exposed to the safelight illumination for one minute, your safelight is *not* safe. Next determine which film you can first see fogging—this will indicate the time that is safe for your film to be exposed to the safelight.

If your safelight is not safe you must do the following things to correct the problem:

1. Replace the bulb with one of lower wattage.
2. Raise the safelight lamp higher from the working surface.
3. Check the filter—the filter may be damaged or broken. (Replace red-lacquered bulbs—they are unsafe.)

Chemistry of Processing

Processing involves chemical reactions which, like all chemical reactions, are critical and require careful attention to details. The sequence of the processing procedure is as follows:

Development—Rinse—Fixation— Wash—Dry

In most darkrooms the developer will be in the left-hand tank as you face the tank, the water bath in the center, and the fixer in the right-hand tank. In strange darkrooms, the developing solutions can be identified by its slippery feeling, the fixer by its vinegary odor when fresh.

We will first consider the purpose of the required solutions, their chemical composition, and how they work.

Developer Process

A photographic developer is a complex chemical system. Its function is to distinguish between those silver halide (bromide) grains which have not received an exposure and those which have. All exposed grains are reduced by the developer to small particles of black metallic silver which form the radiographic image (See Figure 8-11). The extent to which this reduction of silver halide to metallic silver depends upon *time, temperature,* and *concentration* of the developer (See Figure 8-12). Concentration of the developer is affected by the number of films processed and oxidation of the developer by exposure to air.

An x-ray developer contains five basic types of ingredients:

1. Solvent
2. Developing agents or the reducer
3. The accelerator or activator (alkali)
4. Preservative
5. Restrainers

SOLVENT

Water is the solvent used in the de-veloper. It provides a means for the chemicals in the developer for ionization. Water also helps in softening the gelatin emulsion.

DEVELOPING OR REDUCING AGENTS

A developing agent is a chemical compound that is capable of changing the *exposed* grains of silver bromide into metallic silver. At the same time it produces no appreciable effect on the unexposed grains in the emulsion—that is, if the films are not overdeveloped.

The removal of the bromide from the metallic silver is known chemically

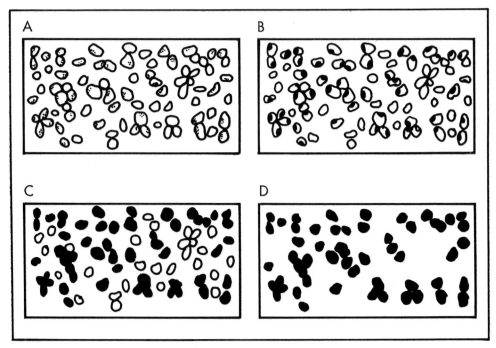

Figure 8-11. Diagrams of processing action in x-ray film emulsions: (A) Schematic distribution of silver bromide crystals. The gray areas indicate latent image produced by exposure—the silver bromide crystals that have been exposed to x-radiation. (B) Partial development begins to produce metallic silver (black) in exposed grains. (C) Development completed. The greater the action of the rays on the film, the greater will be the amount of metallic silver left. (D) Unexposed silver bromide crystals have been removed by fixing. The fixing solution dissolves the excess silver salts and fixes the metallic silver upon the film by stopping the action of the developer. (Courtesy of Eastman Kodak Co.)

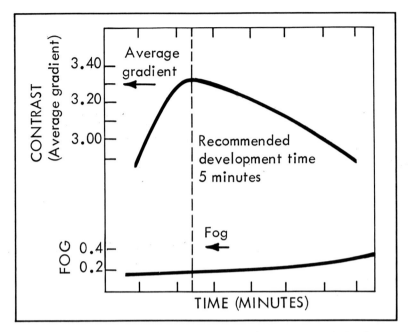

Figure 8-12. This graph illustrates that fact that overdevelopment of the film will cause "chemical fog" on the film. However, remember that a properly exposed film cannot be overdeveloped. The contrast of the film will not be affected in a reasonable amount of time. (10 minutes)

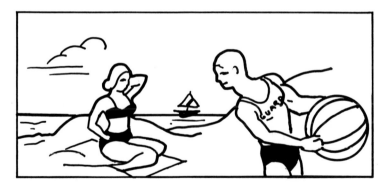

Figure 8-13. The reducing or developing agents must be able to distinguish between exposed and unexposed silver bromide salts. It should be remembered, though, that all reducing agents will begin to develop unexposed parts after a period of time, producing a condition called chemical fog. All developing agents have a definite fogging time beyond which bromide will be freed in unexposed areas.

as "reduction." Chemical reducers have an affinity for oxygen, and must liberate the metals from their salts; so developing solutions contain chemical reducers. Reducing agents used in the developer must be able to reduce the exposed silver bromide, but without affecting unexposed silver bromide, so that their affinity must be within narrow bounds (See Figure 8-13).

Reducing agents commonly used in x-ray developers are hydroquinone and elon (metol).

1. Hydroquinone: 1,4-C_6H_4 $(OH)_2$, (p-d hydroxybenzene) derived from benzene, a coal-tar distillate.
2. Elon (metol): monomethyl para-aminophenol sulfate, a by-product of the manufacture of dyes, treated with methyl alcohol.

These agents have different actions during the period of development, and must be used together to produce all of the steps of grays and the jet blacks in the radiograph.

Hydroquinone brings out the sharp contrast in the radiograph. It works slowly in a maximum efficiency range (65-70°F) and is inactive in cold solution (50°F and below). It is weak and unstable.

The Elon brings out the soft warm tones (grays) in the radiographic image.

It is strong and stable and works quickly over a wide range of temperatures (60-80°F).

If they were used individually the Elon would produce a film with indistinct contrast and the hydroquinone would show just harsh black and whites. A combination of the two brings out all of the steps of grays and the jet blacks for a better result.

Reducers are not stable in the presence of oxygen, for they can readily absorb it from the air or the water. This is why the developer tank should have a cover to prevent oxidation.

ACCELERATOR OR ACTIVATOR (ALKALI)

The developing agents (hydroquinone and Elon) will not develop when used alone. The activity of these chemicals requires the presence of an alkaline solution. Also, an alkali is added to soften and swell the gelatin of the emulsion so the developing agents can diffuse into the gelatin emulsion and attract the exposed silver bromide crystals. In other words, the alkali in effect "opens the

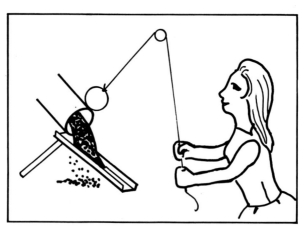

Figure 8-14. Alkali "opens the door" and permits developing agents to enter the pores of the emulsion.

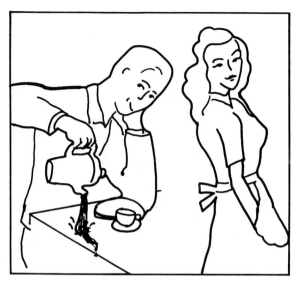

Figure 8-15. The natural attraction of sodium sulfite for oxygen. The affinity is so great, that, when added to a developing solution, sodium sulfite actually reduces oxidation by air of the other components.

door" and permits the developing agents to enter the pores of the emulsion (See Figure 8-14).

Sodium carbonate (Na_2CO_3) and sodium metaborate are the two alkalines most frequently used in the developer.

The regular x-ray developer contains sodium carbonate, which has one disadvantage in its use. If films are developed in a warm solution containing sodium carbonate, tiny bubbles of CO_2 will form when the films are transferred to the cool rinse bath. These bubbles form tiny pits in the film emulsion, which break up the normal radiographic image. This causes blistering of the finished radiograph. Therefore, to combat this disadvantage always be sure that the developer, rinse, and fixer solution temperature is approximately the same.

The rapid x-ray developers contain sodium metaborate, a highly alkaline chemical activator. It does not cause gas bubbles when films are removed from a developer with high temperature and emersed into a cooler fixer.

PRESERVATIVE

Sodium sulfite (Na_2SO_3), an antioxidant, is used to prevent rapid oxidation of the developing agents, especially hydroquinone, by oxygen. As mentioned previously, the developing agents react rapidly with oxygen and if allowed to continue would weaken the action of these agents. Sodium sulfite retards oxidation of the developing agents because it has a natural attraction for oxygen, which prolongs the life of the developing solution (See Figure 8-15).

RESTRAINER

Postassium bromide is used to restrain the developing agents from causing fog. After a certain period of time, the developing agents will begin to deposit silver in the unexposed crystals of the emulsion. This will cause a silver deposit (fog) on the film. Chemical fogging (nondiagnostic radiographic densities) can be retarded by Potassium Bromide, which restrains the action of the developing agents on the unexposed crystals of the emulsion.

However, the development action is slowed down by the silver bromide. Therefore, there must be a proper balance in the proportion of potassium bromide added. If too much is added, the development time will be increased. Too little potassium bromide will result in chemical fogging of the finished film (See Figure 8-16).

Rinsing Process

As already mentioned, bromide is removed from the film emulsion during development, and the restrainer also contains bromide. Therefore, as each film is developed, more bromide or restrainer is added, which theoretically increases the developing time unless the solution strength is maintained by the addition of a refresher. The refresher solution contains a stronger alkali and a higher concentrate of developing agents than the original developer. The restrainer or KBr is either entirely omitted or used in much smaller quantity, since it is continually being removed from films during development. In most dental offices, though, the need for a refresher is eliminated by changing the solution every 3 to 4 weeks depending upon the amount of films developed and whether the solutions have been covered adequately. The developer should be changed by all means when it shows signs of oxidation (a brownish color) and when it will no longer bring up the blacks on the film.

When the film is removed from the

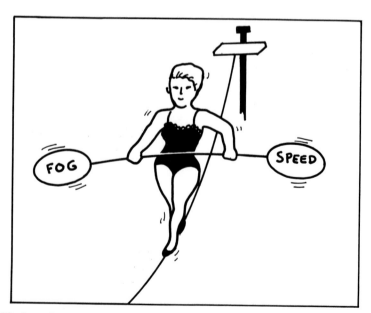

Figure 8-16. Just the proper proportion of potassium bromide is used to balance the chemical fog and speed of development.

developer the gelatin emulsion is swollen and contains several soluble chemicals. The bulk of these chemicals are removed by placing the film into a water bath. By rinsing the film in the water bath the soluble chemicals are removed, the development reaction is stopped, and the alkalinity of the residual developer is neutralized.

The film should be thoroughly rinsed for 15 to 20 seconds in a bath of fresh running water. The temperature of this rinse water should be as close as possible to the temperature of the developer and fixer. If this step were omitted, the alkaline developer retained by the film would soon neutralize the acid of the fixer. The fixing and hardening action of the fixer solution would be impaired and as a result, stains might be produced on the radiograph.

Fixing Process

The fixing process is a chemical treatment which removes the residual undeveloped silver bromide crystals without damaging the image. It also serves to harden the gelatin emulsion.

If these unwanted silver bromide crystals are not removed, the resultant film will discolor when exposed to light. If the film is only partially fixed, the film will turn a brown color with age.

The gelatin coating must be hardened so the film will resist abrasion. The gelatin is animal matter and will decompose if it is not properly cured or tanned.

Like the developer, the fixer is composed of several basic ingredients, each of which will be discussed separately:

1. Solvent
2. Clearing agent
3. Hardening agent
4. Acidifier
5. Preservative

SOLVENT

Sodium thiosulfate ($Na_2S_2O_3$) or hyosulphite of soda (hypo) is the silver bromide solvent or clearing agent. The function of the clearing agent is to change the undeveloped silver bromide crystals into soluble silver salts (silver thiosulfate) so they may be removed in the water bath. Of course, this must be accomplished without destroying the silver image.

Sodium thiosulfate (hypo) is the clearing agent used in powder fixers, and ammonium thiosulfate is used in liquid fixers. It will take approximately 1 to 2 minutes in the fixer to clear the film. When the film is cleared the black silver image produced by the developer will become clearly discernible. The white lights of the darkroom should not be put on until the clearing action has taken place.

The fixer should be changed when it takes an excessively long time (over 3 minutes) to clear the unexposed area, or when it no longer hardens the emulsion.

The developer and fixing solutions normally appear clear. If the solutions appear cloudy one should suspect that something has gone wrong—exhausted or contaminated solutions.

HARDENING AGENT

Because x-ray films may be scratched or distorted quite easily when the gelatin is swollen, a hardening agent is required. Potassium alum or potassium aluminum sulfate $KAl(SO_4)_2$ is the chemical agent of choice. It hardens and toughens the softened gelatin so it may withstand the abuse of normal handling.

The hardening process requires an acid pH in a range between 4 to 6.

ACIDIFIER

In order for the hardening process of potassium alum to act on the swollen gelatin, acetic acid (CH_3COOH) is added to the fixer solution to provide the required acid pH. The acetic acid also does the following:

1. Stops development by neutralizing the developing agent.
2. Prevents contamination of the fixer by neutralizing the alkaline developing solution which is carried over into the fixer solution.

PRESERVATIVE

Sodium thiosulfate of the fixer separates into an insoluble sulfur in an acid medium. Sodium sulfite (Na_2SO_3) is added to the fixer to prevent this decomposition of the sodium thiosulfate.

The total fixing time includes the duration of time needed to clear the film and the time required to harden the film. A safe rule to follow is to allow films to remain in the fixer three times the length of time needed for them to clear. The film may be viewed in white light after the film has cleared, but additional fixing is needed to perserve the image and harden the emulsion properly. It is recommended, therefore, that if films are viewed wet, they should be returned to the fixer and allowed to remain for the recommended time. Although radiographs may be safely left in the fixer over the specified time, it is not wise to let them stay for long periods of time. It will take longer to wash them free of residual silver.

Final Wash

The purpose of the final wash is to remove residual processing chemicals (especially thiosulfate) and silver salts from the film.

Because hardners are used in x-ray fixing solutions it becomes difficult to remove small quantities of the fixer retained by the gelatin. If these chemicals are not removed, the image will discolor or fade and the entire film may deteriorate. Normally, x-ray films should be washed in running water so circulated that the entire emulsion area, as well as every portion of the wash tank, will receive frequent change. Proper washing time for x-ray films depends principally upon the frequency with which the water is changed. The rate of flow of the water should be adjusted so that the water in the tank changes completely at least 10 times each hour. To determine the rate at which the water changes in the wash tank measure the time it takes to fill the tank once. If this is 6 minutes, the tank volume will be replaced ten times in an hour. Under these conditions, films should be washed at least 20 minutes, the time being computed from the moment the last of the group of films is placed in the wash tank. A temperature of approximately 70°F is recommended. If the temperature difference between fixer and wash water exceeds 15°F, there is a possibility of unequal swelling of the emulsion, commonly referred to as reticulation (orange peel appearance). Also, prolonged washing tends to make the emulsion soft, especially if left in the wash overnight.

Drying

In most offices, films are dried by merely hanging a rack in the darkroom above a drip tray designed to catch the run-off excess water. Other offices use an ordinary fan to dry the film. However, the fan should not blow directly on the films.

Cabinet dryers are available which are equipped with a fan and heating elements. Usually this type of dryer should be vented to the outside to prevent moisture condensation in the darkroom. Moderately warm air is preferred to hot air.

It should be remembered that wet films are subject to damage from scratching and abrasion if not handled properly. If there is dust in the air, dirt will become easily embedded within the emulsion. Do not remove wet radiographs from their hangers until they are completely dry.

Films can be rapidly dried by two methods:

1. *Wetting agents* will decrease the drying time and prevent drying marks. It works by reducing the surface tension of water on the film so the water will drain more rapidly from the film after washing. There are a number of wetting agents on the market such as Kodak's Photo-Flo® and General Electric's Super-mix Wetner®. The wetting agents are actually detergents. A small amount of the wetting agent is placed in the final rinse water. After 30 seconds in the final rinse, the radiograph is placed in the dryer. This will decrease the normal drying time of the film.

2. *Alcohol:* This method is used when a dry film is needed in an emergency situation. Use a 70% concentration by volume of any good grade denatured alcohol. Thoroughly drain the films after the final wash and emerse the films in a tray of alcohol with the temperature under 70°F for 2 minutes. Rock the tray to make sure the films do not stick to the bottom of the tray and so both sides of the films are thoroughly bathed. Remove and place films in a second tray of alcohol. This will remove the last remnants of the

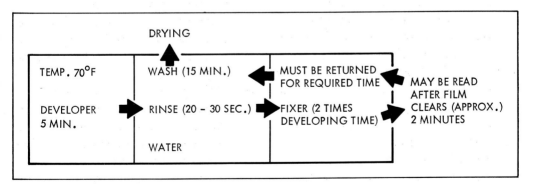

Figure 8-17. Basic steps in processing x-ray film manually.

water. After draining the films, hang the films up for drying. The alcohol will evaporate quickly leaving a dry film.

Summary of Tank Processing

The steps employed in tank processing x-ray films are summarized in the following paragraphs (See Figure 8-17).

1. *Stir solutions:* Stir developer and fixer solutions to equalize their temperature. (Use separate paddle for each to avoid possible contamination.) There is a tendency for the temperature at the bottom of the tank to be less than the upper areas.

2. *Check the solution level* of the developer—if it is low, the correct level should be maintained by adding fresh developer or replenisher. Keep a bottle of fresh developer solution on hand for this purpose. Don't add water to developer to maintain proper level. This practice will dilute the developer and slow down the developing action on the films.

3. *Check temperature* of the solutions and adjust, if possible, to 70°F before development. Never place ice in the solutions to cool them down —this will dilute the solution. One way to cool the solutions in warm weather would be to place ice cubes in a rubber glove and then place in solutions. Be sure to stir the solutions, though, in order to equalize the temperatures in the solutions after cooling.

4. Exclude all white light in processing room and turn on safelights. (Use only safelights with Wratten

6B filters for screen film. This includes the panoramic films.)

5. Remove exposed film from its packet and clip into processing hangers (See Figure 8-18).

6. Set the interval timer so it will ring at end of desired time of development. Consult the manufacturer's table. It is based on the temperature of the developer. When employing regular x-ray developer, the time of development is 5 minutes at 70°F. If rapid x-ray developer is used, the development time is 3 minutes at 70°F.

7. Immerse the film smoothly into the developer solution and start the timer. Agitate film hanger by raising and lowering it several times to break up residual air bubbles and permit the solution to bathe both surfaces of the film. Agitating the film will also drive away the accumulated bromide ions that form near the surface of the film and prevent the developing agents from getting to the film emulsion. Don't crowd film in the developing tank—films may rub together and become stuck. Allow at least 1 inch of space between films.

8. Remove hanger from developer when bell rings indicating the termination of the development period. Don't remove films from the developer tank too rapidly because excess solution is carried away from the tank. Allow 5 seconds for the excess solution to drain back into the developing tank.

9. Immerse the film in the circulating rinse water and agitate. This will

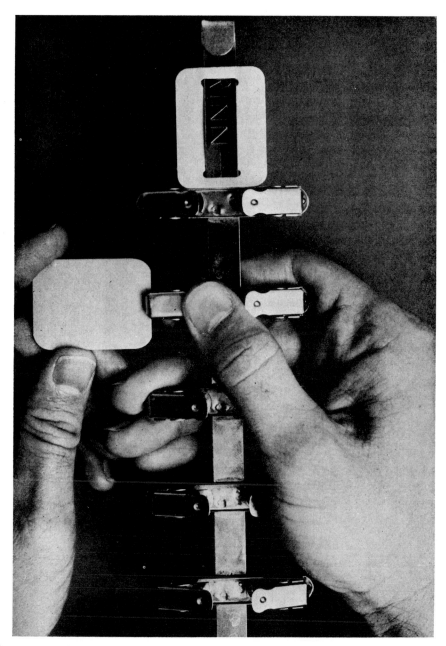

Figure 8-18. After the name of the patient has been placed on the hanger tab, the film is removed from the film packet and placed in the clip of the film hanger. Avoid finger marks, scratches and film bending.

take approximately 15 to 20 seconds.

10. After rinsing, place the film in the fixer solution and agitate until fixer has thoroughly bathed both film surfaces. *Do not expose to white light until the film has cleared.* A film has cleared when its milky look has disappeared. It takes approximately 1 to 2 minutes to clear a film in the fixer. It is possible to view the radiograph in white light at this point, but additional fixing is needed to preserve the image and

to harden the emulsion properly. If the films are viewed wet, they must be returned to the fixer and allowed to remain for the recommended time. The films *must* be fixed for approximately 2 times the development time.

11. Upon completeion of fixation, remove film to the washing compartment. Let it remain until it is completely washed in circulating water. Allow adequate time for thorough washing (15-20 minutes).

12. Remove film from final wash—al-

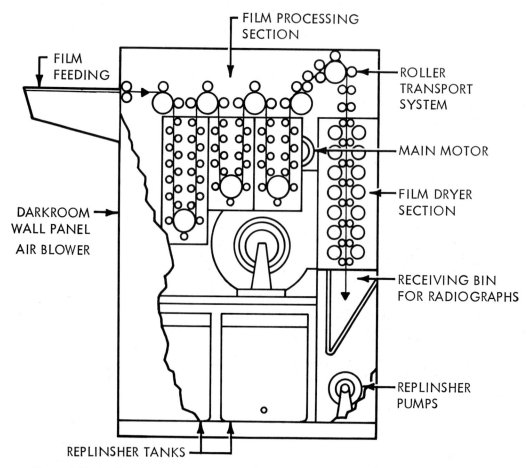

Figure 8-19. Section through a Kodak "X-O-Mat" automatic processor model. (Courtesy of Eastman Kodak Co.)

low films to drain for two or three seconds after being lifted from the wash water.

13. Hang up films to dry, or place in a dryer that supplies circulating, clean dry air.

14. Remove the dry radiographs from the hanger by opening the clips which release their grip on the film. Do not pull film from clips since clips may be broken or portions of film remain to clog them later when another film is to be processed.

15. Place films into special film mounts.

Automatic Processing

Automatic processing is gradually replacing manual processing. In automatic processing, the film is fed into one end and it comes out the discharge end completely processed and dried in 1½ to 7 minutes (depending on the type of processing unit you have).

The advantages of automatic processing are listed below:

1. Rapidity of operation (1½ to 7 minutes dry to dry operation)
2. Uniformity of results (standardized quality)
3. Less floor space required
4. No wet films to be handled; no spilling of solutions during processing

In most automatic processors, a series of rollers carries the film through the four basic stages of developing, fixing, washing and drying (See Figure 8-19).

Processing solutions used in automatic processors differ from those used in manual processing. The developer has a special formula adapted to use with high-speed rollers. It functions at high temperatures (80 degree range) which short-

ens the developing time considerably. In the rapid automatic processors (90 seconds dry to dry), the system is based on chemicals operating at 103°-106°F range and upon special rapid processing x-ray film. It also contains a hardener (glutaraldehyde) which starts the hardening process at the time of the developing procedure. This is done in order to prevent the films from sticking to the rollers. This would cause the films to jam and stop the transport of the films through the processor.

The film is transported directly from the developing solution into the fixing solution. It is here that the films are rapidly cleared and hardened.

From the fixer, the films go into the water wash section and subsequently into the drying section. The films are dried quickly by jets of heated dry air similar to procedures used in an automatic car wash. The entire procedure takes approximately five minutes in the dental automatic processor. Two of the better dental automatic processors on the market today are Pennwalt's Auveloper® (See Figure 8-20) and Profexray's P-6 Automatic Processor® (See Figure 8-21).

X-Ray Checker

The analysis of film quality can be done rather simply by use of a "x-ray checker" as devised by Wainwright and Villanyi in 1960 (See Figure 8-22). The three parts of the "x-ray checker" are as follows:

Lead (total absorber) ($\frac{1}{32}$" thick, $\frac{9}{16}$" × 1¼" in size) clear area used to analyze fog.

2. *Aluminum* (specific absorber) (4mm thick, $\frac{9}{16}$" × 1¼" in size) gray area used to analyze density changes.

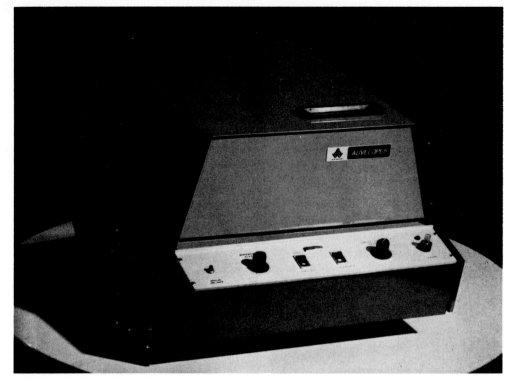

Figure 8-20. The Pennwalt (SSW) Auveloper Dental Automatic Processor. (Courtesy of Pennwalt Corp.)

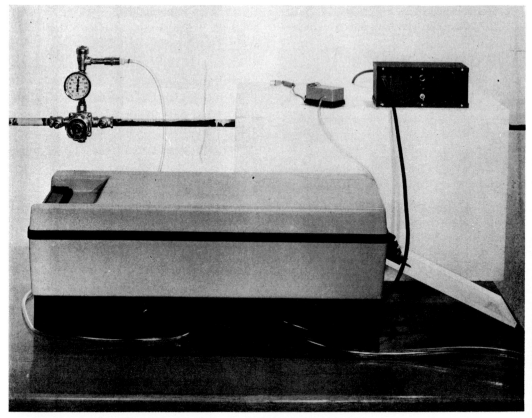

Figure 8-21. The Profexray (Litton) Dental Automatic Processor. (Courtesy of Profexray Div., Litton Medical Products, Inc.)

3. *Acetate* (air absorber) ($\frac{1}{32}$″ thick, $1\frac{1}{4}$″ × $1\frac{3}{4}$″ in size) black area to analyze developing technic.

In order to obtain a standard radiograph using the Wainwright X-ray Checker, place the "x-ray checker" over a #2 regular film and bring the tip of your x-ray cone 1″ from the film. Expose the film for the same amount of time you normally use for the lower molar region. Process the film with your regular processing technique. If you cannot get a good standard film with your technic, take your "X-ray Checker" to another dental office known for producing good films and have them expose and process a film for you. This will give you a standard film to compare with radiographs taken by you from time to time. Proper use of the "X-ray Checker" will aid you in "trouble-shooting" for problems associated with your exposure and processing technics (See Figure 8-22).

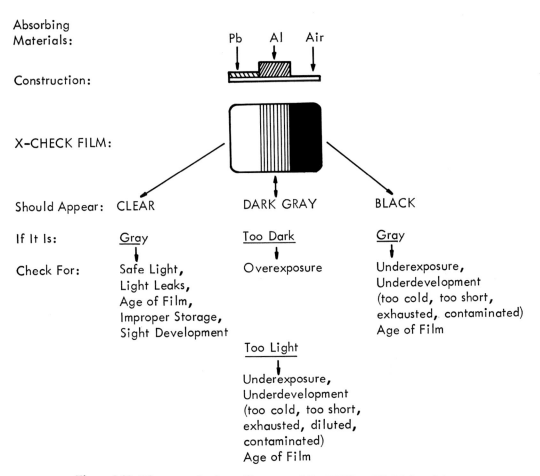

Figure 8-22. The x-ray checker. (Courtesy of Dr. William W. Wainwright.)

Cleanliness of Darkroom and Equipment

Cleanliness is very important in the darkroom. It is a necessity in the production of high-quality radiographs. Spots, streaks, fog and other artifacts usually can be traced to poor darkroom conditions. Often a dirty tank contaminates the processing solutions and decreases film contrast.

It is a recommended practice to sponge off routinely the outside and inside of solution tanks insert covers. Always replace tank covers when tanks are not in use to minimize oxidation and contamination.

Wiping dirty, stained areas in the darkroom with a damp cloth will in most cases be sufficient to prevent contamination of films and solutions from dust. If liquid solutions spilled on the work bench are not wiped dry, the solutions will evaporate leaving a chemical residue on the working bench which will contaminate and stain radiographs.

Whenever chemicals are changed, it is good darkroom procedure to clean the processing tanks by using a stiff brush with soap and water. Then rinse well and wipe dry with a cloth. However, deposits often form on the walls of the developer tanks because of the action between the mineral salts dissolved in the water and the carbonate in the developing solutions. These deposits may be removed by using a dilute solution of muriatic acid (28-38% Hydrochloric acid, commercial grade) as follows:

Run a little cold water into the tank. Add 1½ oz of muriatic acid for each gallon of tank capacity. Fill the tank with warm water, cover it, and let the acid solution stand for at least one half hour. Drain the tank and rinse the walls well with fresh water. Wipe the tank out with a clean cloth, after which a new developer may be mixed. If necessary, the procedure should be repeated with a less dilute solution.

Film hangers should be washed thoroughly after use, so that the solutions through which they have passed will be completely rinsed off and not allowed to dry and crystallize. Particular attention should be paid to the clips. If they are not thoroughly cleaned, they may cause streaks on the film.

Stain Removal

Both the developer and the fixer solutions will stain clothing. Stains due to the developer are yellow or brown. Stains due to the fixer are yellow, brown, or black due to the formation of silver sulfide from decomposition of the hypo.

When developer and fixer solutions have been splashed on clothing, the garment should be rinsed as soon as possible in cold water. The stain can be prevented entirely if the chemicals are removed thoroughly before they have a chance to decompose. Even if the stains have formed the garment should be rinsed thoroughly before laundering to prevent possible intensification of the spots. Usually the developer stains can be removed by the usual laundering process or by soaking the material in a weak 5% solution of sodium hypochlorite bleach (commercial laundry bleach). Any bleach should be applied with caution to colored fabrics because some dyes can be affected by the bleaching process.

If the spilled chemicals (whether developer or fixer) have dried out or have gone unnoticed for any length of time, however, the stained fabric can be treated with a solution made up as follows:

Sodium hypochlorite
bleach (5% solution)   ½ oz (15 cc)
Acetic Acid, 5%
(vinegar)   ½ oz (15 cc)
Water about 100°F   1 gal (3.8 liters)

Soak the stained portion of the uniform in this solution for about 5 to 10 minutes. Then soak the stained portion in *fresh* fixer. Rinse in plain water and dry. Small stains can be removed by touching the stain with iodine, then by fresh hypo, followed by a plain water rinse. Do not use the above techniques with colored fabrics. Use of iodine-hypo cleaner is not recommended with nylon because the resulting iodine stains are difficult to remove. However, the sodium hypochlorite-acetic acid treatment is satisfactory with nylon.

There is a commercially- available fixer stain remover called "Fix-Off®." The Fix-Off stain remover is used by saturating the stain thoroughly and then laundering the garment as usual. The application is repeated for heavy fabrics or aged stains.

Chemical Dermatitis from Processing Solutions

Persons with extremely sensitive skins occasionally may experience a severe skin reaction from processing solutions. The skin becomes sore and cracked. Usually it is from the alkaline in the developing solution. It is a good suggestion to wash your hands thoroughly after processing or wear rubber gloves. However, if you wear rubber gloves when loading films on hangers, it may result in artifacts on the film.

Mounting Dental Radiographs

The following are reasons why dental radiographs should be mounted:

1. There is less chance for an error in interpretation because each film is mounted in normal anatomic relation to each other.

2. It prevents finger marks, scratches and abrasions because radiographs are not handled as much.

3. Repeated study and comparison of single radiographs with each other is time-consuming. It results in inefficiency and confusion.

4. Mounts exclude illumination around the individual radiographs. This is an aid in interpretation as it prevents glare.

5. Radiographs in mounts are easy to file. Therefore, they are instantly available for study during an operative procedure and consultation.

6. It has a psychological effect on patients. The impression that mounted radiographs have upon the patient is in itself sufficient reason for mounting them. It cannot be expected that a handful of small radiographs which are shuffled in and out of an envelope will be valued very highly.

Identification of Films

Right or Left Side of Mouth

When the slower single-coated films were used, the emulsion side (dull by reflected light) of the film is always facing the teeth and tissues, and the non-emulsion (shiny) side is away from the teeth. Thus, when the viewer looked at the film with the shiny side toward him, he was viewing from the lingual aspect, as though he were inside of the mouth looking out. Conversely, if he held the dull side toward himself, he was viewing the radiographs from outside the oral cavity.

The faster double-coated films have two emulsions, hence two dull sides. The single-coated films are not available today. For identification purposes the double-coated films have a raised, embossed dot. The raised, or convex side of the dot is always placed toward the cone of radiation and, therefore, is the side of the film toward the teeth. The concave side of the dot denotes the side of the packet which is away from the teeth, corresponding to the shiny side of the older single-coated film.

Extraoral films are double-coated and do not have the embossed dot for identification purposes. Therefore, they must be marked at the time of exposure by placing a lead letter *R* or *L* on the tube side of the film holder.

Tooth Area

A particular tooth area on the radiograph is readily recognized by identifying the teeth—therefore, it is important for you to know normal radiographic anatomy (See Figures 8-23, 8-24, 8-25, 8-26, and 8-27).

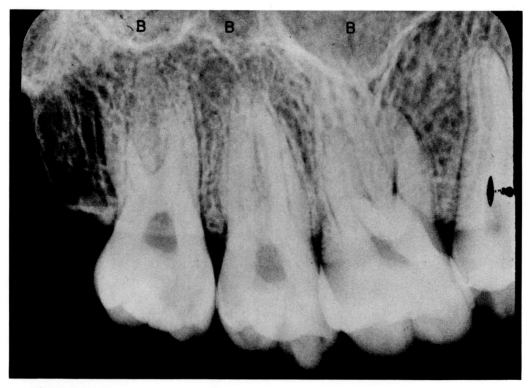

Figure 8-23. Radiograph of maxillary molar region. (A) Maxillary tuberosity. (B) Maxillary sinus.

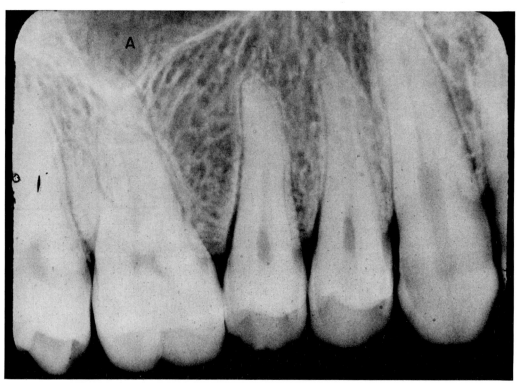

Figure 8-24. Radiograph of maxillary premolar region. (A) Maxillary sinus.

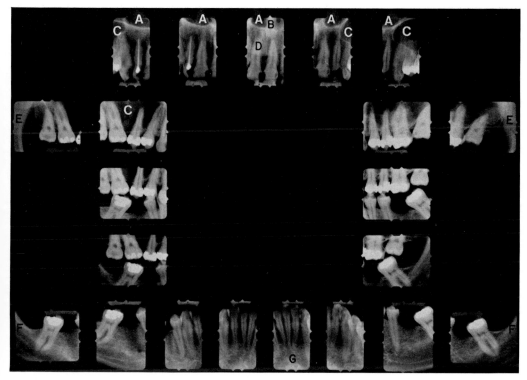

Figure 8-25. *Complete Mouth Survey.* (A) Nasal fossa. (B) Anterior nasal septum. (C) Maxillary sinus. (D) Cartilage of the nose. (E) Coronoid process. (F) Anterior border of ramus. (G) Genial tubercles.

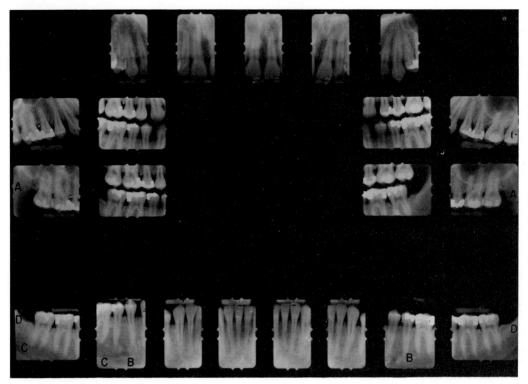

Figure 8-26. *Complete Mouth Survey*. (A) Coronoid process. (B) Mental foramen. (C) Mandibular canal. (D) Anterior border of ramus.

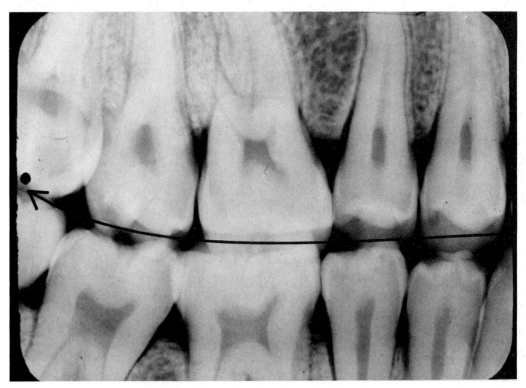

Figure 8-27. Posterior bitewing illustrating that "Curve of Spee" curves upwards from an anterior to posterior direction.

Anatomic Landmarks

Maxillary Molar Area:
   a. posterior wall of the maxillary tuberosity
   b. hamular process
   c. coronoid process of mandible
   d. maxillary sinus
   e. malar process

Maxillary Premolar Area
   a. maxillary sinus

Maxillary Incisor Area
   a. incisive foramen
   b. cartilage of nose
   c. nasal septum
   d. nasal fossae

Mandibular Molar Area
   a. external oblique line
   b. mylohyoid ridge
   c. mandibular canal

Mandibular Premolar Area
   a. mylohyoid ridge
   b. mental foramen

Mandibular Incisor Area
   a. mental ridge
   b. lingual foramen
   c. genial tubercles

Aspect for Viewing

The radiographs can be mounted for viewing two ways:

1. The radiographs may be mounted with all of the shiny surfaces (single-coated films) or the depressed or concave sides of the embossed dots (double-coated films) toward the viewer. The viewer, then, is observing the radiographs from the lingual aspect, with the tube side of the film toward the back of the mount. This is as though you are inside the patient's mouth looking out. The reasons given for mounting the films this way are two-fold: (1) objects nearing the film during exposure record sharper images than those farther from it; thus, the true relation of the objects is best seen by viewing from the lingual aspects since the lingual aspect of the teeth are closer to the film; (2) it is easier to visualize the effect of angulation by viewing from an opposite direction to that which the x-rays travel.

2. The radiographs are mounted with all of the dull surfaces (single-coated films) or the raised or convex sides of the embossed dots (double-coated films) toward the viewer. The viewer, then, is observing the radiographs from the facial aspect with the tube side toward the viewer. This is as though the viewer is looking directly at the patient. The films are mounted in this way at Louisiana State University because it is easier to view the radiographs in the same direction that the rays were projected. Another advantage is that the films are mounted in the same relationship as the teeth are recorded on the examination chart. This makes for less chance for error. However, it depends upon previous training and preference as to which method of mounting radiographs is used. If you do not like the way the films are mounted, just turn the mount over.

REFERENCES

A Look at X-ray Film Processing. Milwaukee, General Electric Company, X-ray Department.

Beck, James O.: *Syllabus of Oral Radiology.* University of Minnesota School of Dentistry, 1970.

Bloom, William L.; Hollenbach, John L., and Morgan, James A.: *Medical Radiographic*

Technic, 3rd ed. Springfield, Ill., Charles C Thomas, 1969.

Cahoon, J. B.: *Formulating X-ray Technics.* Durham, N. C., Duke University Press, 1953.

Carr, J. D., and Norman, R. D.: Effective use of the darkroom. *Dent Clin North Am,* July, 1961, pp. 363-370.

Darkroom Technique for Better Radiographs. Wilmington, Delaware, Photo Products Department, E. I. du Pont de Nemours and Co.

Du Pont's Darkroom Technique. Wilmington, Delaware, Photo Products Department, E. I. du Pont de Nemours and Co.

Ennis, LeRoy; Berry, Harrison; and Phillips, James E.: *Dental Roentgenology,* 6th ed. Philadelphia, Lea and Febiger, 1967, pp. 307-320.

Fuchs, Arthur W.: *Principles of Radiographic Exposure and Processing,* 2nd ed. Springfield, Ill., Charles C Thomas, 1967, pp. 224-258.

Herz, R. M.: *The Photographic Action of Ionizing Radiations.* New York, Wiley-Interscience, 1969, pp. 396-399.

Jacobi, Charles A.: *X-ray Technology,* 2nd ed. St. Louis, C. V. Mosby, 1960, p. 65.

McCall, John, and Wald, Samuel: *Clinical Dental Roentgenology,* 4th ed. Philadelphia, W. B. Saunders, 1957, pp. 113-128.

Peterson, Shailer: *Clinical Dental Hygiene.* St. Louis, C. V. Mosby, 1959, pp. 240-252.

Radiology Specialist. Washington, D. C., U. S. Government Printing Office, Department of the Air Force, pp. 8-15.

Simpson, Clarence O.: The advantages of mounting dental radiographs. *Dent Radiogr Photogr,* No. 1, 1937.

Stafne, Edward: *Oral Roentgenographic Diagnosis,* 3rd ed. Philadelphia, W. B. Saunders, 1969, pp. 380-386.

Sweet, A. Porter: Processing technic. *Oral Surg,* May, 1950.

Sweet, A. Porter: Safelights reconsidered. *Dental Radiogr Photogr,* No. 2, 1962.

Sweet, A. Porter: X-ray processing solutions. *Dent Radiogr Photogr,* No. 2, 1955, p. 27.

The Fundamentals of Radiography, 10th ed. Rochester, N. Y., Medical Division, Eastman Kodak Co., 1960.

Wainwright, William W., and Villanyi, Andrew A.: The simplest radiographic analyzer: The x-ray checker. *J So Calif Dent Assoc,* 28:122-125, No. 4, April, 1960.

X-rays in Dentistry. Rochester, N. Y., X-ray Division, Eastman Kodak Co., 1962, pp. 66-80.

CHAPTER 9

COMMON CAUSES AND CORRECTIONS OF UNSATISFACTORY RADIOGRAPHS

FILMS LACKING in diagnostic quality should be avoided for the following reasons.

1. Retakes expose the patient to unnecessary radiation.

2. Retakes waste the time of the dentist and his auxiliaries.

3. Retakes waste film which cost money.

4. Faulty radiographs interfere with accurate interpretation.

The three major causes of faulty radiographs are errors in exposure, projection, and processing technics.

The following is a list of common errors and their corrections. Hopefully, this list will help those who take radiographs eliminate the causes of the errors.

I. PROJECTION ERRORS

Error	Cause	Correction
1. *Apical ends of teeth "cut off"* (See Figure 9-1).	Film is placed too close to teeth in maxillary arch in paralleling technic.	Move film away from the teeth.
	Too flat a vertical angulation which causes elongation.	Increase vertical angulation (especially shallow vaults).
2. *Overlapping of teeth* (See Figure 9-2).	Plane of film not parallel with lingual surface of teeth or incorrect horizontal angulation of cone.	Place film horizontally parallel to lingual surface of teeth and direct central ray of the x-ray beam perpendicular to the facial surfaces of the teeth.
3. *All of specific region not showing* (See Figure 9-3).	Faulty film placement.	Center the film over teeth to be radiographed.
4. *Crowns of teeth not showing* (See Figure 9-4).	Not enough film showing below or above the crowns of the teeth.	Increase amount of film showing below and above the crown of the teeth (approximately ⅛" showing).
	Vertical angulation too steep.	Decrease vertical angulation.
5. *Partial image "cone cut"* (See Figures 9-5 and 9-6).	Cone of radiation not covering area of interest.	Make sure vertical and horizontal position of cone covers film.
6. *Shape Distortion* a. Foreshortening (See Figure 9-7 A & B).	*Bisecting Technic:* Vertical angulation of cone too acute.	Reduce vertical angulation.
	Paralleling Technic: Film not paralleling with long axes of teeth.	Place film parallel to long axes of teeth—it is difficult in shallow palatal vault case.
	Paralleling Technic: Long cone is not positioned correctly.	Position long cone so CR strikes film at right angle.

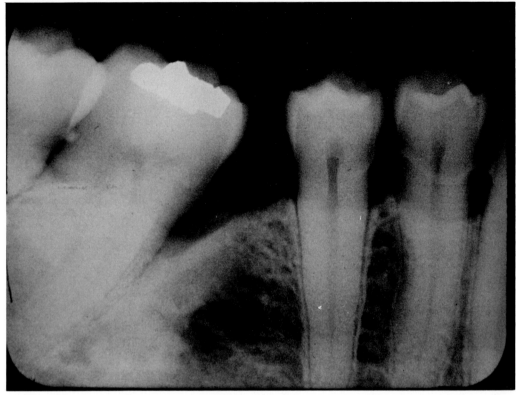

Figure 9-1. Radiograph of apices of roots of mandibular premolars "cut off."

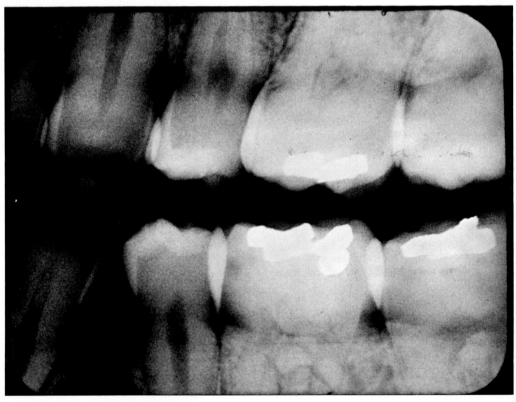

Figure 9-2. Radiograph with overlapping of contact points.

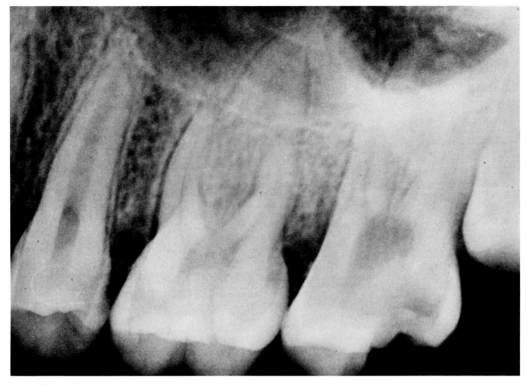

Figure 9-3. Common projection error of not depicting all of specific region on the film. In this radiograph of the maxillary molar region the third molar has been "cut off."

Error	*Cause*	*Correction*
b. Elongation (See Figure 9-8 A & B).	*Bisecting Technic:* Vertical angulation of cone is too flat.	Increase vertical angulation of cone.
	Paralleling Technic: Film not positioned parallel to long axes of teeth.	Place film parallel with long axes of teeth.
	Paralleling Technic: Long cone not positioned correctly.	Position long cone so CR strikes film at right angle.
c. Image Distorted (See Figure 9-9).	Film is bent as patient bites on film holder, bite block or as patient holds film in mouth.	Use a film backing.
7. *Herring-bone effect* (See Figure 9-10).	Printed back side of film placed toward cone of radiation.	Place pebbled or front side of film toward cone of radiation.
8. *Black dot in apical area* (See Figure 9-11).	Manufacturers identifying mark on film placed toward apical area of teeth.	Place black dot on film toward the occlusal or incisal surfaces of teeth.
9. *Artifacts on Radiograph*		
a. Writing lines on radiograph (See Figure 9-12).	Writing on film packet with ball point pen or lead pencil.	Use a crayon-type pencil to mark on film packet.
b. Black marks on radiograph (See Figure 9-13).	Moisture contamination (failure to blot film packet).	Blot film packet immediately after removal from patient's mouth.
c. Black lines on radiograph (See Figure 9-14).	Routine bending of film to reduce patient discomfort.	Avoid unnecessary film bending.

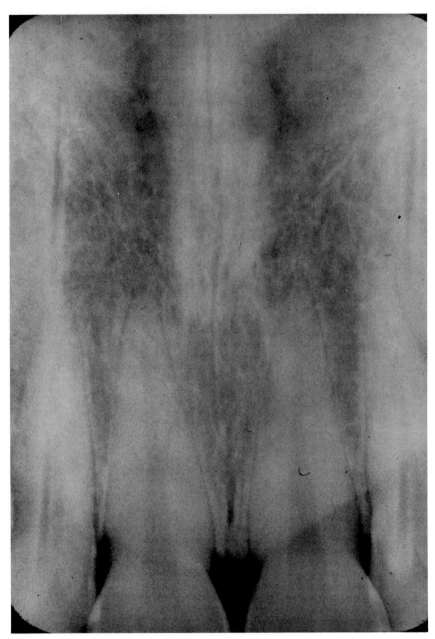

Figure 9-4. Radiograph showing only a "partial image" of the crown of the maxillary incisors.

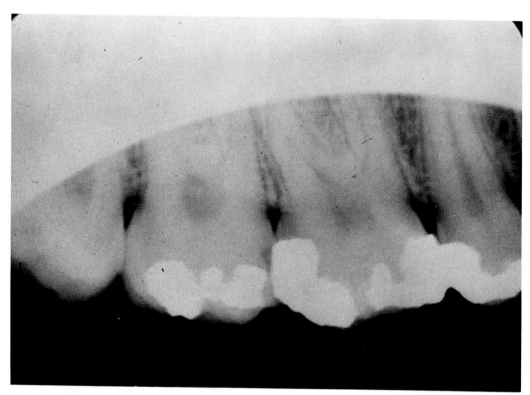

Figure 9-5. Radiograph with vertical "cone cut" of apices of maxillary molars.

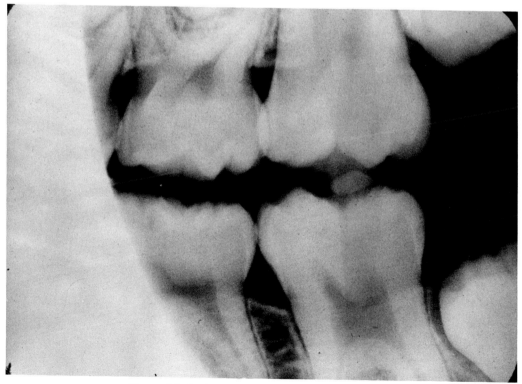

Figure 9 6. Radiograph with horizontal "cone cut."

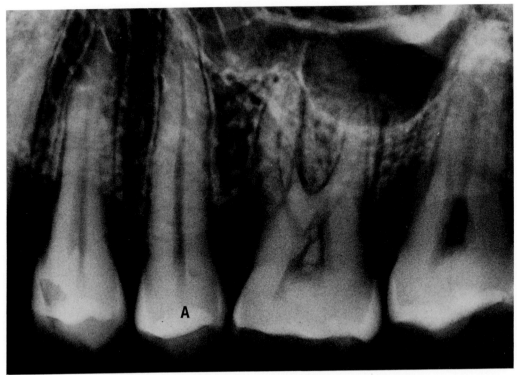

Figure 9-7A. Accurate projection of maxillary premolar region.

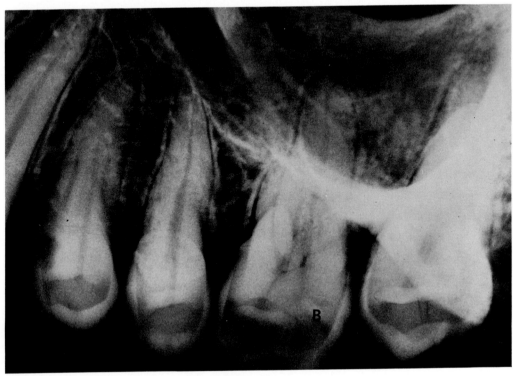

Figure 9-7B. Foreshortening of radiographic images of same maxillary premolar region as shown in 9-7A.

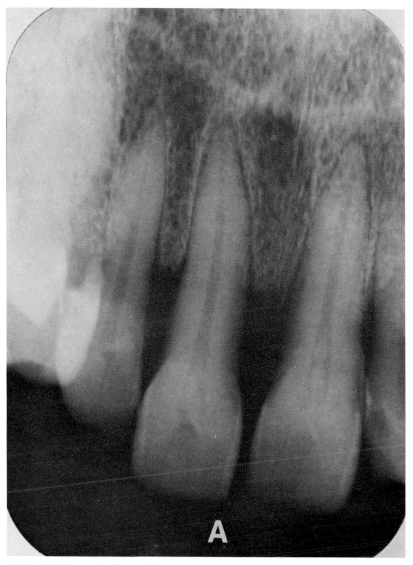

Figure 9-8A. Radiograph illustrating elongation of radiographic image. Elongated maxillary centrals.

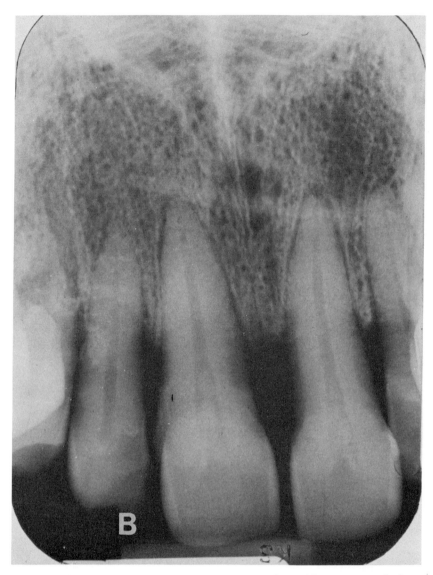

Figure 9-8B. Same teeth as seen in figure 9-8A taken with accurate technic.

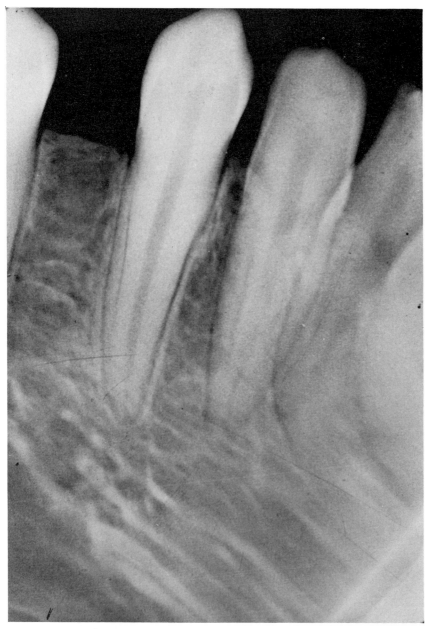

Figure 9-9. Radiographic distortion from film bending.

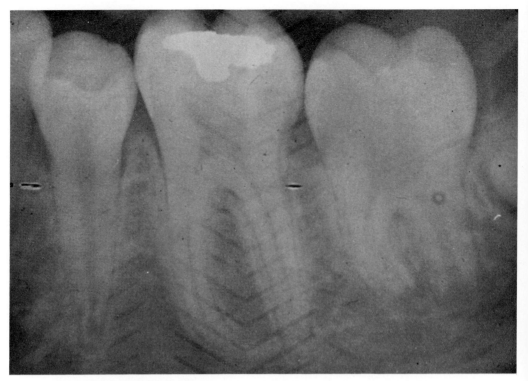

Figure 9-10. Herring-bone effect: Film placed backwards in mouth.

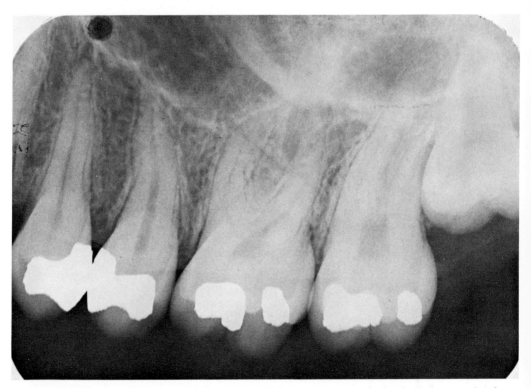

Figure 9-11. Manufacturers raised dot should be placed toward the incisal or occlusal surface of the teeth during exposure of a periapical film. The dot is shown here superimposed over the apical end of the maxillary 1st premolar periapical region.

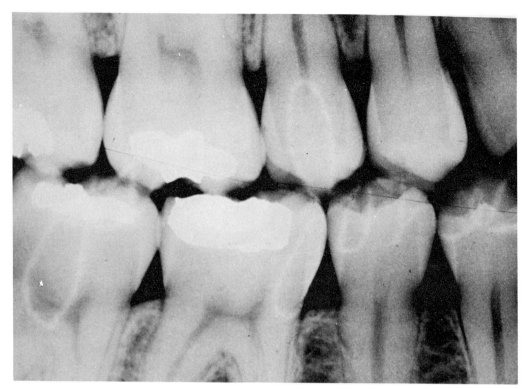

Figure 9-12. Do not write on the film packet with a pencil or ball-point pen as the writing will show through on the developed radiograph.

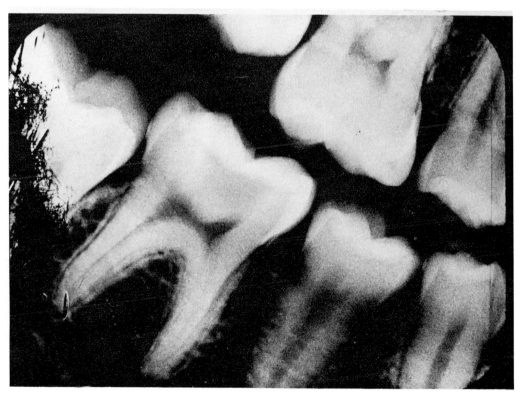

Figure 9-13. Moisture contamination from failure to blot the film after removal of film from patient's mouth. The black protective paper surrounding the film becomes attached to film emulsion.

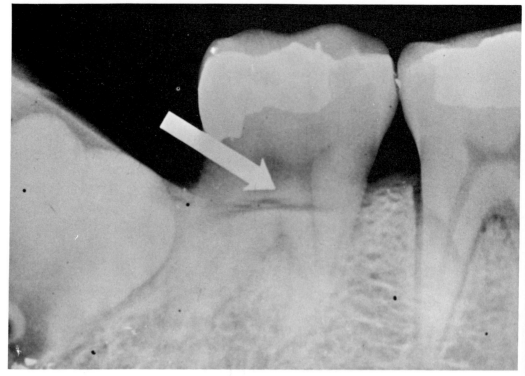

Figure 9-14. Bending the film excessively will cause a break in the emulsion with resultant black lines on the radiograph.

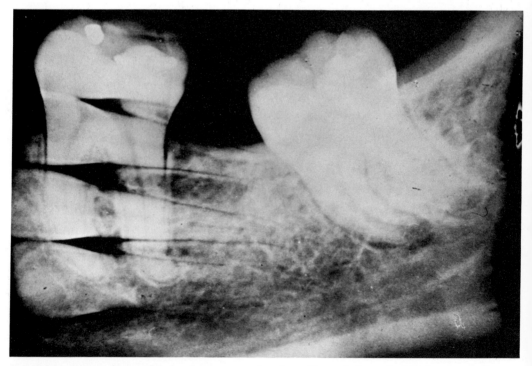

Figure 9-15. A film which has been exposed twice will result in a double image on the radiograph. (Courtesy of Eastman Kodak Co.)

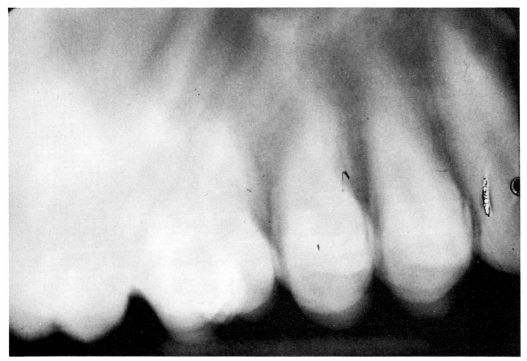

Figure 9-16. If there is movement of the film, patient or tubehead, it will result in a radiograph with a blurred image.

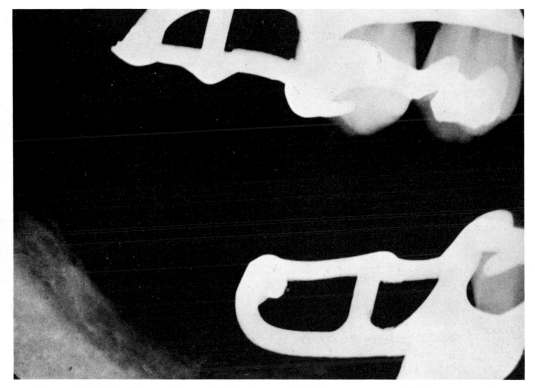

Figure 9-17. Metallic appliances left in the mouth during exposure will be seen on the processed film as shown in this bitewing radiograph.

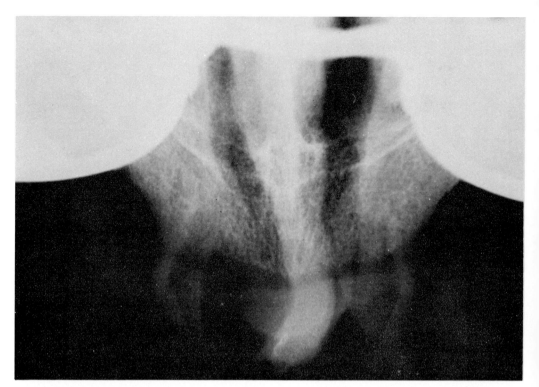

Figure 9-18. Remove the patient's glasses before exposure or they may reveal themselves in the resultant radiograph as shown in the occlusal radiograph of an edentulous maxillary arch.

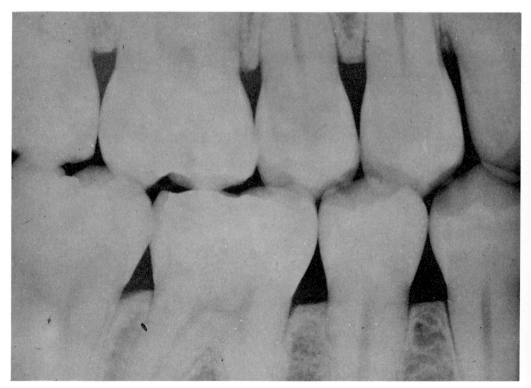

Figure 9-19. Low density or light radiographs can be caused by several factors. Usually the cause is from "too short of an exposure time."

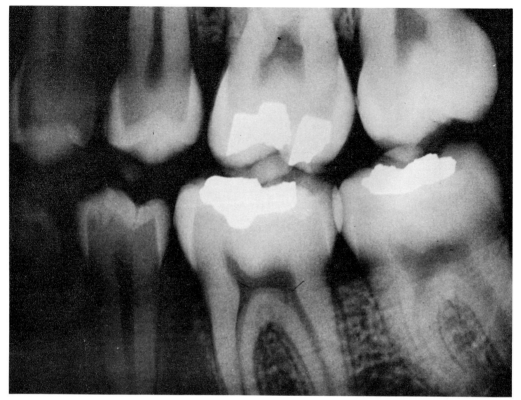

Figure 9-20. High density or dark radiographs are caused by a number of factors. Usually it is from the use of excessive exposure times.

Error	Cause	Correction
10. *Double images on radiograph* (See Figure 9-15).	Film exposed twice to radiation.	Place exposed film in receptacle.
11. *Blurred image on radiograph* (See Figure 9-16).	Movement of film, patient or tube during exposure.	Instruct patient properly; immobilize patient and tube. Re-do radiograph if you notice patient moving during exposure.
12. *Radiopaque artifacts on radiograph* (See Figures 9-17 and 9-18).	Leaving dental appliance in mouth and/or glasses on person.	Instruct patient to move dental appliances and glasses before exposure.

II. EXPOSURE AND PROCESSING ERRORS

Low Density Films (See Figure 9-19.)	*Underexposure* a. Too short exposure.	Set exposure time correctly, and/or check calibration of exposure time.
	b. Source-film distance too great.	Check source-film distance.
	c. Too low kVp.	Increase kVp by approximately 5 kVp.
	d. Too low mA.	Increase mA or exposure time (mAS is one factor).
	e. Film packet placed backward in mouth.	See herring-bone effect error (See 9-10).

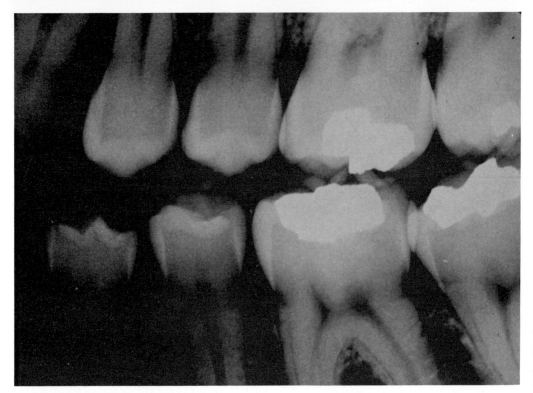

Figure 9-21. Radiograph with high contrast. Exposure technics utilizing low kVp usually produce high contrast films.

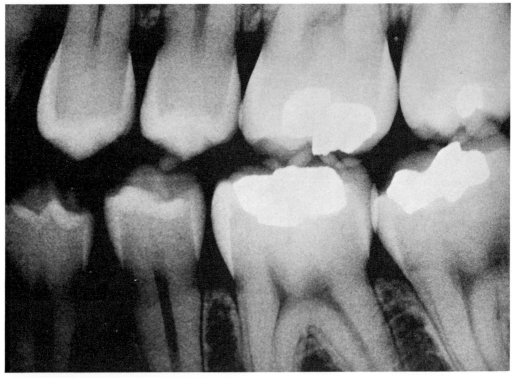

Figure 9-22. Radiograph with low contrast. High kVp technics produce films with low contrast; however, these radiographs have "long scale contrast," which is preferred by many dentists.

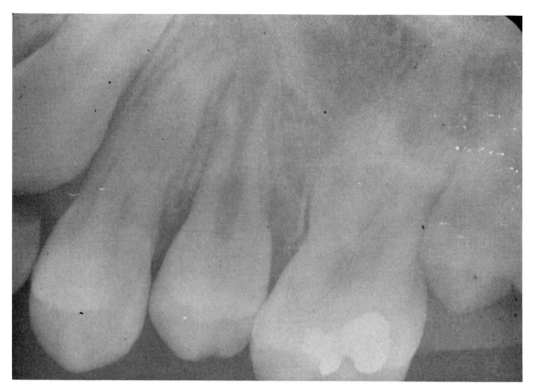

Figure 9-23. Fogging of film can be a result of several factors. The most important cause is from light leaks and unsafe "safelight" in the darkroom.

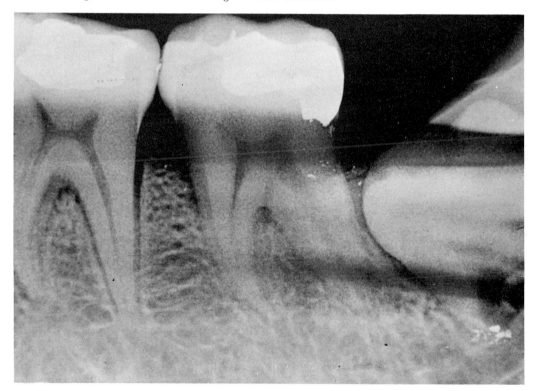

Figure 9-24. Black streaks on the film from unclean film hanger clips. The fixer chemicals adhere to the clips and dissolve in the developer the next time the hanger is used to cause the black streaks on the processed films.

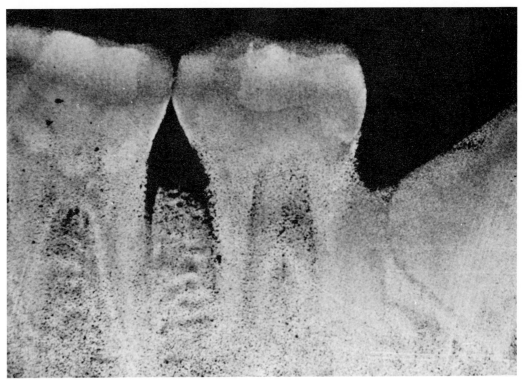

Figure 9-25. Reticulation (orange peel effect) which is caused by sudden extreme temperature changes in processing. (Radiograph courtesy of Dr. William Updegrave.)

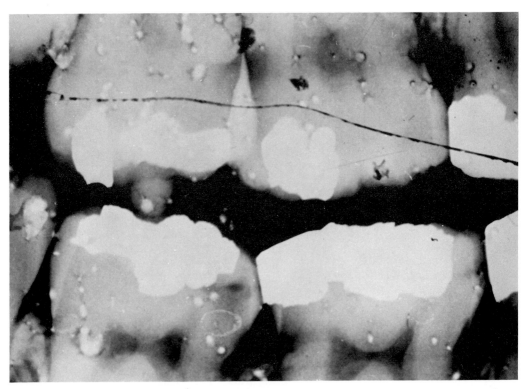

Figure 9-26. Air bubbles trapped on the film surface will prevent film development and result in white spots on the film called air bells.

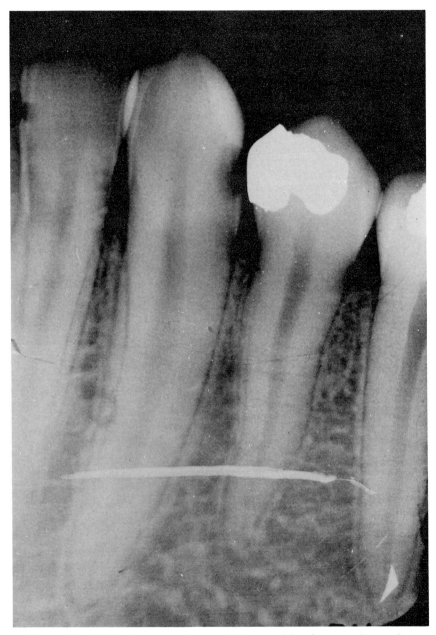

Figure 9-27. White lines caused by scratching emulsion in processing tanks.

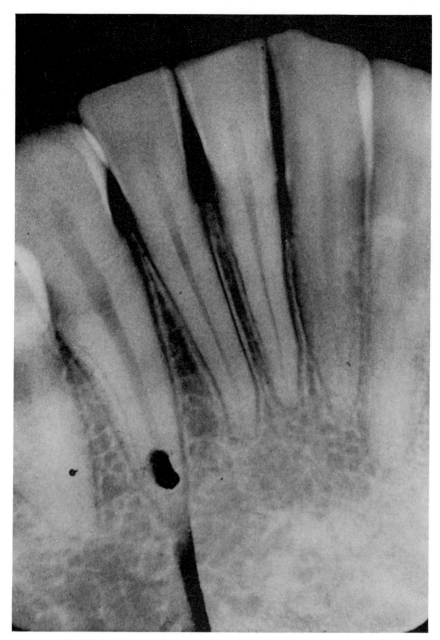

Figure 9-28. Black spots on film caused from developer solution contamination.

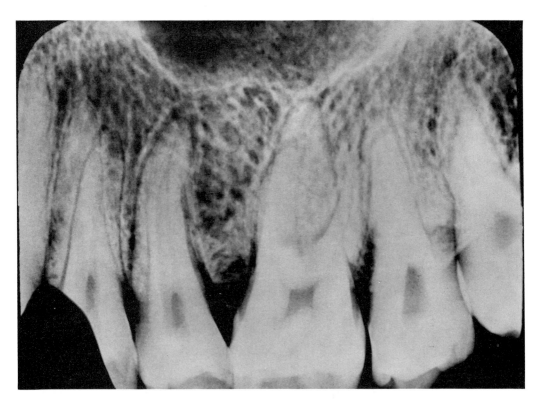

Figure 9-29. Black spot on film caused by films touching each other in the fixing solution. Black spot resulted because fixer could not react on area of film in contact with the other film.

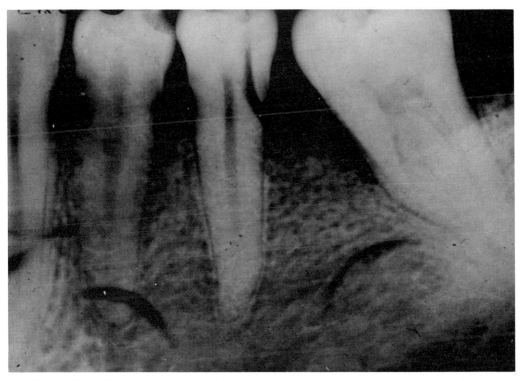

Figure 9-30. Black crescents caused by rough handling of the film during opening of the film packet.

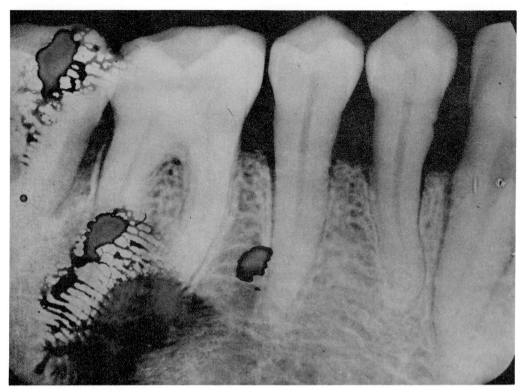

Figure 9-31. Black smudge marks from fingerprints on the radiograph before processing.

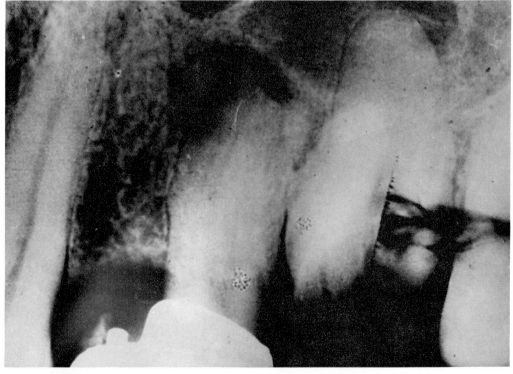

Figure 9-32. Static electricity will cause black lines on the film from rapidly removing film from its film packet in air with dry humidity.

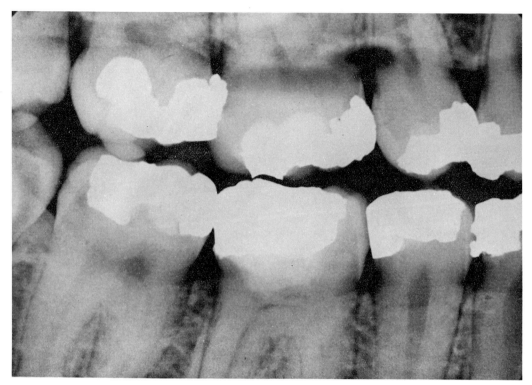

Figure 9-33. Brown stain on film caused from insufficient rinsing of film between developing and fixing.

Error	*Cause*	*Correction*
	f. Drop in line voltage.	
	(1) Elevators, furnaces, blowers, etc. on same circuit as x-ray unit.	Use separate circuit for x-ray units.
	(2) Insufficient size of power line.	Increase size of power line and/or transformers.
	Underdevelopment	
	a. Improper development.	
	(1) Time too short.	Set darkroom timer correctly (check accuracy).
	(2) Low developer temperature.	Raise temperature to 70°F.
	(3) Inaccurate thermometer.	Replace thermometer.
	b. Exhausted and/or contaminated developer.	Replace developer.
	c. Diluted developer.	
	(1) Water added to raise level of developer solution.	Add replenisher or replace developer.
	(2) Insufficient developer solution added to water.	Add more developer solution.
High Density Films (See Figure 9-20.)		
	a. Exposure time too long.	Set timer correctly and/or reduce exposure time.

Error	*Cause*	*Correction*
	b. kVp too high for exposure time.	Reduce kVp.
	c. Source-film distance too short for exposure time.	Measure source-film distance and adjust exposure time accordingly.
	d. Timer inaccurate.	Check timer with spinning top and adjust exposure time accordingly.
	e. mA too high for exposure time.	Reduce mA or exposure time.
	Overdevelopment	
	a. Developing time too long.	Use time-temperature method with darkroom timer.
	b. Developer temperature too high.	Lower developer temperature to 70°F.
	c. Combination of a. & b.	
	d. Inaccurate thermometer.	Replace thermometer.
	e. Overstrength developer.	Check tank capacity and mixing directions (See Chapter 8 under processing tanks).
High contrast (See Figure 9-21.)	a. Insufficient penetration	Increase kilovoltage.
	b. Overdevelopment	See correction above (underdevelopment).
	c. Use of film and/or intensifying screens of too high contrast.	Use lower contrast film or slower-speed screens.
	d. Too long exposure.	Timer inaccurately set, or timer out of calibration.
Low Contrast (See Figure 9-22.)	a. Excessive penetration.	Decrease kilovoltage.
	b. Underdevelopment.	See correction above underdevelopment.
	c. Use of film having insufficient contrast and/or cassettes with too slow intensifying screens.	Use of higher contrast films or higher speed screens.
	d. Scattered radiation.	Check diaphragm size and use suitable cone.
Fog (See Figure 9-23.)	*Light*	
	a. Light leaks in darkroom.	Check doors and walls for leaks.
	Improper safelight.	Reduce wattage of bulb.
	Improper filter in safelight.	Check type of filter and examine for cracks in filter (Wratten 6B type for screen film).
	b. Turning overhead (white) light on too soon.	Fix films 1-2 minutes before turning on the white light.
	c. Prolonged exposure of films to safelight.	Reduce exposure time of films to safelight.
	Radiation	
	a. Insufficient protection.	Store unexposed film in lead receptacles.
	Chemical	
	a. Developer temperature too high.	Reduce temperature of developer to manufacturer's optimum temperature (70°F).
	b. Overstrength developer.	Check tank capacity and mixing directions.
	c. Prolonged development.	Develop by time-temperature method.
	d. Contaminated developer.	Clean developer tank periodically.

Error	Cause	Correction
	Deterioration of film.	
	a. Temperature of storage area too high.	Store film in a cool place (70°F) or use refrigerator for storage of film.
	b. Humidity of storage area too high.	Store films in dry place (50% relative humidity. Use refrigerator).
	c. Strong fumes (ammonia, paint).	Keep films away from fumes.
	d. Outdated film.	Limit supply and use older films first.
Streaks on film	a. Failure to agitate film during development.	When first immersed in developer, agitate films.
	b. Undue amount of inspection of film during development. When films are held in front of safelight during development, the developer solution runs across the films producing uneven reduction of emulsion.	Use time-temperature method of development. This reduces the need to inspect film during development.
	c. Chemical deposits on hanger clips (See Figure 9-24).	Keep hanger clips clean.
	d. Excessive drying temperature.	Reduce air flow over films.
	e. Insufficient fixing.	Usually the fixing time is twice the development time.
	f. Dirty or contaminated wash water.	Wash films in fresh running water.
	g. Premature exposure of film to white light before fixing process is complete.	It usually requires approximately 2 minutes of clear film in fixing solution.
Blisters on film.	a. Unbalanced processing temperatures.	Control the temperature of water bath, which in turn controls temperature of processing solution.
	b. Excessive acidity of fixer.	Replace fixing solution.
	c. Films not agitated when first immersed in fixer.	Agitate.
Reticulation (orange-peel appearance) (See Figure 9-25).	a. Sudden extreme temperature changes in processing.	Maintain uniform processing temperature.
	b. Weakened fixer solution.	Replenish or replace fixer solution.
Frilling.	Hot processing solution.	Maintain correct processing solution (70°F).
Air Bells (See Figure 9-26).	Air bubbles trapped on film surfaces preventing uniform reduction of emulsion.	Agitate films upon immersion into developer.
White spots and lines on film.	a. Grit or dust present on films or upon screens.	Keep darkroom clean to prevent dust and dirt particles from settling on films. Periodically clean screens with commercial screen cleaner.
	b. Emulsion tears from rough handling of films in processing tank (See Figure 9-27).	Do not rub films up against sides of tanks or on other film hangers.
Black spots on film.	a. Grit or dust in contact with undeveloped film.	Prevent fine particles of developer coming in contact with film (dry chemicals).

Error	Cause	Correction
	b. Film splashed with developer before being placed in developer tank (See Figure 9-28).	Careful handling of solutions *and* clean work area.
	c. Films touching during fixing (See Figure 9-29).	Films should not touch in processing tanks.
Artifacts from processing. a. Black crescents (See Figure 9-30).	Rough handling of film.	Handle film by edges only.
b. Black smudge marks (See Figure 9-31).	Fingerprints or finger abrasions.	Have fingers dry when handling film (processing *and* mounting).
c. Black lines (See Figure 9-32).	Static electricity.	Too rapid removal of x-ray from pocket in air with dry humidity.
Stains on film. a. Yellow or brown (See Figure 9-33).	Exhausted developer. Oxidized developer. Prolonged developer. Insufficient rinsing.	Replace developer solution. Keep developer covered. Use correct development time. Rinse films 15-20 seconds in fresh running water.
	Exhausted fixer solution.	Replace fixer solution frequently.
b. Dichroic (Showing two colors).	Old or exhausted developer. Nearly exhausted fixer. Developer containing small amounts of scum or fixer. Film partially fixed in weak fixer, exposed to light, and washed. Prolonged intermediate rinse in contaminated rinse water.	Replace developer solution. Replace fixer solution. Remove scum and/or replace fixer solution. Replace fixer solution: follow recommended processing cycle. Use fresh, running water and recommended cycle.
Deposits on film.	Contaminated solutions (oil, impurities). Chemical deposits on hangers. Grit from dirty water. Metallic deposits (oxidized products from developer). Fixer contains excessive amounts of silver. White deposits: use of fixer which has milky appearance. This is caused by excessive amounts of precipitated aluminum sulfite. Excessive amounts of developer carried into fixer on film emulsion.	Mix new solution. Clean clips and hanger tops. Use fresh, running water. Replace developer solution. Replace fixer solution. Follow manufacturer's recommendations for mixing fixer solution. Use premixed liquid solution. Rinse properly and allow developer solution to drip into water a few seconds before placing film in fixer.
Brittleness of finished radiograph.	Excessive drying temperature. Excessive drying time; incoming air too humid and cold air velocity too low. Excessive fixer acidity.	Reduce dryer temperature. If use dryer, reduce drying time and adjust incoming air. Use a wetting agent prior to placing films in dryer. Replace fixer solution.
Faded image on finished radiograph.	Exhausted fixer. Inadequate fixing. Insufficient final wash.	Replace fixer solution. Fix films three times the clearing time. Wash film in fresh, running water for a minimum of 15-20 minutes.

OPERATORS' TROUBLESHOOTING GUIDE

(For Dental Automatic Processors*)

Section I—Film Density Problems

Error	Cause	Correction
1. *Decrease of film density (overall light films).*	a. Developer temperature low.	Increase heat in the developer. NOTE: Check the temperature of the developer solution with a thermometer of known accuracy.
	b. Developer reaching exhaustion.	Drain and thoroughly clean tank; install new developer solution.
	c. Developer contamination—the most likely reason for contaminated developer is fixer solution splashed or dripped into the developer.	Drain and thoroughly clean tank and rack; install new developer solution.
	d. No agitation in developer tank.	Be sure the agitator paddle drive belt is in the proper position in the pulleys.
2. *Increase in film density (overall dark films).*	a. Developer temperature too high.	Water turned off. Check temperature of incoming water supply and adjust from 75° to 78°F. Decrease the heat in the developer solution. NOTE: Check the temperature of the developer solution with a thermometer of known accuracy.
3. *Fogged film.*	a. Developer solution contaminated with fixer.	Drain and thoroughly clean tank and rack; install new developer solution.
	b. Processor light leaks.	Be sure processor cover is secured firmly in place.
	c. Light leaks in other areas.	Check light tightness of darkroom.
	d. Improper safelight.	Use 7½ watt frosted bulb in safelight with proper filter, mounted no closer than 4 feet from working area.
	e. Heat fog.	Make sure film storage area is not excessively hot.
	f. Excessively high developer temperature.	Readjust developer thermostat and water to proper temperature.

Section II—Film Drying Problems

1. *Films are not dry.*	a. Depleted fixer.	Install new fixer solution.
	b. Insufficient water flow (film not properly washed).	Check incoming water lines and valves. NOTE: The incoming water flow must be a minimum of ½ gallon-per-minute—or a maximum of 1 gallon-per-minute.
	c. Dryer temperature setting too low.	Increase dryer temperature.
	d. Chemical imbalance (either developer or fixer).	Replace with new solution.

---

* From Profexray's Automatic Dental Film Processor's Manual.

Error	Cause	Correction
	e. Improper type of film for time cycle of processor.	Check with dealer for information regarding proper type of film. (It is not recommended for film with acetate film base or any other film not designed for automatic processing.)

Section III—Abnormal Film Surface Marks

Error	Cause	Correction
1. *Peeling of film emulsion.*	a. Developer temperature too high.	Reduce developer temperature to proper level.
	b. Improper fixer strength or depleted fixer.	Replace fixer solution.
	c. Heavy developer deposits on developer rack rollers above solution level.	Be sure to follow the recommended housekeeping and cleaning procedures.
	d. Improper film.	Check with dealer for information regarding proper type of film.
2. *Pressure marks.*	a. Foreign material or rough spot on roller.	Clean rollers and/or remove rough area on roller.
	b. Rough handling or excessive hand pressure on film before processing.	Film emulsions are extremely sensitive, particularly after exposure and before processing. Good habits in gentle handling of film must be practiced.
3. *Cloudy or smudge appearance on film surface (greenish or yellowish)*	a. Depleted fixer.	Replace fixer solution.
	b. Improper type of film for time cycle of processor.	Check with dealer.
4. *White cloudy appearance over film surface.*	a. No water in wash tank.	Check incoming controls and lines. Be sure drain plug in wash tank is inserted in drain outlet.
5. *Scratches on film surface.*	a. Foreign material on roller (s).	Clean rollers.
	b. Improper handling of film before processing.	Proper, gentle handling of film must be practiced.
	c. Damaged or defective film.	Hand develop film (s) of the same batch or box. This may pick up defects that could be characteristic of the particular box or batch of film.
	d. Stalled or sticking roller.	Inspect racks, gears, and gear mesh. Correct as required.
6. *Drying pattern on film surface.*	a. Dryer too hot.	Reduce dryer temperature.
	b. Characteristic of film.	Process film of same box through other processor and chemicals to determine consistency of pattern.

REFERENCES

A Look At X-ray Film Processing. Milwaukee, X-ray Department, General Electric Co.

A Textbook of Selective X-ray Tcehnique. Rochester, New York, Ritter, pp. 136-138.

Bloom, William L.; Hollenbach, John L.; and Morgan, James A.: *Medical Radiographic Technic,* 3rd ed. Springfield, Ill., Charles C Thomas, 1969, pp. 127-128.

Darkroom Technique for Better Radiographs. Wilmington, Delaware, Photo Products Department, E. I. du Pont de Nemours and Co.

Du Pont Guide for Dental X-ray Darkrooms. Wilmington, Delaware, Photo Products Department, E. I. du Pont de Nemours and Co.

Fuchs, Arthur W.: *Principles of Radiographic Exposures and Processing,* 2nd ed. Springfield, Ill., Charles C Thomas, 1958, pp. 199-258.

McCall, John, and Wald, Samuel: *Clinical Dental Roentgenology,* 4th ed. Philadelphia, W. B. Saunders, 1957, pp. 124-126.

Peterson, Shailer: *Clinical Dental Hygiene.* St. Louis, C. V. Mosby, 1959, pp. 239-247.

Radiodontic Pitfalls. Rochester, N. Y., Eastman Kodak Co., X-ray Division.

CHAPTER 10

SPECIAL RADIOGRAPHIC TECHNICS

THE EXPOSURE technics listed are only approximate values and vary depending on the many factors involved.

OCCLUSAL RADIOGRAPHY

Maxillary Topographical Projection

Purpose: To observe a much larger area of the maxilla than can be observed with the intraoral periapical radiographs (See Figure 10-1C).

Head Position: Line from tragus of ear to ala of nose is horizontal, and parallel to the floor. The mid-sagittal plane is perpendicular to the floor.

Film Retention and Placement:

Film placed in mouth with longer axis of film running laterally from side to side. Place the pebbled side against the maxillary teeth and insert posteriorly as inner vestibule will permit. Patient bites down gently to hold in position. If edentulous, have patient use thumbs to hold film against edentulous ridges (See Figure 10-1B).

Projection of the Central Ray:

The principle involved is the same as that used in the bisecting angle technic in intraoral radiography. The central ray of the beam of radiation is directed through, or at the level of, the apex of the maxillary incisor teeth so that it is

perpendicular to the bisector of the angle formed by the film and the long axes maxillary incisor teeth.

Direct the *central ray* at a vertical angle of +65 degrees, through a point in the mid-sagittal plane between the tip of the nose and the nasal bridge, to the center of the packet (See Figure 10-1A).

Radiographic Factors:

FILM: Kodak® Ultra-Speed Occlusal Film.

SOURCE—FILM DISTANCE: 10 inches (short cone).

Exposure Factors	*Adult*
65 kVp 10 mA	½ second
90 kVp 15 mA	⅒ second

(Reduce exposure time by approximately one fourth in edentulous patients.)

Mandibular Cross-Sectional Projection

Purpose: The projection shows the relationship of an object to the teeth in horizontal plane and thus provides the information which, when coupled with that obtained from the intraoral periapical survey, accurately localizes the position of an object within the mandible. It is also very important in the diagnosis of sialoliths in the submandibular gland duct (Wharton's) and of calcifications within the gland itself (See Figure 10-2).

Head Position: Head tipped backwards until occlusal plane of maxillary

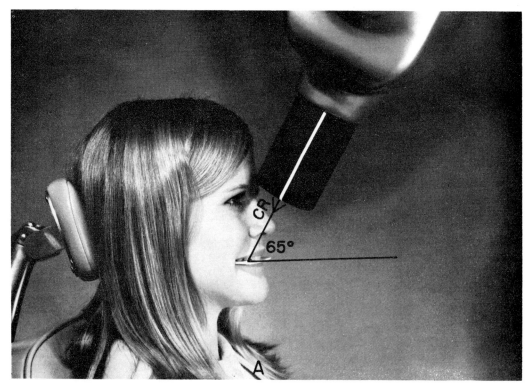

Figure 10-1A. Maxillary occlusal. Cone and film placement, lateral view.

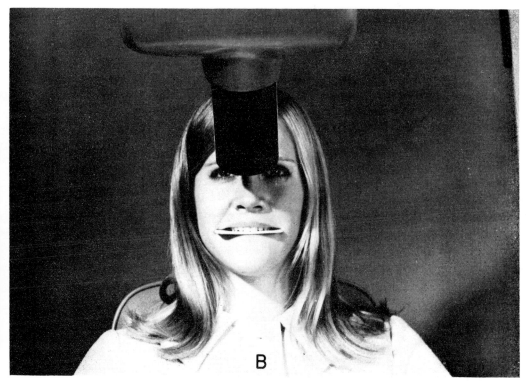

Figure 10-1B. Frontal view.

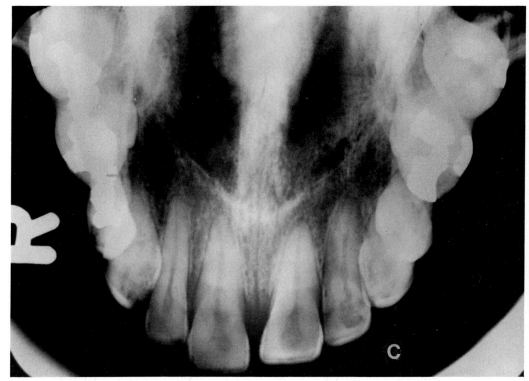

Figure 10-1C. Radiograph of maxillary occlusal projection.

teeth is vertical and at right angles to median plane.

Film Retention and Placement:

Occlusal packet inserted with pebbled side adjacent to mandibular occlusal surfaces; short center axis coincident with mid-sagittal plane; posterior edge of packet against anterior aspect of rami. Patient slowly closes on packet with gentle end-to-end bite. Edentulous patients should hold film against ridge with their forefingers.

Projection of the Central Ray (CR):

The central ray enters beneath the chin, approximately one inch posterior to the mental symphysis at the midline. The central ray is directed perpendicular to the occlusal film (See Figure 10-2A).

Radiographic Factors:

FILM: Kodak Ultra-Speed Occlusal
SOURCE—FILM DISTANCE: 10 inches (short cone)

Exposure Factors	Adult
65 kVp 10 mA	½ second
90 kVp 15 mA	⅒ second

(Reduce the exposure by one-fourth in edentulous patients.)

Mandibular Symphysis Projection

Purpose: To get an enlarged view of the mandibular incisor region (See Figure 10-3B).

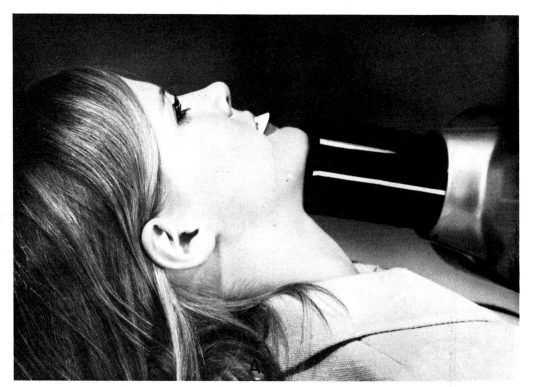

Figure 10-2A. Mandibular cross-sectional radiograph. Cone and film placement.

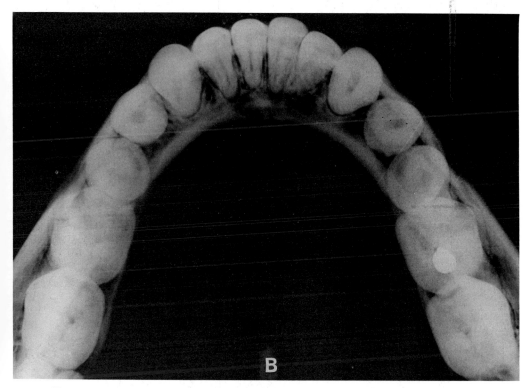

Figure 10-2B. Resultant radiograph of mandibular cross-sectional occlusal projection.

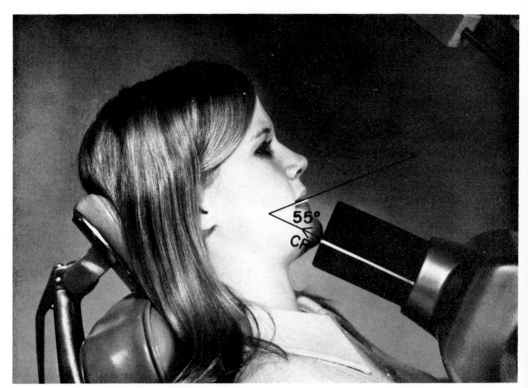

Figure 10-3A. Mandibular symphysis radiograph. Cone and film placement.

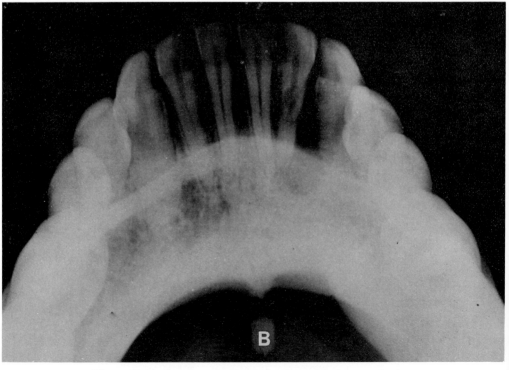

Figure 10-3B. Resultant radiograph of mandibular symphysis.

Head Position: Tilt chair backwards until occlusal plane of the maxillary teeth forms an angle of 55° to the horizontal plane. The mid-sagittal plane should be perpendicular to the floor.

Film Placement and Retention:

Occlusal packet inserted with pebbled side adjacent to mandibular occlusal surfaces. Long center axis coincident with mid-saggittal plane. Patient slowly closes down on packet with gentle end-to-end bite.

Projection of the Central Ray:

Use a −20° *vertical angulation* of the cone and direct the central ray parallel to the sagittal plane through the symphysis to the approximate center of the packet. The film packet and the central ray should form an approximate angle of 55° (See Figure 10-3A).

Radiographic Factors:

FILM: Kodak Ultra-Speed Occlusal Film.

SOURCE—FILM DISTANCE: 10 inches (short cone).

Exposure Factors	Adult
65 kVp 10 mA	½ second
90 kVp 15 mA	$\frac{1}{10}$ second

ANTERIOR PROFILE AND LATERAL JAW TECHNICS

Anterior Profile or "Tangential" Projection

Purpose: To aid in the buccolingual localization of maxillary canine impactions to maxillary incisors. It can also be used to obtain a modified anterior profile of patient (See Figures 10-4 and 10-5).

Head Position: Line from tragus of ear to ala of nose is horizontal.

Film Placement and Retention:

Patient holds pebbled side of film against the cheek parallel to the mid-saggital plane and centered over the canine region of interest. The long axis of the film should coincide with the mid-sagittal plane.

Projection of the Central Ray (CR):

The central ray is directed from the other side of the face through the apices of the teeth of the maxillary or mandibular anterior region perpendicular in both the horizontal and vertical planes to the center of the film.

Radiographic Factors:

FILM: Kodak Ultra-Speed Occlusal Film (a #2 regular periapical film may be used).

SOURCE—FILM DISTANCE: 13 inches (short cone).

Exposure Factors	Adult
65 kVp 10 mA	2-2½ seconds

Lateral Jaw Projections (Body and Ramus Views)

Purpose: The lateral jaw projection is used to view the mandible laterally from the angle of the ramus forward to the symphysis and the maxilla from the pterygoid plates to the 1st premolar (See Figures 10-6 and 10-7).

Head Position: The teeth are placed in occlusion with occlusal plane parallel to the floor. The mid-sagittal plane should be perpendicular to the floor.

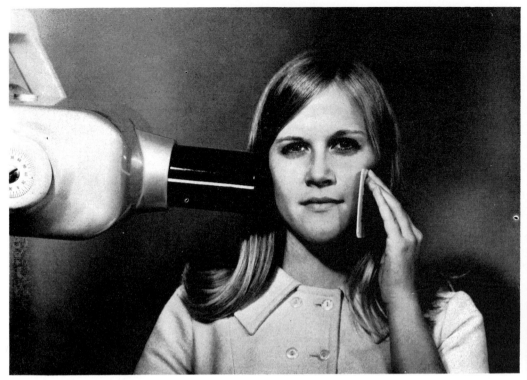

Figure 10-4. Anterior profile or "Tangential" projection—position of head, cone and film.

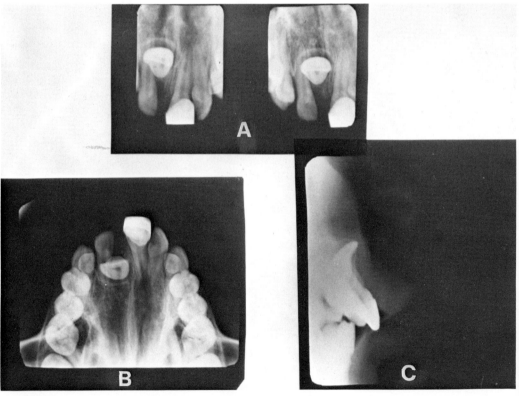

Figure 10-5. Three radiographs. (A) Periapical radiographs. (B) Maxillary occlusal radiographs. (C) Anterior profile or "Tangential" projections.

This is only a starting position, which standardizes the head position for subsequent steps. With the teeth still in occlusion, the chin is thrust out. This throws the mandible out away from the cervical vertebrae. If the patient is permitted to keep his chin in the normal position, the vertebrae will be superimposed over the ramus of the mandible and the resultant radiograph.

The long axis of the head is tilted at an angle of about 15° toward the side being radiographed. This position will move the opposite side of the mandible up out of the way from the side of the mandible being radiographed. The tilt should be kept at a minimum in order to minimize the distortion.

Film Placement and Retention:

The long axis of the film holder or cassette is placed horizontally and centered over the area of interest. The lower border of the film holder should be parallel to the floor and extend approximately one inch below the lower border of the mandible. The ideal position would be to have the long axis of the film holder exactly perpendicular to the floor, but this is impossible in some patients because of the contour of the face. The patient holds the film holder between the heel of the hand and the malar bone, with the fingers resting on the skull, thus keeping the lower border of the film holder away from the face. This retains the film holder in a perpendicular position with the floor. However, if the film holder is retained too far away from the face the resultant radiograph will include distorted images.

In the lateral jaw body projection, ro-

tate the patient's head until the nose is approximately touching the film holder. When taking the ramus projection do not rotate the head as much. The chin should be slightly raised.

Projection of the Central Ray:

Vertical Angulation:

The vertical angulation will vary with the tilt of the head of the patient. If the tilt of the head is approximately 15 degrees, use −10 degrees. This gives an aggregate angle of 25 degrees.

If the patient's head does not have to be tilted, a vertical angulation of −17 degrees (upward angulation) is used. A low angle is preferred with patients with short necks and wide shoulders. With these types of patients the head will have to be tilted slightly (15 degrees).

Horizontal Angulation:

This is determined by aligning the top edge of the x-ray tube parallel with the top edge of the film holder.

Point of Entry:

This is located ½ inch posterior and inferior to the mandible on the opposite side of the mandible to be radiographed.

Point of Emanation:

The *Central Ray* is directed at a point just superior and anterior to the area of interest. There are separate projections for the ramus, body and anterior regions.

Radiographic Factors:

Film: 5 x 7 Kodak No-Screen Film® or 5 x 7 Screen Film. (No-Screen film has a thick emulsion and is sensitive to x-radiation. The thicker emulsion is advantageous from two aspects: (1) Less radiation is needed to produce the desired film density, and (2) a greater range of densities or shades of grey can be obtained in the finished radiograph. A 50 percent increase in developing, fixing, and washing time is recommended because of the thick emulsion. Develop the film for 8 minutes at 70 degrees F and fix for 15 minutes.

R & L MARKERS: R and L lead markers must be used to identify which side of the patient was examined. Place the marker just above the orbits of patient.

FILM HOLDER: 5 x 7 cardboard film holder or metal cassette. The cardboard film holders are inexpensive. This is very desirable, as more often than not, two exposures of any one patient are needed. Two exposures are advisable in most instances, not only to accurately locate and depict a lesion, but also to compare one side of the jaw with the other side. The cardboard film holder is lightweight which is desirable when lateral jaw radiographs are taken of children and the elderly.

Exposure Factors	*5 × 7 Film Holder*	*Adult*	*Seconds Child*
65 kVp—10 mA	Cardboard holder	2½	1¼
65 kVp—10 mA	Metal cassette	¼-³⁄₂₀	⅛-¹⁄₁₀
90 kVp—10 mA	Metal cassette	¹⁄₁₅	¹⁄₂₀

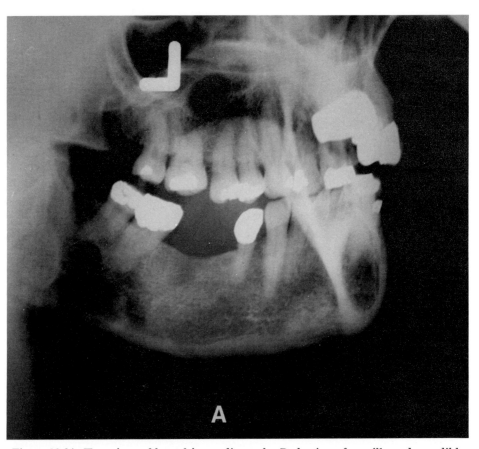

Figure 10-6A. Two views of lateral jaw radiographs. Body view of maxilla and mandible.

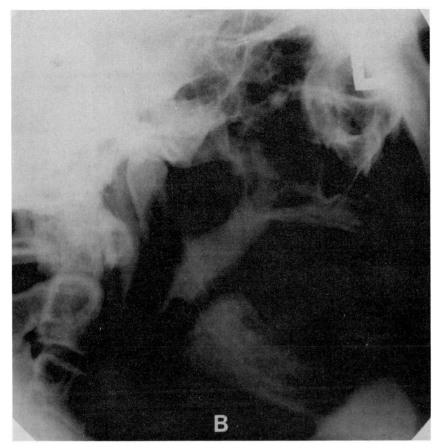

Figure 10-6B. Ramus view of mandible.

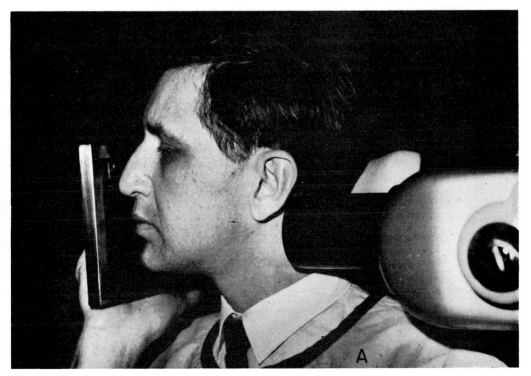

Figure 10-7A. Positioning the patient for lateral jaw—body projection.

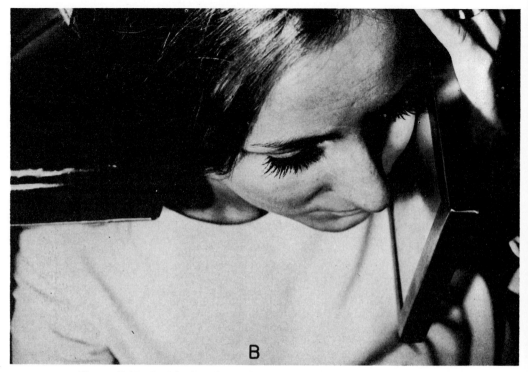

Figure 10-7B. Positioning the patient for lateral jaw—ramus projection.

SOURCE-FILM DISTANCE: Short cone (approximately 20″).

FILM AND CASSETTES: No-Screen film with cardboard film holder or screen film with metal cassette and high speed screens.

PARANASAL SINUS RADIOGRAPHY

The routine sinus x-ray examination includes a lateral view and two axial views (the Waters and Caldwell views). Sometimes the infracranial (submento-vertex) view is especially useful in depicting the sphenoid sinus.

Anterior Lateral Face
(Lateral Maxillary Sinus)

Purpose: It not only shows the antero-posterior position of objects or lesions in the antral area, but also reveals the condition of the bones of the face (especially bones of the nose). The antero-posterior view of all the sinuses should be revealed in this projection (See Figure 10-8).

Head Position: Line from tragus of ear to ala of nose is parallel to the floor; mid-sagittal plane is perpendicular to the floor. Jaws should be in normal occlusion.

Film Holder Placement and Retention:

A film holder containing screen film is placed vertically (long axis of holder vertical) against the lateral aspect of head, with the lower edge resting on shoulder and the zygomatic arch centered on the cassette. The front edge of the film holder should be parallel to the mid-sagittal plane. If a cassette holder is not used, have the patient hold the film holder steady in the correct position with his hand.

Projection of the Central Ray:

POINT OF ENTRY: It is at the point of intersection of two lines, one drawn from the ala of the nose and parallel to the floor, and one drawn from the corner of the eye and perpendicular to the floor.

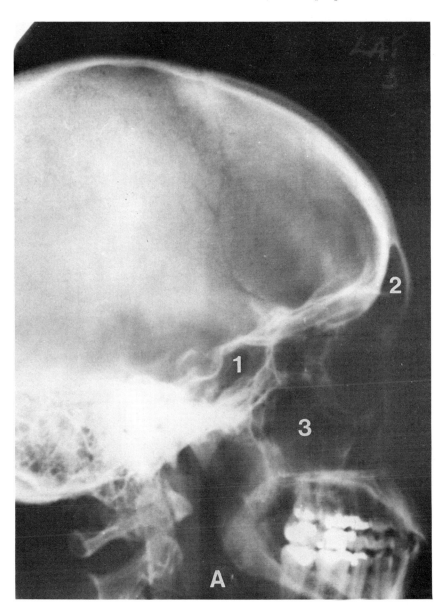

Figure 10 8A. Lateral face radiograph. Lateral maxillary sinus radiograph. (1) Sphenoid sinus. (2) Frontal sinus. (3) Maxillary sinus.

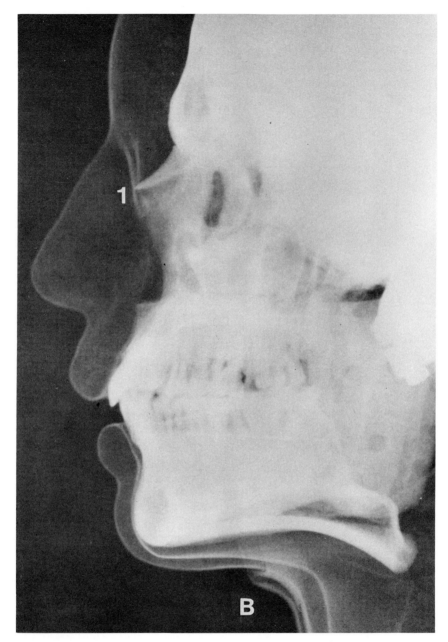

Figure 10-8B. Lateral face profile radiograph. (1) Anterior nasal spine.

The central ray is directed vertically and horizontally perpendicular to the point of entry and center of film holder. The point of exit will be the same point on the face as the point of entry, but *on* the other side of the face adjacent to the film holder.

Radiographic Factors:

FILM: 8 x 10 Screen film.

FILM HOLDER: 8 x 10 film cassette with high speed screen. Place R & L markers away from boney structures of interest.

EXPOSURE FACTORS. 65 kVp and 10 mA. Use *Short Cone,* a source-film distance of 36" and expose the film for approximately .5 seconds.

Note: (If you are interested in obtaining a facial profile of face, direct the CR horizontally and laterally perpendicular through the anterior nasal spine to the center of the film. Reduce the exposure to .3 seconds.)

Waters Projection for the Paranasal Sinuses, Posteroanterior View of Paranasal Sinuses

Purpose: The Waters position is essential to the study of the nasal accessory sinuses and facial bones. Before the introduction of this view of the cranium the occipitofrontal projection of Caldwell was used routinely, but superimposition of the shadows of the petrous portions of the temporal bones frequently prevented visualization of the maxillary antra in their entirety. Therefore, Waters and Waldron in 1915 introduced a projection which allows visualization of the frontal and maxillary sinuses and many of the ethmoid cells with little or no interference by shadows of structures within the cranium, particularly the petrous portions of the temporal bones. Better visualization of the superior portions of the frontal sinuses is obtained in the Caldwell position, especially when the sinuses extend superiorly for a greater than average distance. The maxillary sinuses are best revealed with the Waters view (See Figure 10-9).

Head Position: This view is preferably obtained with the patient in the head-upright position in order to detect fluid levels in the sinuses. If it is impossible to place the patient in this position, the examination is done with film in horizontal position on top of a table.

The film holder is placed vertically in the cassette holder. The sagittal plane of the skull is perpendicular to the film holder. The chin is placed against the film holder with the head tilted back sufficiently to prevent the nose from touching (2-3 cm off the film cassette). The junction of the nose and the upper lip is centered at the middle of the film, and the head is so positioned that the orbitomeatal line makes an angle of 45° with the film and/or the central ray. Therefore, the chin touches the cassette and the nose is 2-3 cm from the cassette.

Projection of the Central Ray:

The central ray is directed perpendicular in both the horizontal and vertical planes to the film along a line extending from the lambda (sagittal-lamboidal suture juncture) to the inferior margin of the base of the nose. The conventional Waters view is obtained with the film vertical.

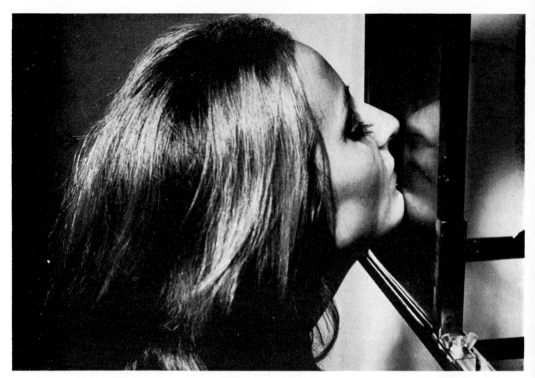

Figure 10-9A. Waters' projection. Central ray directed through lambda of skull. (1) 8 x 10 cassette. (2) Cassette holder.

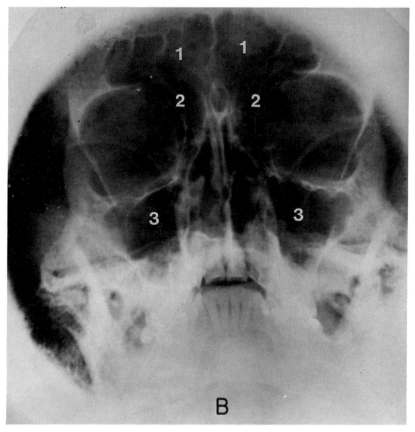

Figure 10-9B. Waters' radiograph of paranasal sinuses. (1) Frontal sinuses, (2) Ethmoidal sinuses, and (3) Maxillary sinuses.

Radiographic Factors:

FILM HOLDER: 8 x 10 x-ray cassette with high speed screens.

FILM: Screen Film.

CONE: Short Cone   SFD 24 in

EXPOSURE FACTORS:

kVp-mA 65-10 3 sec
80-10 2 sec

IDENTIFICATION: Use lead letters.

Caldwell Position for Paranasal Sinuses (See Figure 10-10)

Purpose: Caldwell described an occipitofrontal projection of the nasal sinuses in an article published first in 1906 and reprinted in 1918. This projection is superior to others for demonstration of the frontal sinuses and the superiorly located ethmoid cells. The superior portion of the maxillary sinuses is usually blocked by the petrous bone, but the alveolar region is usually seen (See Figure 10-10).

Head Position: The 8 x 10 or 10 x 12 cassette is placed vertically in the wall cassette holder. The patient is positioned in a sitting posture with the *nose* and *forehead* against the film and the glabella at its center. The patient's head is adjusted so that the sagittal plane is positioned perpendicular to the film so that the cantho-meatal line (outer canthus of the eye to the tragus of the ear) is perpendicular to the plane of the film. Therefore, the nose and forehead touch the cassette.

Projection of the Central Ray:

The central ray is centered to the glabella and angled toward the feet ap-

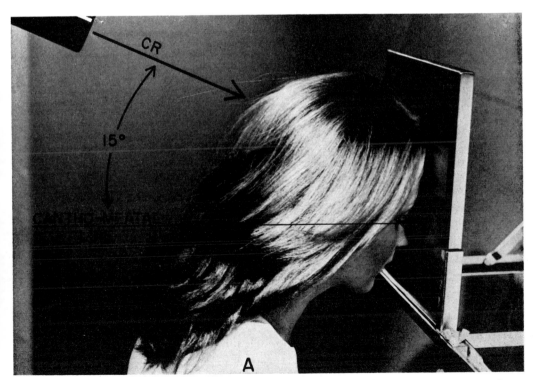

Figure 10-10A. Caldwell projection for frontal and ethmoidal cells. Head, cassette and cone positioning.

proximately 15 degrees with respect to the cantho-meatal line. The downward projection of the x-ray beam assures a clearer view of the orbits.

If the frontal bone is the region of major interest, a straight postero-anterior view of the frontal bone is obtained without angulation of the tube. The central ray of the x-ray tube is positioned perpendicular to the film and coincides with the cantho-meatal line. The posterior instead of the anterior cells of the ethmoidal sinuses will be seen in this view, and the dorsum sellae is seen as a curved line extending between the orbits just above the ethmoids.

Radiographic Factors:

FILM HOLDER: 8 x 10 or 10 x 12 Cassette with High Speed Screens (Use R or L markers).

FILM: Screen Film.

TARGET-FILM DISTANCE:

24 seconds (short cone)

EXPOSURE FACTORS:

65 kVp—10 mA   3 sec
80 kVp—10 mA   2 sec

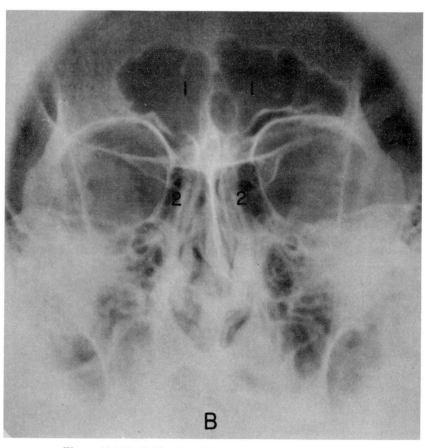

Figure 10-10B. Caldwell radiograph of paranasal sinuses.

TEMPORO-MANDIBULAR RADIOGRAPHY

TMJ radiography is probably the most difficult technic for a dentist to perform. The anatomic location of this joint is the primary cause of this difficulty. The following boney structures are located adjacent to the TMJ and superimposed over the joint unless special technics are utilized:

1. *Petrous portion of temporal bone:* medially and superiorly to joint.
2. *Mastoid process of temporal bone:* posterior to joint.
3. *Zygomatic process of maxilla:* anterior to joint.

These special technics utilize the conventional dental units or more sophisticated x-ray equipment found in institutions or hospitals. Some of the more specialized technics include tomography, cephalometry, arthrography, cinefluorography and panoramic radiography. The dental x-ray unit is used to take three basic views:

1. Lateral Oblique Transcranial View
2. Anteroposterior Transcranial View
3. Infracranial and Bregma-Menton Views

The Lateral Oblique Transcranial Technic

Purpose: It is used primarily to view the condyle in lateral relation to the glenoid fossa. (This is usually the method of choice.)

This is a modification of Lindblom's technic first proposed in 1936 (without an angle board) (See Figure 10-11).

Head Position: Position the mid-sagittal plane perpendicular to the floor and the tragal-ala line parallel to the floor.

Film Placement and Retention:

A 8 x 10 cassette film holder is placed with the long axis of the film perpendicular to the floor. Use a leaded rubber mat to block one side of the film. Take right and left projections on one 8 x 10 film. The head of the condyle to be radiographed is centered on the film holder. The film holder is positioned against the zygomatic arch, the superior temporal crest, and the ear. To show a second view of the articulation on the same film, the film holder is shifted and the other half of the film is masked by the leaded rubber blocker. The anterior edge of the film holder should be parallel to the mid-sagittal plane of the patient.

Projection of the Central Ray:

VERTICAL ANGULATION: Initially at 25 degrees downward.

POINT OF ENTRY: In order to pass the x-ray beam tangentially to the head of the condyle, a point of entry of the central ray of the x-ray beam is found by first measuring $2\frac{1}{2}$ inches vertically above the superior edge of the external auditory meatus and then 1 inch posteriorly. (This is to prevent the superimposition of the petrous portion of the temporal bone over the head of the condyle.)

POINT OF EMINENCE: Head of condyle on the side projected.

HORIZONTAL ANGULATION: It is selected so that the central ray will emerge at the articulation to be examined. The centering of the beam horizontally on the TMJ is examined first from the front and then from the side of the patient.

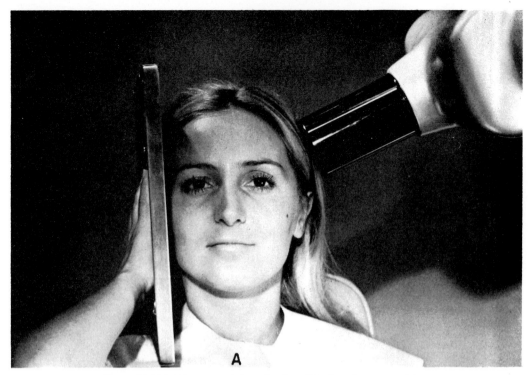

Figure 10-11A. Transcranial projection. Head and cone position.

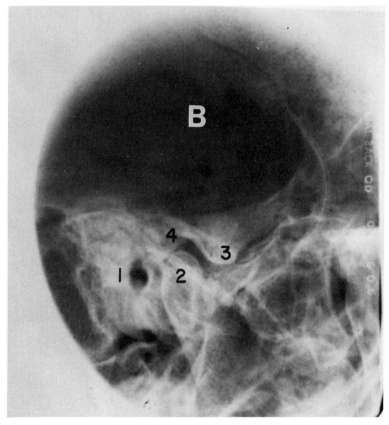

Figure 10-11B. Resultant radiograph. (1) Internal auditory meatus. (2) Head of condyle. (3) Articular eminence. (4) Glenoid fossa.

Radiographic Factors:

FILM HOLDER: 8 x 10 cassette with lead blockers (High-Speed Screens).

FILM: Screen Film.

SOURCE-FILM DISTANCE: Short Cone adjacent to the skull at point of entry.

EXPOSURE FACTORS:

65 kVp—10 mA   1½ sec
90 kVp—15 mA   ⅔ sec

Lateral TMJ Transpharyngeal Technic*

Head Position: The mid-sagittal plane is positioned parallel to the cassette film holder which is perpendicular to the floor.

---

* This is a modification of the original technic advocated by McQueen in 1937.

Film Placement and Retention:

A 5 x 7 or 8 x 10 film holder is placed in a cassette holder or it may be held by the patient. If you use a 8 x 10 film holder, a lead blocker should be utilized. The lead of the condyle to be radiographed is centered on the film holder. Position the film holder against the zygomatic arch and the external auditory meatus (See Figure 10-12).

Projection of the Central Ray:

VERTICAL ANGULATION: Direct the x-rays at a −10° vertical angulation through the sigmoid notch toward the opposite condyle.

HORIZONTAL ANGULATION: Direct the x-rays posteriorly 10 degrees toward the opposite condyle.

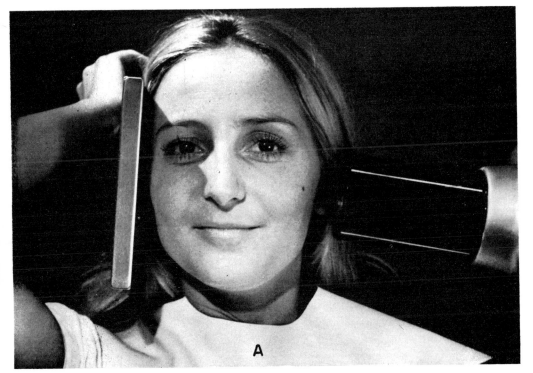

A

Figure 10-12A. McQueen or lateral TMJ articulation technic. Head and cone position.

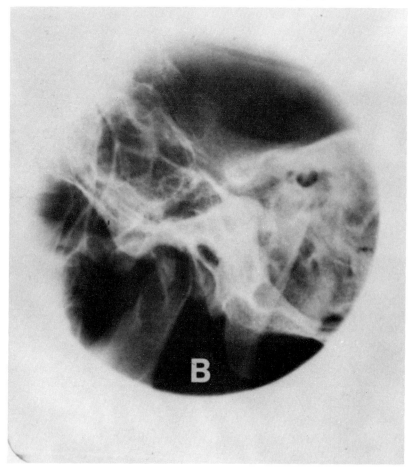

Figure 10-12B. Resultant radiograph (McQueen Technic).

POINT OF ENTRY: The point of entry is the sigmoid notch, which is just inferior to the zygomatic arch.

POINT OF EMINENCE: Head of condyle on the opposite side.

Radiographic Factors:

FILM HOLDER: 8 x 10 or 5 x 7 cardboard film holder.

FILM: Kodak No-Screen Film.

SOURCE-FILM DISTANCE: Short Cone against the point of entry.

EXPOSURE FACTORS: 65 kVp—10 mA 2½ sec

Lateral or Oblique Transcranial Technic for Projection of Temporomandibular Joints Using Updegrave Angle Board*

This technique utilizes a dental x-ray unit and a specially constructed 15° angle board, with a protractor-rod assembly to assist in duplication of the head position.

A plastic side tunnel with a leaded rubber mat is provided which permits

---

* This technic was advocated by Updegrave in 1953.

multiple exposures without changing the position of the patient's head. (A 6-exposure technic takes an open, closed, and rest position of the TMJ articulation.) A filter-collimator-retainer is used to provide a shorter source-film distance which will eliminate structures that are superimposed over the TMJ by magnifying and distorting them. The diaphragm is made of $\frac{1}{8}$-inch lead, and the round center opening is from 1 to $1\frac{1}{2}$ inches in diameter (See Figure 10-13A).

Head Position: Patient is seated facing the angle board and the head is positioned with the external auditory meatus of the side being examined. The ear positioner is made of plastic. The head is supported at three points, the auditory

meatus, zygoma, and the angle of mandible. The tip of the patient's nose is aligned on the horizontal level of the side positioning rod. The head position is recorded (See Figure 10-13B).

Projection of the Central Ray:

With the conventional cone replaced by a modified cone-collimator-filter combination, the x-ray machine is brought into contact with the patient's head and aligned with the positioning rods at the side and top of board. The tube head reading should be 0 or 90 degrees (See Figure 10-13C).

Film Placement and Retention:

A loaded 8 x 10 wafer cassette is placed in the plastic tunnel with the

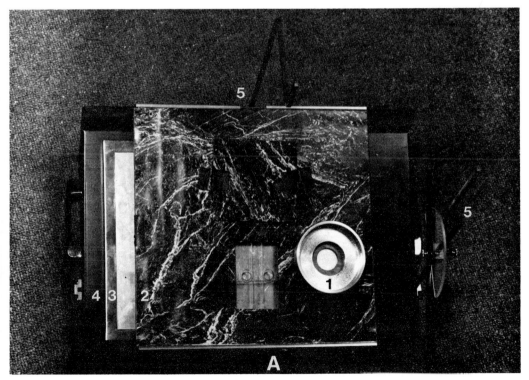

Figure 10-13A. Updegrave angle board. (1) Filter-diaphragm-retainer. (2) Leaded shield. (3) 8 x 10 Wafer cassette. (4) 15° angle board. (5) Alignment rods.

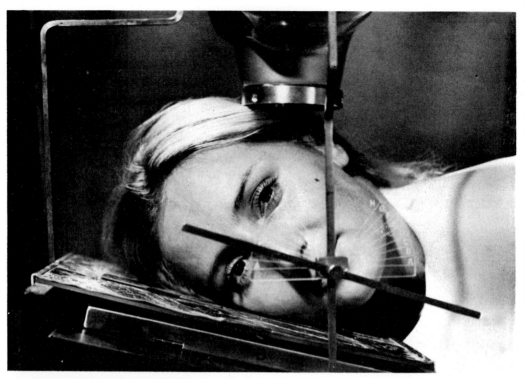

Figure 10-13B. Side view of Updegrave angle board, alignment rods and patient's head.

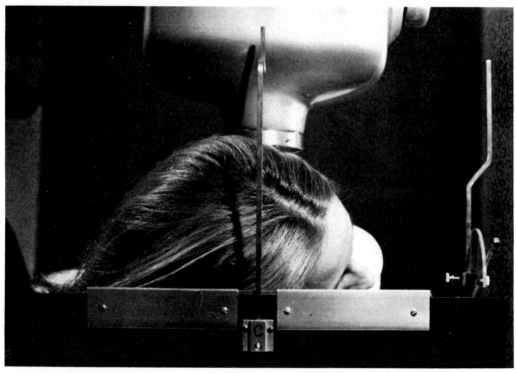

Figure 10-13C. Front view of Updegrave angle board and patient's head.

opening in the rubber shield placed over the region of the threaded plastic ear positioner. Multiple exposures of condylar function can be made without changing the head position of the patient simply by moving the cassette in the side tunnel. Six exposures are made on one 8 by 10 inch film. It is usually advisable to make the first exposure with the teeth in centric occlusion to assure a firm head position, and then to shift the cassette and make the next exposure in the rest position. The third position is the open position. Use a mouth prop to open the patient's mouth about one inch.

For the *centric position,* have the patient say "Mississippi" and then close their teeth together. This is the "lip-closed, teeth-together position." In the *rest position,* have the patient swallow and then relax his lower jaw. This is the "lips-closed, teeth-apart position." (See Figure 10-14.)

Radiographic Factors

FILM HOLDER: 8 x 10 wafer cassette with high speed screens.

FILM: Screen Film.

SOURCE-FILM DISTANCE: Approximately 10 inches. Use a specially designed modified filter-collimator-retainer attachment in place of conventional cone.

EXPOSURE FACTORS: 65 kVp—10 mA, 1 second.

Anteroposterior (Transorbital) Temporo-Mandibular Projection

Purpose: This is an excellent film for lateral movements of the condyle, frac-

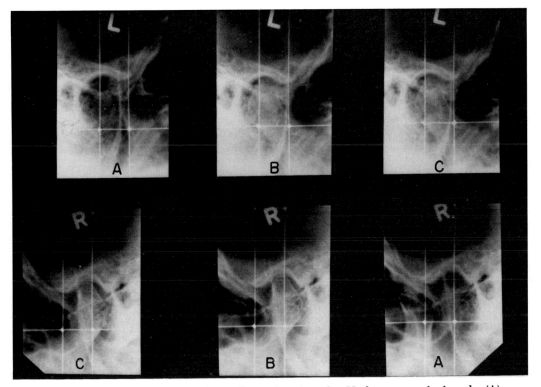

Figure 10-14. Lateral transcranial radiograph using the Updegrave angle board. (A) Open. (B) Centric relation. (C) Closed position.

tures of the condylar neck and the zygoma. This radiograph gives a medio-lateral view of articular eminence, relation of condyle to articular eminence, and neck of condyle* (See Figure 10-15).

Head Position: An 8 x 10 cassette is placed behind the patient perpendicular to the floor. Occlusal plane should be parallel to the floor. One-half of the cassette is shielded with a lead rubber mat which will permit two exposures on one film. Use a mouth prop to maintain the mandible at a maximum opening. Rotate the head twenty degrees toward the side being examined.

* This technic is based on the work of Zimmer (1941), Norgaard (1947), and Grant and Lanting (1953). This is an open-mouth technic.

Projection of Central Ray:

The central ray is directed 35 degrees caudally through the orbit and condyle. Alternate method: Keep the patient's head erect with the mid-sagittal plane perpendicular to the floor. The central ray is directed caudally 30 degrees and laterally 20 degrees from the mid-sagittal plane.

The rubber lead mat is moved for the second projection to protect the exposed film. Of course, the patient and film must be repositioned for examination of the opposite condyle. Be sure to use R and L lead markers on the film.

Radiographic Factors:

FILM HOLDER: 8 x 10 cassette with high speed screens.

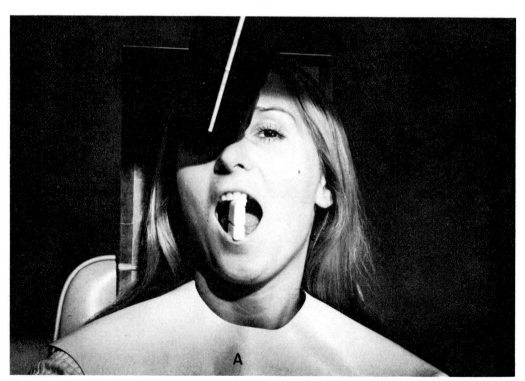

Figure 10-15A. Anteroposterior or transorbital TMJ projection. View of extension cone, patient's head and cassette.

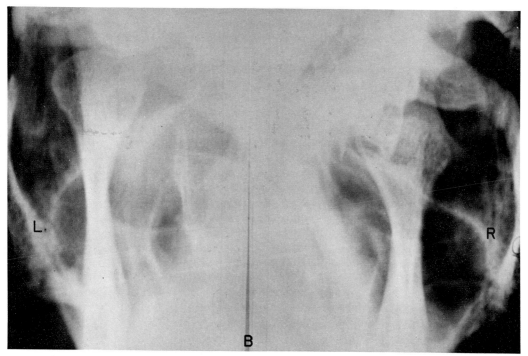

Figure 10-15B. Resultant radiograph (Transorbital TMJ projection).

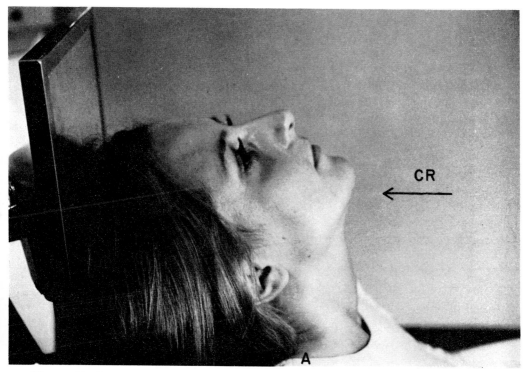

Figure 10-16A. Infracranial temporomandibular projection. View of patient's head, cassette and central ray.

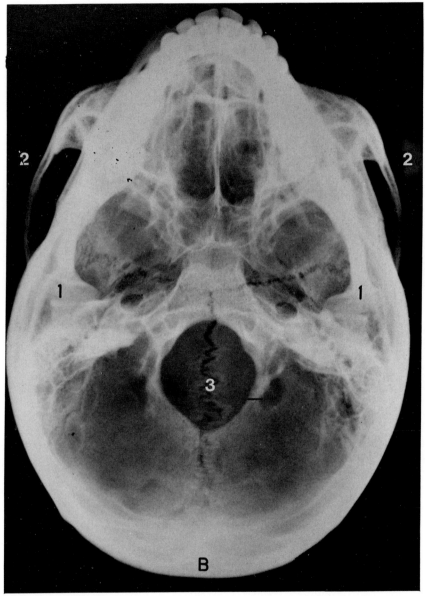

Figure 10-16B. Resultant infracranial TMJ radiograph. (1) Mandibular condyle, (2) Zygomatic arch, and (3) Foramen magnum.

FILM: Screen Film.

SOURCE-FILM DISTANCE: 22-24 inches long cone.

EXPOSURE FACTORS: 65 kVp—10 mA, ¾ second.

Infracranial and Bregma-Menton Views

These are alternate projections for the transorbital technic, and are used in patients with limited mandibular move-ments. These technics are utilized to reveal lateral movements of the condyles, displacement of the condyles heads following fractures, and depressed fractures of the zygoma.

Infracranial Technic

Head Position: The cassette is placed behind the patient who leans backwards in order to touch the top of his head on

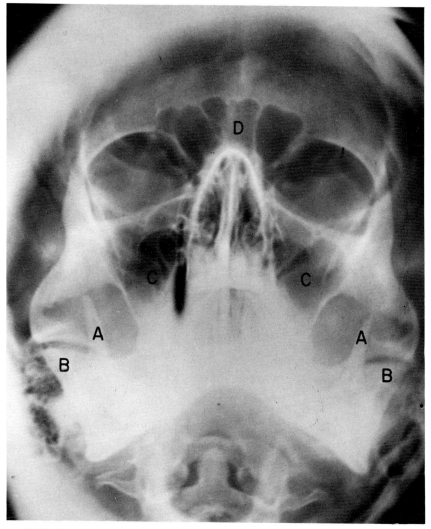

Figure 10-17. Bregma-Menton projection radiograph. (A) Coronoid process. (B) Condylar process. (C) Maxillary sinus. (D) Frontal sinus.

the cassette. The tragal-ala line should be perpendicular to the floor (See Figure 10-16).

Projection of the Central Ray:

Direct the central ray perpendicular to the film through a point midway between the mandibular rami. Exposures are made with the teeth in occlusion.

Radiographic Factors:

FILM HOLDER: 8 x 10 with high speed screens.

FILM: Screen Film.

SOURCE-FILM DISTANCE: 18 inches with short cone.

EXPOSURE FACTORS: 65 kVp—10 mA, 2½ seconds. (Reduce the exposure time if fractures of the zygomatic arches are suspected.)

Bregma-Menton Technic

Head Position: The cassette is placed flat on a metal table. The patient's chin is centered on the cassette. In order to accomplish this, the patient's neck should be extended. Use a lead apron in patient's lap (See Figure 10-17).

Projection of the Central Ray;

Direct the central ray through the bregma of the skull to the menton (lowest point of the chin). The bregma is the junction of the coronal and sagittal sutures.

Radiographic Factors:

FILM HOLDER: 8 x 10 cassette with high speed screen.

FILM: Screen Film.

SOURCE-FILM DISTANCE: 24 inches (short cone). (A short cone placed adjacent to the patient's scalp.)

EXPOSURE FACTORS: 65 kVp—10 mA, 2½ seconds.

PA MANDIBLE AND SKULL PROJECTIONS

Posteroanterior Mandible Technic

The technic is especially useful in the showing fractures of the necks of the condyles. Also, it will reveal fractures of the coronoid process and the body of the mandible (See Figure 10-18).

Head Position: Center the nose and chin of the patient on an upright cassette. The mid-sagittal plane of the patient's head should be perpendicular to the cassette. The patient's mouth may be opened or closed. An open position will produce a clearer view of the condyles. Of course, in fracture cases this may be impossible.

Projecion of the Central Ray:

Direct the central ray through the mid-sagittal plane at the level of the angles of the mandibular rami. An alternate method is the Reverse Towne Technic. In this method, the patient is positioned in the nose-forehead position with the cantho-meatal line perpendicular to the cassette. The central ray is directed through the mid-sagittal plane with a 30° upwards projection through the top of the patient's head.

Radiographic Factors:

FILM HOLDER: 8 x 10 cassette with high speed screens.

FILM: Screen Film.

SOURCE-FILM DISTANCE: 36 inches (short cone). An alternate method is to use a 24-inch source-film distance. A shorter source-film distance will avoid cervical spine superimposition by overly

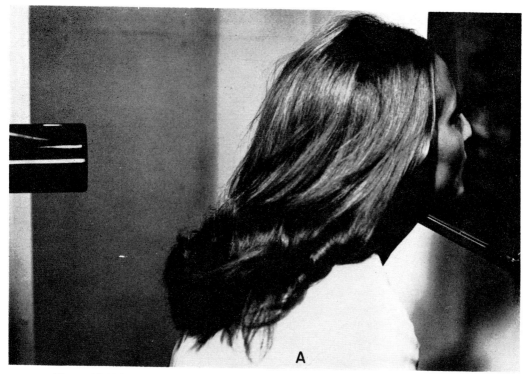

Figure 10-18A. Posteroanterior mandible. (A) Position of head, cone and cassette.

distorting these structures on the resultant radiograph.

EXPOSURE FACTORS: 65 kVp—10 mA, 1½-2½ seconds.

Lateral Skull Radiography

The lateral radiograph reveals all the osseous structures of the skull in a lateral view. The images of the structures of the left and right sides of the skull are superimposed over each other. The structures on the side of the skull toward the film will be less magnified. The lateral radiograph will reveal changes in the size, shape, and mineral content of the cranial bones. The facial bones are better visualized when less exposure is used (See Figure 10-19).

Head Position: The cassette is placed vertically perpendicular to the floor. The patient's head is positioned against the cassette. The tragal line should be parallel to the floor. The jaws should be in centric relation.

In evaluating the lateral skull radiograph, the two halves of the mandible should be superimposed over each other. If there is a considerable discrepancy between the two halves of the mandible, the radiograph should be repeated.

Projection of the Central Ray:

Direct the central ray perpendicular to the film in both the horizontal and vertical planes. The central ray should pass through a point one inch above the midpoint of the line joining the outer canthus of the eye with the tragus of the ear (cantho-meatal line). This will ordi-

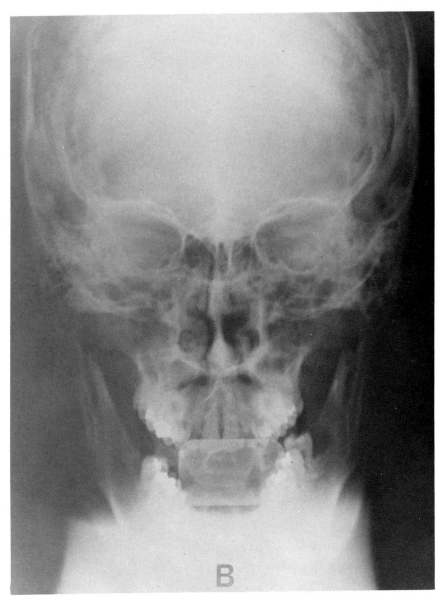

Figure 10-18B. Resultant radiograph with mouth open. (PA Mandible)

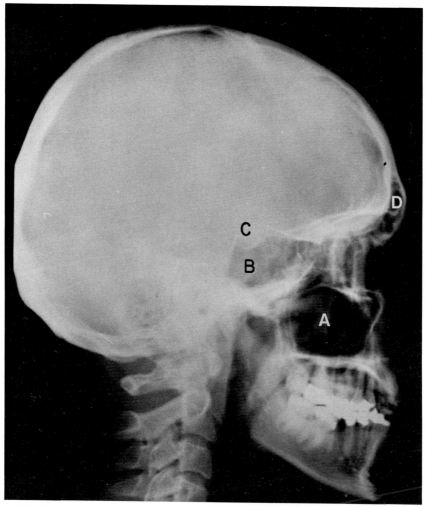

Figure 10-19. Lateral skull radiograph. (A) Maxillary sinus. (B) Sphenoid sinus. (C) Sella turcica. (D) Frontal sinus.

narily fall immediately over the sella turcica.

Radiographic Factors:

FILM HOLDER: 8 x 10 or 10 x 12 cassette with high speed screens.

FILM: Screen Film.

SOURCE-FILM DISTANCE: 36 inches, short cone.

EXPOSURE FACTORS: 65 kVp—10 mA, 2-3 seconds.

Cephalometric Radiography

Cephalometric radiography is used almost exclusively by orthodontists. Pucini (1922) was the first to introduce this technic for growth and development studies of the skull. However, it took Broadbent (1931) of the United States and Hofrath (1931) of Germany to make the technic a practical diagnostic method in orthodontics. They both advocated headholding devices. Cephalometrics is a

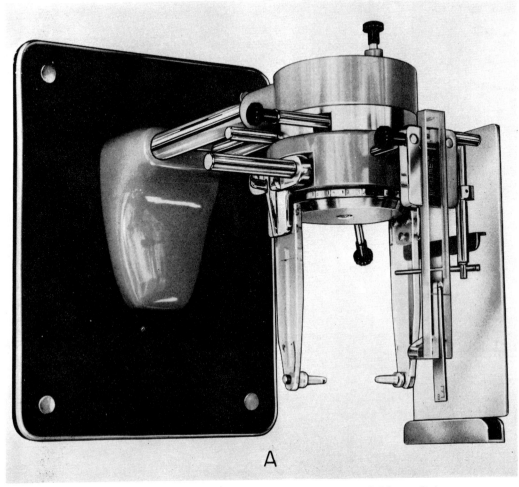

A

Figure 10-20A. Wehmer Cephalostat. (Courtesy of B. F. Wehmer Co.)

radiographic technic for obtaining head measurements from skull radiographs. A headholding device called a cephalometer or cephalostat is used to place the patient's head in a standardized position. This device allows the operator to place the patient's head in almost the same position on successive exposures. Two views are used: the lateral and the posteroanterior (PA) views (See Figure 10-20).

Lateral Cephalometric Technic

Head Position: Usually, the lateral view is taken first. Immobilize the patient's head in the head holder by means of the nasion positioning rod and the ear plugs. The patient's head is positioned in the Frankfort plane horizontal by use of infraorbital marker. The midsagittal plane should be parallel to the vertically placed cassette (See Figure 10-21).

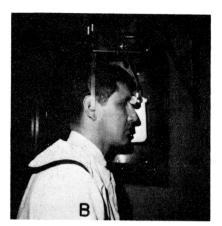

Figure 10-20B. Positioning of head for lateral cephalometric radiograph.

PROJECTION OF THE CENTRAL RAY:

Direct the central ray perpendicular to the cassette through the central axis of the ear rods and the auditory canals.

RADIOGRAPHIC FACTORS:

Film Holder: 10 x 12 (phototimer cassette) with high speed film and stationary grid.

Film: Screen Film (RPL 54 Kodak).*

Source-Film Distance: 60″ (5 ft.).

Exposure Factors: 80 kVp—100 mA, .3 seconds (Rotating anode and phototimer).

Posteroanterior Cephalometric Technic

Head Position: The patient's head is positioned with the patient facing the film. This allows for less distortion of the facial structures which are the most important to the orthodontist. The patient's head is immobilized in the head holder by means of the nasion positioning rod, the infraorbital marker and the ear plugs. The patient's mid-sagittal plane should be perpendicular to the plane of the cassette (See Figure 10-21).

PROJECTION OF THE CENTRAL RAY:

The central ray is directed perpendicular to the cassette through the budge of the nose at the nasion (frontonasal suture).

RADIOGRAPHIC FACTORS:

Film Holder: 10 x 12 phototimer cassette with high speed screens and stationary grid.

Film: RPL 54 Kodak Film.®

Source-Film Distance: 5 feet.

Exposure Factors: 80 kVp—100 mA, .5 seconds (Rotating anode and phototimer).

FACTORS IN EXTRAORAL RADIOGRAPHY

In extraoral radiography, the many variables of the exposure must be kept in mind. The most important are kVp, mAS, Source-Film distance, type of screens, type of film, and whether a grid is used or not.

* This is the film used by L.S.U. School of Dentistry Department of Orthodontics.

FACTORS FOR CONVERTING EXPOSURES
FOR CHANGES MADE IN kVp
(Direct Exposures Only)

Original kVp	*New Kilovoltage*						
	60	65	70	75	80	85	90
60	1.0	0.77	0.6	0.47	0.37	0.29	0.25
65	1.29	1.0	0.77	0.61	0.48	0.37	0.32
70	1.66	1.29	1.0	0.79	0.62	0.48	0.42
75	2.1	1.63	1.26	1.0	0.79	0.6	0.52
80	2.66	2.06	1.6	1.26	1.0	0.76	0.66
85	3.48	2.69	2.0	1.65	1.3	1.0	0.87
90	4.0	3.1	2.4	1.9	1.5	1.15	1.0

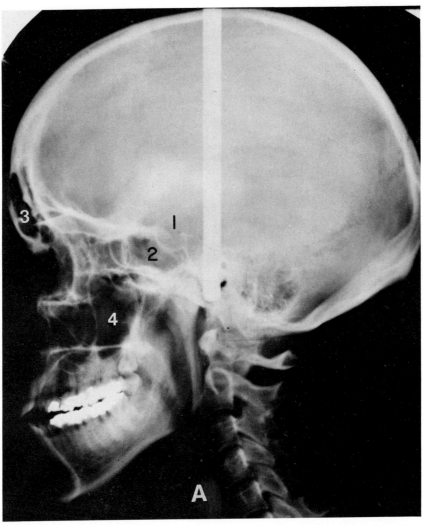

Figure 10-21A. Lateral cephalometric radiograph (1) sella turcica, (2) sphenoid sinus, (3) frontal sinus, (4) maxillary sinus.

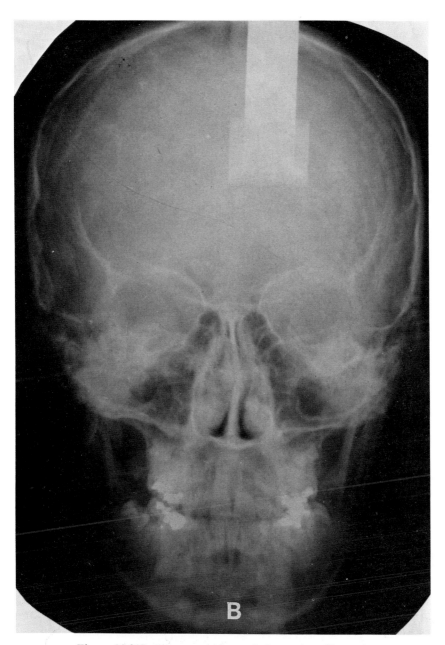

Figure 10-21B. Posteroanterior cephalometric radiograph.

Exposure Factors for Changing Screens. Decrease mAS by 25 percent when changing from medium to high speed screens.

Exposure Factors in Changing Source-Film Distance. The time-distance factors are related to the inverse-square rule.

To produce a given density a different distance then, it is necessary to vary the exposure directly as the square of the distance. The formula is written:

$$\frac{\text{New Time}}{\text{Original Time}} \qquad \frac{\text{New Distance}^2}{\text{Original Distance}^2}$$

TECHNICS FOR MAXILLARY AND MANDIBULAR THIRD MOLARS

Maxillary Third Molar Technic

The distal oblique projection is recommended for the maxillary unerupted or impacted third molars. The distal oblique projection should show the distal half of the first molar, the second molar, and all of the third molar regardless of its position in the tuberosity. The tuberosity, the distal wall and a portion of the floor of the maxillary sinus, the hamular process of the sphenoid bone, and the coronoid process of the ramus of the mandible should be in evidence also. Usually the contacts will be closed because of the distal projection of the x-ray beam.

The Rinn Snap-a-Ray® and the Fitzgerald hemostat film holder are the instruments of choice. If the third molar is erupted, its inclination is used as the guide in film positioning. Generally, the alignment of the long axis of the third molar is tipped more bucally than the second molar; therefore, it is necessary to also take a lateral projection to establish the true relationship of the second and third maxillary molars. If the third molar is not erupted, it is routine practice to incline the film packet to a greater degree in order that all of the maxillary tuberosity will be completely in evidence on the radiograph.

While the distal portion of the film is positioned against the opposite tuberosity, the mesial portion of the film forms an angle with the midpalatal suture (See Figure 10-22). In order to counteract the increased object-film distance in this projection, the long extension cone is recommended.

The correct vertical angulation is determined by the vertical inclination of the film. The operator can estimate this angulation after the patient has closed down on the bite block. The range of the vertical angulation varies from a plus 20° to a plus 36°. A plus 30° vertical angulation usually is a good starting angle to use.

The long extension cone is directed downward and forward so the x-ray beam is directed just under the notch of the inferior border of the zygomatic arch. The notch is about a finger's width anteriorly to the mandibular condyle.

The x-ray beam is directed toward the apices of the third molar. Parallel the film with the open face of the extension cone to minimize distortion.

Mandibular Third Molar Technic

Occlusal Technic: The occlusal film technic was developed to show buccolingual relationships within the jaws. However, the standard occlusal technic often does not reproduce all of the crown of the impacted mandibular third molar. This is because the ramus of the mandible often times prevents

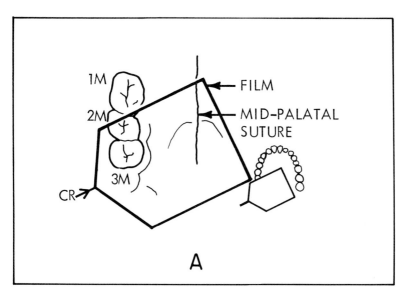

Figure 10-22A. Disto-oblique projection. Position of the film in relation to the mid-suture line, third molar and opposing tuberosity.

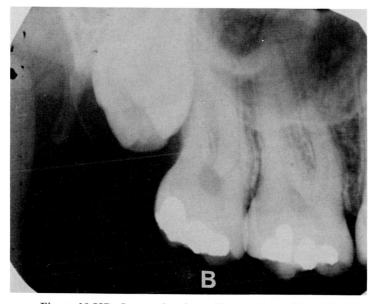

Figure 10-22B. Conventional maxillary molar radiograph.

the distal extension of the film to cover all of the impacted third molar. Substitution of the standard periapical film for the occlusal film has routinely failed to give improved coverage (See Figure 10-23).

MODIFIED OCCLUSAL TECHNIC:

A modified occlusal technic was advocated by Donovan (1952) to remedy this problem (See Figure 10-24). Donovan recommended two changes: (1) a change in the position of the film packet

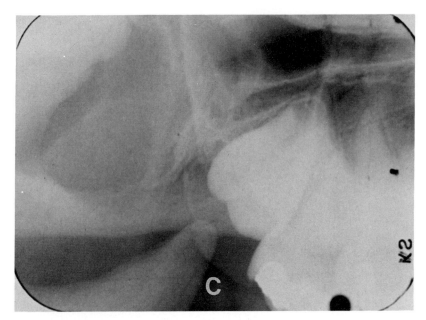

Figure 10-22C. Disto-oblique radiograph of maxillary third molar.

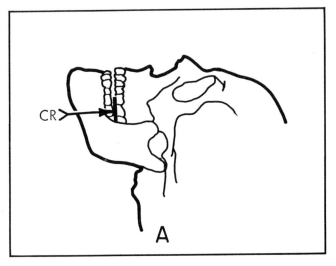

Figure 10-23A. Standard occlusal radiograph of mandibular third molar.

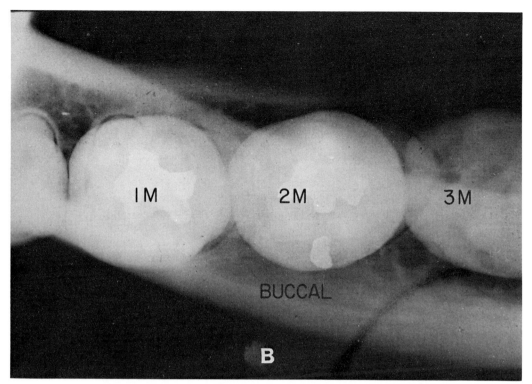

Figure 10-23B. Occlusal radiograph of mandibular third molar.

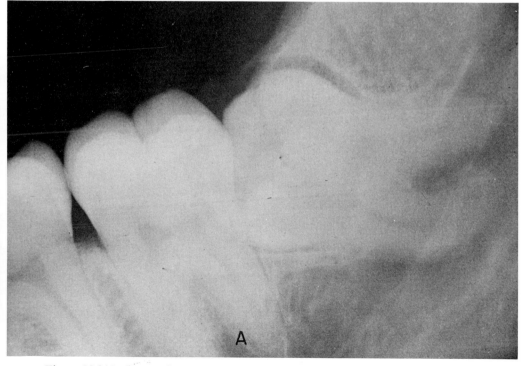

Figure 10-24A. Conventional lateral periapical view of the mandibular third molar.

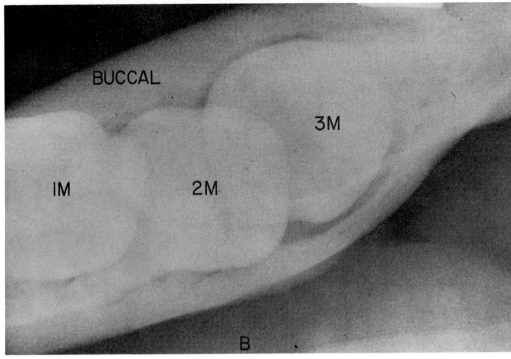

Figure 10-24B. Occlusal view of mandibular third molar using Donovan Technic.

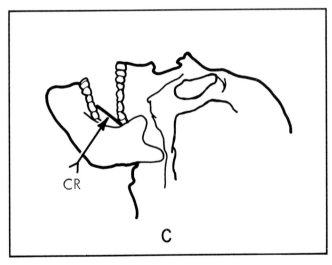

Figure 10-24C. Diagram showing position of the film packet and central ray using Donovan's Technic.

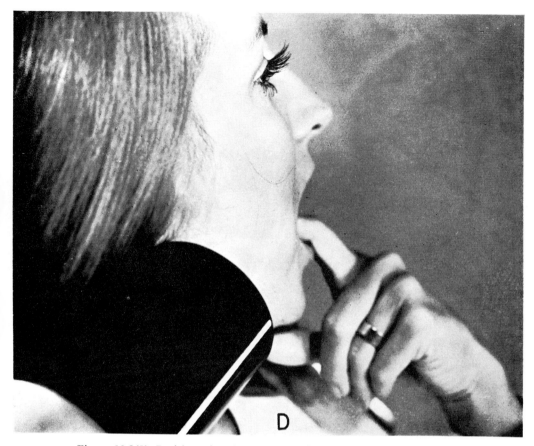

Figure 10-24D. Position of patient's head and cone. (Donovan's Technic)

and (2) a change in the direction of the central ray.

The mouth remains open in this technic, with the periapical film packet permitted to ride up on the edge of the mandible. The film packet is held in place by the patient's index finger at a point where the film packet touches the occlusal surface of the mandibular teeth. The film should not be allowed to bend. If desired, the larger occlusal film may be used. The central ray is again directed at right angles to the film packet, but in this improved technic the patient's head must be rotated away from the x-ray head so the short cone may come in close proximity to the angle of the mandible.

Periapical Radiography of Mandibular Third Molars

In the past, most textbooks have recommended a vertical angulation ranging from 0 to −15 degrees. However, when the anatomy of the third molar is examined, it will be discovered that the third molar in most cases has a lingual inclination of between 0 to 15 degrees. Therefore, in order to avoid distortion, the vertical angulation of the cone

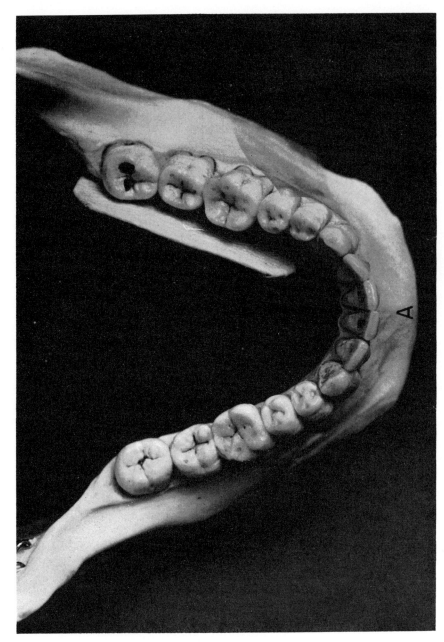

Figure 10-25A. Periapical radiograph of mandibular third molar. In most cases, a periapical film placed in the mandibular third molar region will flare lingually.

should have a positive angulation of between 0 to 15 degrees rather than the negative angulation recommended. A positive angulation of 15 degrees is a good starting point (See Figure 10-25).

The film is placed in the Rinn Snap-a-Ray® and inserted into the mouth until the anterior border of the film is opposite the middle third of the mandibular first molar. Have the patient close on the bite block. Rapid and shallow breathing usually overcomes the

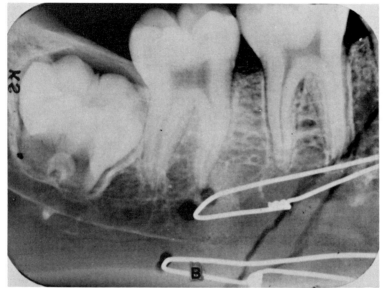

Figure 10-25B. Impacted third molar taken by using a —5° vertical angulation.

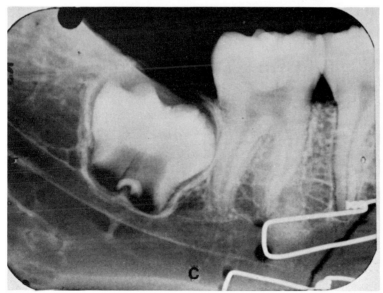

Figure 10-25C. The same impacted third molar taken by using a +15° angulation. Notice the superimposition of the buccal and lingual cusps of both the 2nd and 3rd molars.

tendency to gag. The film should always be placed far enough posteriorly to include the distal roots; low enough to show a small amount of structure past the apices; and high enough to show the relationship of the ascending ramus.

If the patient tends to gag, or if tenderness due to infection or other causes prevents placement of the periapical film intraorally, a lateral jaw radiograph of the mandible or a panoramic film may be indicated.

RADIOGRAPHY OF EDENTULOUS JAWS

Past studies have shown that approximately one out of four edentulous patients have residual roots, unerupted and supernumerary teeth, cysts, residual areas of infection, and foreign bodies. Four types of edentulous surveys are available:

1. A mixed occlusal-periapical survey.
2. An occlusal-lateral jaw survey.
3. A complete periapical survey.
4. A panoramic radiograph.

Mixed Occlusal-Periapical Survey

The mixed occlusal-periapical survey consists of the following film:

One maxillary topographical occlusal film.

One mandibular cross-sectional occlusal film.

Four molar standard (#2) periapical films.

The occlusal films give an excellent bucco-lingual view of the major portions of the jaws (See Figure 10-26). However, the occlusal film does not, in most cases, give the detail to edentulous ridges that the periapical survey will give. The most posterior areas which are difficult for the occlusal films to cover are taken by

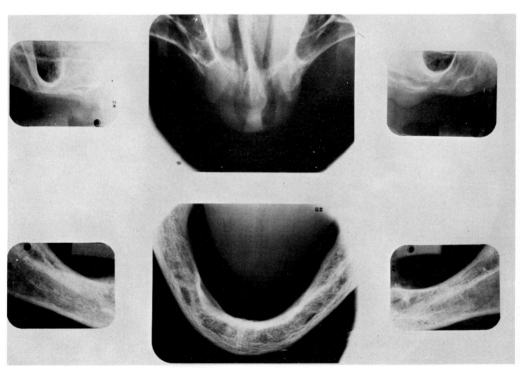

Figure 10-26. Mixed occlusal periapical edentulous survey.

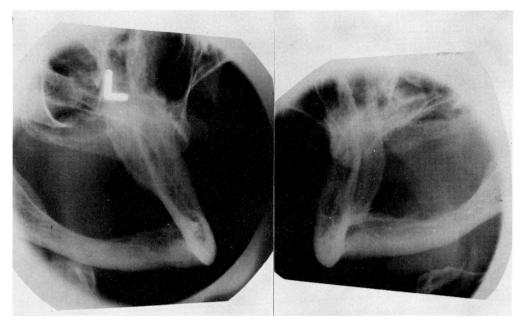

Figure 10-27. Lateral jaw edentulous radiographs (left and right).

means of four periapical films. This type of survey is usually indicated in new patients who have worn dentures for a number of years. It is rapid and covers the jaws quite adequately.

Occlusal-Lateral Jaw Survey

This survey consists of the following radiographs:

One maxillary topographical occlusal film.

One mandibular cross-sectional occlusal film.

Two lateral jaw films (right and left side).

This survey may be substituted for the mixed occlusal-periapical survey when the patient will not tolerate intraoral molar periapical films (See Figure 10-27).

Periapical Edentulous Survey

This is usually the edentulous survey of choice and may be taken by either the modified paralleling or bisection of the angle technic (See Figure 10-28).

RECOMMENDED EDENTULOUS PERIAPICAL SURVEY

Exposure Time (Seconds)

Technic	No. of Films	Region	Maxilla	Mandible	Vertical Angulation Maxilla	Mandible
Modif. Paralleling	4	Molar	1½	1	+30	−10
Modif. Paralleling	4	Premolar	1	1	+35	−10
Bisecting Angle	6	Anterior	1	1	+55	−25

Radiographic Factors: kVp—65, mA—10
  Film: #2 Standard, Kodak Ultra-Speed
  Cone: Long (extension)
  Film Holder: Rinn Snap-a-Ray, Rinn XCP instruments with cotton rolls

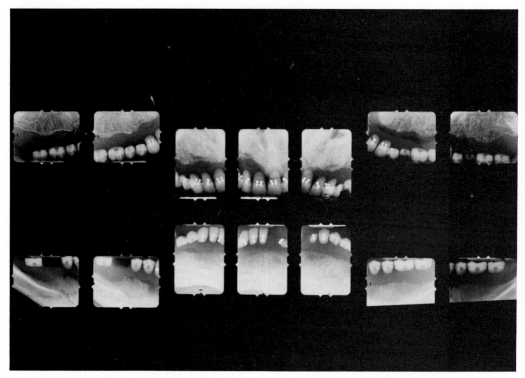

Figure 10-28. The ten film periapical edentulous survey. The patient's dentures were not removed in this case. This is an acceptable technic, as the acrylic dentures do not impede the passage of the x-ray.

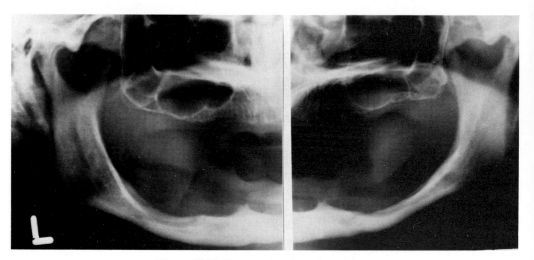

Figure 10-29. Panoramic edentulous survey.

Modified Paralleling Technic Using the Rinn Snap-a-Ray

Place film in the Snap-a-Ray holder and have the patient hold the film parallel to the residual ridge with the fingers of the opposing hand (use the hand of the same side to take the weight off the forearm and holding the film holder). Direct the cone of radiation perpendicular to both the residual ridge and the film. The film may have to be inclined toward the ridge more than usual and the vertical angulation of the cone increased in cases where the edentulous ridges have become exceptionally flat.

The Rinn XCP® instruments can be used in edentulous surveys by utilizing cotton rolls on each side of the bite block.

Panoramic Radiography

The panoramic technic produces an edentulous survey which provides exceptional coverage of both jaws on one radiograph. It has the disadvantage of not having the clarity of detail as revealed on the periapical radiograph (See Figure 10-29).

LOCALIZATION TECHNICS

The dental radiograph is a two dimensional picture of a three dimensional object and lacks perspective depth. Localization by the use of dental radiographs must be interpreted by comparison of views taken at different angles of projection, plus an anatomic knowledge of the regions radiographed.

Localization is indicated in the following instances: foreign bodies, broken needles, broken instruments, filling materials in the alveolar process, retained roots, impacted supernumerary and unerupted teeth, calculi in a gland or duct of salivary glands, fractures of the maxilla and mandible, fracture of condyles, and expansion of the alveolar process in cystic formation. The methods of localization are as follows:

1. Stereoscopic method
2. Clark's method
3. Buccal-Object rule
4. Periapical-Occlusal method (Miller's Technic)

Stereoscopic Method

This method is seldom used at the present time because of the development of more accurate and simplified methods. Stereography is a radiographic procedure of producing a pair of radiographs identical in all respects. The tube is shifted horizontally a distance equal to the distance between the pupils of the eye. The radiographs so produced are viewed by means of a device known as a stereoscope. It is very difficult to duplicate the position of the film and the cone for two separate exposures. Also, it is difficult to mount the radiographs accurately in the stereoscope and train the eye to view them.

Clark's Method

This method was first described by C. Clark (1909). It is used to determine the buccolingual relationship of foreign objects, and impacted or unerupted teeth within the jaws. The method requires two periapical radiographs of the area in question. The vertical angulation is fixed for each exposure while the horizontal angulation is varied (See Figure 10-30). If the foreign object moves in an opposite direction to the horizontal shift of the tube, the object is buccal or labial to the remaining teeth within the jaws.

If the foreign object moves in the same direction as the horizontal tube shift, the object is lingual to the remaining teeth within the jaws.

Buccal-Object Rule

This method of localization was suggested by Richards (1952) as a means of localizing the mandibular canal. In general, the x-ray image on a radiograph can be shifted relative to a lingual object by projecting the x-ray beam in that direction (whether it be mesially or distally, superiorly or inferiorly). Therefore, a buccal object will move with the change in angulation of the cone (whether up or down or left or right).

With this technic the relation of the apices of the mandibular third molar with the mandibular canal can be estimated.

Two radiographs are needed. The first radiograph is a routine view of the mandibular third molar. The second radiograph is taken with −20° change in vertical angulation. If the mandibular canal is buccal to the apices of the mandibular third molar, the mandibular canal image will move superiorly to the image of the mandibular apices in the resultant radiograph. If the mandibular canal is lingual to the apices of the mandibular third molar, the mandibular

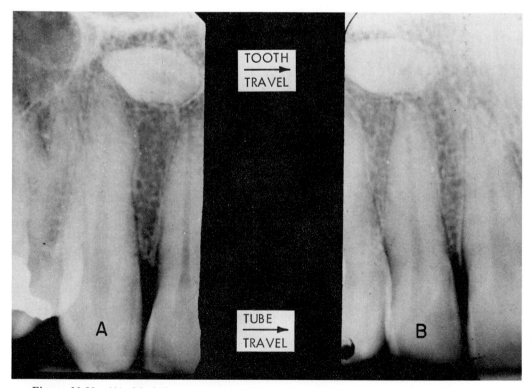

Figure 10-30. (A) Mesiodens (extra tooth) is situated between maxillary canine and lateral incisor teeth. (B) Mesiodens has moved in same direction as tube toward the apex of the maxillary lateral incisor. Therefore, the mesiodens is lingual to the incisor teeth.

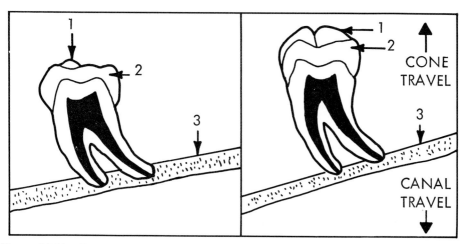

Figure 10-31. (A) Conventional lateral view of mandibular third molar. (1) Lingual cusps. (2) Buccal cusps. (3) Mandibular canal. (B) Radiograph produced with a negative 20° (upward) angulation in x-ray cone. The mandibular canal is lingual to the roots of the 3rd molar because canal moves in opposite direction of movement of cone.

canal will move superiorly, or in the opposite direction the vertical angulation change of the cone (See Figures 10-31 and 10-32).

Periapical-Occlusal Method

While Clark's Method is applicable to many cases where unerupted teeth are to be localized, the likelihood of good results in the region of the mandibular third molar is more predictable with the periapical-occlusal method of localization as first suggested by Dr. Fred Miller (1914) and later popularized by Winter (1926) (See Figure 10-33).

This technic requires two radiographs to be made of the area under investigation which includes (1) a periapical view

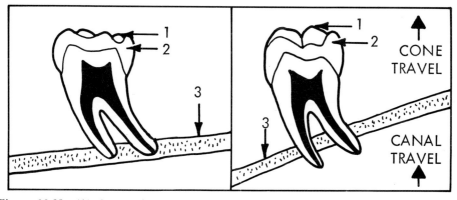

Figure 10-32. (A) Conventional lateral view of mandibular third molar. (1) Lingual cusps. (2) Buccal cusps. (3) Mandibular canal. (B) Radiograph produced with a negative 20° (upwards) angulation of the x-ray cone. The mandibular canal is buccal to the roots of the 3rd molar because the canal moves in the same direction of movement of the cone.

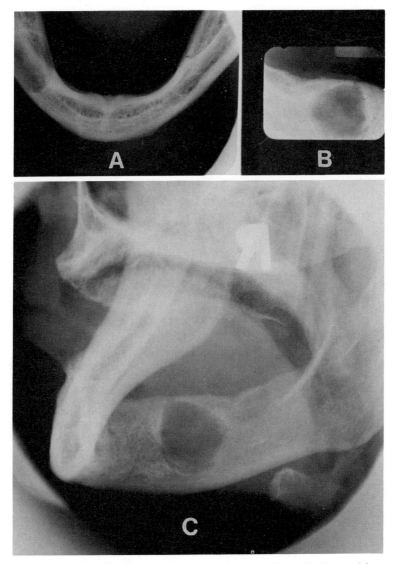

Figure 10-33. Periapical-occlusal-lateral jaw localization technic. Patient with a residual bone cyst. (A) Occlusal cross-sectional radiograph. (B) Periapical radiograph. (C) Lateral jaw radiograph of same patient.

to establish the mesiodistal and superio-inferior relationship between a fixed landmark and the object to be localized and (2) an occlusal view to determine the bucco-lingual relationship (See Figure 10-24 and 10-33).

ENDODONTIC RADIOGRAPHY

In endodontic therapy it is important that the radiograph produced is anatomically accurate.

The paralleling technic is the method of choice. The Rinn paralleling instruments can be used (See Figure 10-34).

Remove the rubber dam to one side. Place the Rinn anterior instrument in the mouth so that the patient bites on a tooth *adjacent* to the tooth with the measuring file in it. Do not place the cotton roll on the same arch unless the patient has teeth of less than average crown-root length and/or patient's with flat vaults. Moreover, it may be advantageous to offset the #2 film in the XCP anterior instrument in order to center the tooth under examination on the radiograph.

For radiographing the buccolingual rooted premolar teeth, use the anterior Rinn XCP instrument or the Rinn Snap-a-Ray instrument if the patient cannot tolerate the Rinn XCP instrument. Off-

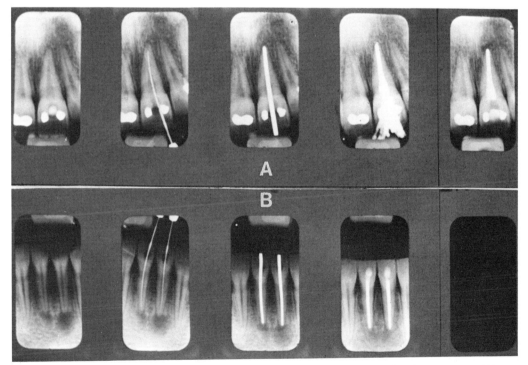

Figure 10-34. Endodontic radiographs using the Rinn XCP Anterior instrument. (A) Series of radiographs used in treating the root canal of a maxillary left central incisor. (B) Series of radiographs used in treating root canals of the mandibular central incisors. (Radiographs courtesy of Dr. Vander Voorde, Moline, Ill.)

set the film in the XCP holder and place the film as if you were taking a canine projection. Direct the central ray in a mesio-oblique 15 degree horizontal angulation. This will separate the buccal and lingual roots of the maxillary first premolar (See Figure 10-35).

For radiographing the tri-rooted maxillary molar teeth, the same procedure is followed as with bucco-lingual rooted 1st premolars. However, the preoperative film should establish the relationship of the lingual root to the mesiobuccal and distobuccal root. If this relationship is unknown from previous radiographs, it

is well to take a standard lateral view, as well as a disto-oblique and mesio-oblique projections. These series of radiographs should give the endodontist an unobstructed view of these three roots. Radiographs taken with files in the roots should be approached from the standpoint of not superimposing the buccal root over the lingual root; therefore, the mesio-oblique, or disto-oblique radiograph will be indicated, depending upon the configuration of the roots.

For illustration of root canal x-ray examination of multirooted teeth see Figure 10-36.

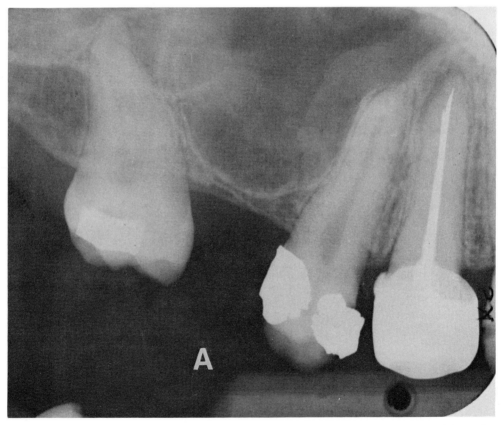

Figure 10-35A. Radiograph of maxillary premolar region showing superimposition of buccal and lingual roots of maxillary 1st premolar.

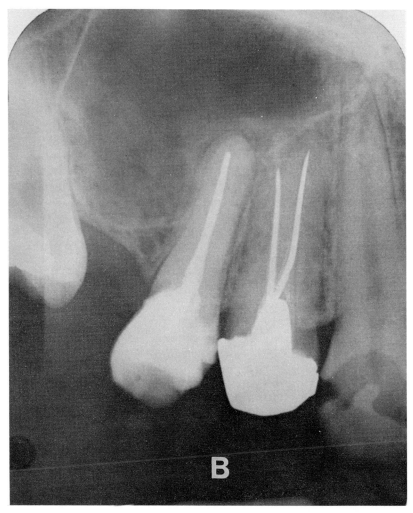

Figure 10-35B. Radiograph taken with distal projection of cone to separate buccal and lingual roots of maxillary 1st premolar.

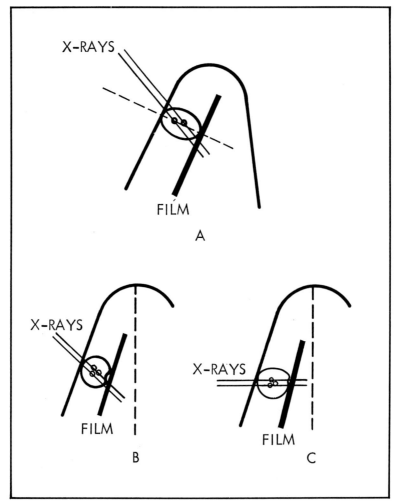

Figure 10-36. Radiographic technics for multirooted teeth. (A) In the conventional lateral radiograph of the maxillary 1st premolar the buccal root is superimposed over the lingual root. To be able to see both roots in the maxillary 1st premolars, direct the x-ray slightly mesiodistally at approximately 15° from the perpendicular. (B) A slight mesial direction of the x-ray will produce an image of the disto-buccal roots of the maxillary molar. (C) The slight distal direction of x-rays will produce a distinct image of the mesio-buccal roots of the maxillary molars.

SIALOGRAPHY

Sialography may be defined as a technic whereby the ducts and the parenchyma of the major salivary glands can be demonstrated radiographically by the introduction of radiopaque contrast material into the main secretory duct of the gland. It is used to study the parotid and submandibular salivary glands.

The most widely utilized contrast media in sialography are Lipiodol®,

Ethiodol® and Pantopaque®.

Lipiodol is a stable iodized poppy seed oil (40% by weight of iodine). Its main disadvantage is its viscosity. It requires slow injection and about thirty days for complete absorption from the gland.

Ethiodol is an ethyl ester of an iodized fatty acid of poppy seed oil (37% organically bound iodine). It has a lower viscosity than Lipiodol.

Pantopaque (ethyl iodophenyl undeylate) is an oil base type of contrast media similar to Lipiodol and Ethiodol, but with a lower viscosity. It flows well and is excreted from the gland within a short period of time.

The basic armamentarium for sialog-raphy includes blunt-ended lacrimal duct dilators, a number of blunt-ended 22 to 26 gauge needles, and a 3 ml syringe.

In all cases, routine radiographs are made prior to sialography to determine the presence of calculi within the ducts and glands. The basic preliminary views are as follows:

1. A cross-sectional mandibular occlusal projection through the floor of the mouth at right angles to the occlusal film. This view will reveal a sialolith (salivary stone) only if it is located toward the orifice of the Wharton's duct.

2. To further localize stones in the

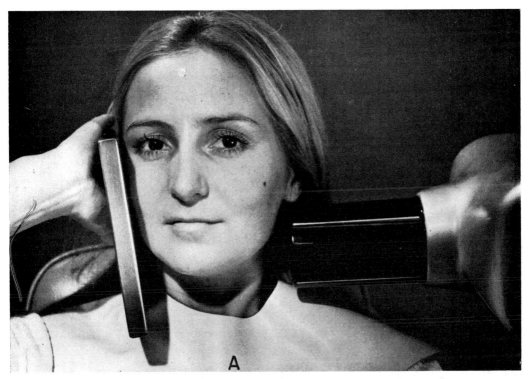

Figure 10-37A. Lateral submandibular gland projection. The head is held erect, the cassette is placed against the face and is held perpendicular to the floor and parallel to the sagittal plane. The x-rays are directed just below the lower border of the mandible at the angle. The exposure time is reduced to bring out the soft tissue of the gland.

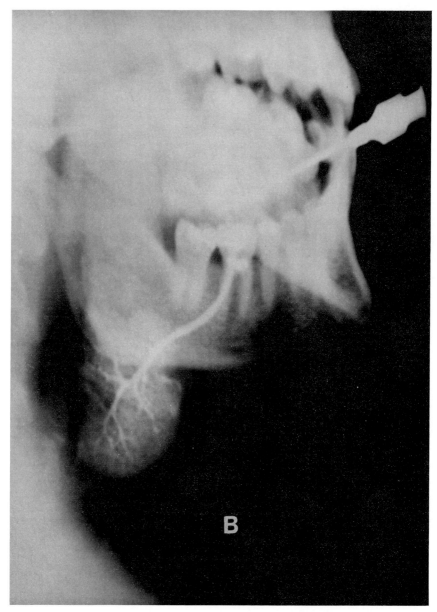

Figure 10-37B. Radiograph of submandibular gland after injection of radiopaque liquid into Wharton's Duct. (Courtesy of Dr. James Quinn, Oschner Clinic, New Orleans, Louisiana.)

salivary glands a true lateral radiograph is of value. This is exposed by directing the central ray perpendicular to a 5 x 7 cassette held by the patient. The patient's head is held erect with the midsagittal plane perpendicular to the floor. The exposure time should be decreased to bring out the soft tissue of the salivary glands.

The orifices of Stenson's duct and Wharton's duct may be easier to find if the patient sucks on a lemon first. Once the orifice is found, it can be dilated by means of the lacrimal probes. Then, insert the blunt-ended needle into the duct for 0.5 to 1 cm. Do not insert the needle very far into Stenson's duct because the duct forms a sharp angle as it is passed through the buccinator muscle. After insertion of the needle, the plunger of the syringe is withdrawn slightly so that the residual saliva in the duct is removed, leaving a space for the liquid to flow. This will relieve the patient from discomfort. The injection is made slowly, and pain or swelling of the gland is an indication that the injection should be stopped. Inject about 1.5 cc into the parotid gland and 1 cc into the submandibular gland. The needle can then be withdrawn and the patient asked to compress the orifice with his thumb and forefinger until the time of the radiographic exposure. Other operators prefer to leave the syringe in position while the radiograph is taken as it controls the leakage of the contrast media into the floor of the mouth.

The true lateral jaw is probably the technic of choice for the salivary glands

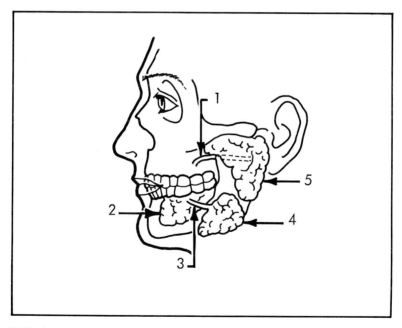

Figure 10-38. Anatomical position of the salivary glands and their relation to the maxilla and the mandible. (1) Stenson's duct (parotid gland). (2) Sublingual gland. (3) Wharton's duct. (4) Submandibular gland. (5) Parotid gland.

(See Figure 10-37). It produces a clearer, undistorted view of each gland. An occlusal radiograph may be useful in depicting calculus in the anterior portion of Wharton's duct. Panoramic radiography has been found to be an excellent technic for demonstrating contrast media in the salivary glands. Pappas (1970) has described a sialographic technic used with the orthopantomograph.

Only one gland should be radiographed at a time. If other glands must be examined, they can be done at a later time. It depends on the time required to eliminate the radiopaque material from the glands. The time required to eliminate the contrast media depends on the viscosity of liquid used. See Figure 10-38 for the anatomical positions of the major salivary glands and their ducts.

Sialography is useful in the demonstration of salivary stones, strictures, and recurrent infections of the salivary glands. It is particularly useful in confirming the presence of a suspected tumor in the salivary gland region. Sialography is contraindicated in acute inflammation of the glands or in patients with a history of sensitivity to radiopaque contrast media.

PEDODONTIC RADIOGRAPHY

Complete mouth radiographs are recommended at the first dental examination of the child. Radiographs will reveal additional dental problems in more than 50 percent of the young patients radiographed. A complete radiographic survey of children will reveal many conditions which cannot be discovered by any other method. They are (1) morphology and related hard tissues; (2) dental caries; (3) environment of the root ends of the primary teeth; (4) extent and quality of the calcification of the crowns of the permanent teeth; (5) dental anomalies (shape, size, number, position, and texture); (6) alterations in the integrity of the periodontal membrane; (7) alterations in the supporting hard structures of the teeth; and (8) injuries to the teeth and supporting structures (trauma, dilaceration, and foreign bodies).

There are certain common-sense rules to follow in taking radiographs of a child and these are suggested for application as the case demands:

1. Acquaint the child with the radiographic apparatus and the contemplated procedure *before* inserting the film. Having the child place his hand at the end of the cone and making a short exposure with the machine turned off will help allay fear and create confidence. Be sure lead apron has been draped over the child's body.

2. Position the machine with the approximate angulation and correct timer setting BEFORE placing the film in the mouth.

3. Try to use the largest film possible for the patient with consideration of the following factors: (a) information sought by the examination; (b) development of the oral structures; (c) age of patient; and (d) cooperation of the patient. If impingement occurs, try to relieve

SURVEY	FILM RETENTION	SIZE AND TYPE OF FILM	NUMBER OF FILMS
A. EARLY ERUPTIVE GROUP -- UP TO 6 YEARS OF AGE (2 to 6 years):			
1. Periapical, Posterior Bite-Wing Survey		All Kodak Ultra-Speed	
a. Periapicals	1) Rinn Snap-a-Ray 2) Ant. XCP with Pedo. backing 3) Stabe Disposable Film Holder	O Child Film	4 Post. (2 Max. & 2 Mand.) 6 Ant. (3 Max. & 3 Mand.)
b. Bite-wings Posterior	Bite-Wing Tab For O Film	O Child Film	2 Post. (L & R)
			TOTAL FILMS - 12
2. Pedodontic Anterior Occlusal, Periapical, Posterior Bite-Wing Survey		All Kodak Ultra-Speed	
a. Occlusal views, ant. max. & mand.	Patient bites gently on film	Standard #2 Size	2 (Max. & Mand.)
b. Periapicals	1) Rinn Snap-a-Ray or 2) Stabe Disposable Film Holder	O Child Film	4 (2 Max. & 2 Mand.)
c. Posterior Bite-Wings	Bite-Wing Tab For O Film	O Child Film	2 Post. (L & R)
			TOTAL FILMS - 8
B. MIXED DENTITION GROUP (6 to 9 years of age):			
1. Periapical		All Kodak Ultra-Speed	
a. Posterior	1) Rinn Snap-a-Ray or 2) Stabe Disposable Film Holder	Narrow #1 Size	4 (2 Max. & 2 Mand.)
b. Anterior	1) XCP with Narrow Film Backing or 2) Stabe Disposable Film Holder	Narrow #1 Size	6 (3 Max. & 3 Mand.)
2. Posterior Bite-Wings	Bite-Wing Tab For #2 Film	Standard #2 Size	2 Post. (L & R)
			TOTAL FILMS - 12
C. PREADOLESCENT GROUP (9 to 12 years of age):			
1. Periapical		All Kodak Ultra-Speed	
a. Anterior	1) XCP with Narrow Film Backing or 2) Stabe Disposable Film Holder	Narrow #1 Size	8 (5 Max. & 3 Mand.)
b. Posterior	1) Rinn Snap-a-Ray or 2) Stabe Disposable Film Holder	Standard #2 Size	4 (2 Max. & 2 Mand.)
2. Posterior Bite-Wings	Bite-Wing Tab For #2 Film	Standard #2 Size	2 Post. (L & R)
			TOTAL FILMS - 14

Figure 10-39. Children radiographic surveys for various age groups.

corners by bending. If this fails, reduce the size of the film. Remember though, that each film of the survey must be of the same size to be properly mounted.

4. For retention of the film, use the *Rinn Snap-a-Ray* or *Stabe* Film holders for posterior areas. Have patient close firmly but gently, using just enough pressure to hold the film holder in place. For the anterior teeth use the Rinn XCP anterior instrument or a Stabe film holder. When using the Standard Size #2 periapical film as a child anterior occlusal film, have the patient bite gently to secure the film.

5. Take the easiest areas first to inspire confidence and gain cooperation. The anterior occlusals, anterior periapicals, and posterior bitewing films are generally the easiest areas, and the posterior periapicals are the most difficult. Remember again that films should be all the same size in each complete survey.

6. Hold the attention of the patient by an upraised finger and an admonition to "hold steady" during the actual exposure.

7. Encourage the patient after each exposure.

See Figure 10-39 for a table of radiographic surveys for various age groups.

CHILDREN'S RADIOGRAPHIC TECHNICS

The Early Eruptive Groups (2 to 6 years)

There are two complete radiographic surveys which are recommended for the 2 to 6 age group. These are the periapical-bitewing complete survey (See Figure 10-40) and the anterior occlusal, periapical and bitewing complete survey (See Figure 10-46). Also, the panoramic radiograph taken with posterior bitewings is an excellent technic for this age group (See Figure 10-50).

A brief description of each technic will be given in outline form.

Head Position: Except when otherwise noted, the standard head position is in the tragal-ala plane parallel to the floor and the mid-sagittal plane perpendicular to the floor. To minimize movement of the preschool child, the dental chair should be adjusted so that the head, back, arms and feet are well supported.

Bite-Wing Technic (for the Early Eruptive Group and the Mixed Dentition Group)

PURPOSE: Caries detection.

FILM: Type 0, #1, or #2 film with bitewing tabs depending on age and size of child. (Use child size type of bitewing tab for type 0 film.)

FILM POSITION: The film should include the distal of the canines. For children 12 and over, take a premolar and molar bitewing radiograph on both sides.

TECHNIC:

Vertical Angulation: 8 degrees downward.

Horizontal Angulation: The front of the x-ray cone is parallel to the buccal surfaces of the posterior teeth.

TYPE OF CONE: Long cone (16″ Source-Film distance).

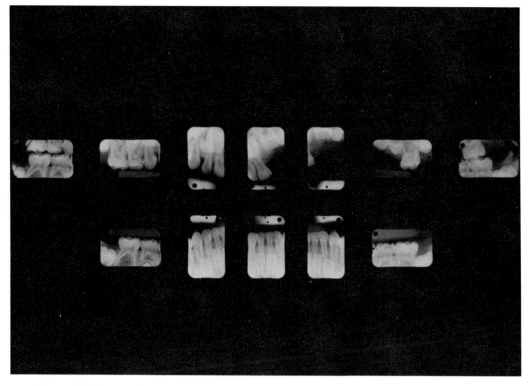

Figure 10-40. Complete mouth x-ray survey of child under 5 years of age using 12 (child size 0 type) films (6 anterior films, 4 posterior films, and 2 posterior bitewings).

ENTRY OF THE CENTRAL RAY: Midpoint of the film.

Anterior Periapical Technic (All Age Groups)

PURPOSE: Caries detection, periapical infection, supernumerary teeth, and missing teeth.

FILM: Type #0, and Type #1 Narrow.

FILM RETENTION: The film is held lingual and parallel with the long axes of the anterior teeth by the anterior XCP instrument with the appropriate backing. The child bites on the holder to secure the film (See Figure 10-41).

CONE: Long (16" Source-Film distance). The **Stabe** disposable periapical x-ray film holder may be used with the child patient. It is made of rigid, non-elastic plastic. It retains the film and prevents film bending (See Figure 10-42). The bite portion of the **Stabe** film holder is perpendicular to the film plane. The film and film holder are retained in position by having the patient bite gently into the bite portion of the film holder. The teeth should indent the plastic, which in turn will secure the film and holder in position (see Figure 10-43). Both the bisecting-angle and paralleling technics may be used with the **Stabe** film holder.

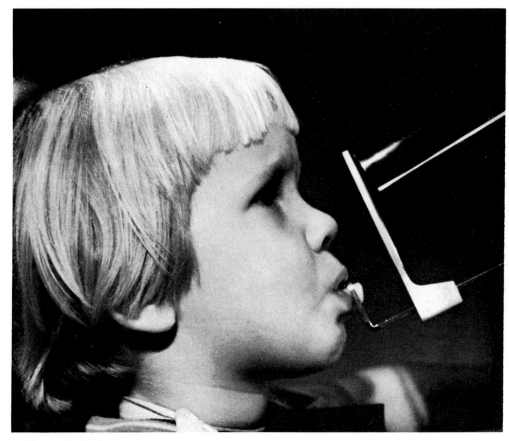

Figure 10-41. Maxillary anterior projection of child under 5 years of age using Rinn XCP instrument.

Posterior Periapical Technic (All Age Groups)

PURPOSE: Caries detection, periapical infection, supernumerary teeth and missing teeth.

FILM: Type #0, #1, and #2 standard.

FILM RETENTION: (a) Rinn paralleling or bisecting instrument, (b) Rinn Snap-a-Ray instrument (See Figure 10-44), (c) **Stabe** disposable film holder, (d) digital bisecting technic (See Figure 10-45).

CONE: Long (16" Source-film distance).

TECHNIC: *Rinn Snap-a-Ray and Stabe Disposal Film Holder:* The film is held lingually and parallel to the long axes of the posterior teeth by the film holder. The child bites on bite block to secure the film.

VERTICAL ANGULATION: Direct the central beam at right angles to the long axes of the teeth and film. Minimize film bending.

HORIZONTAL ANGULATION: The face of the cone should be parallel to the facial surface of the teeth to be radiographed.

DIGITAL METHOD: The film is held

into position by the child's fingers or thumb. The digital method is used when the child cannot tolerate the film holder. The bisecting-angle technic is always used with the digital method of film retention (See Figure 10-45).

The Anterior Occlusal Periapical Complete Survey is a popular survey for children between the ages of 2 to 6.

a. Maxillary Pedodontic Anterior Occlusal Film (Age 2-6 years)

PURPOSE: Caries detection, supernumerary teeth, missing teeth, anterior spacings, heavy frenum, and injuries to the incisor teeth (See Figures 10-46 and 10-47).

FILM: Type #2 standard adult film.

FILM POSITION: The sensitive side of the film faces the maxillary teeth, symmetrical to the mid-sagittal plane with approximately 1/4″ of the packet protruding labially to the central incisors. The child bites gently to secure the film.

TECHNIC:

Vertical Angulation: 60 degrees downward.

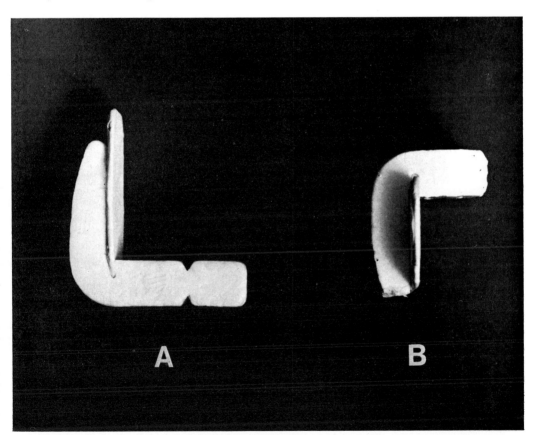

Figure 10-42. (A) The Stabe Disposal Film Holder with a child's size 0 film inserted vertically for an anterior projection. (B) The Stabe Disposal Film Holder with a 0 size film placed horizontally for the posterior projections. The film holder is soft and may be altered to accommodate itself in the small mouths of children under 5 years of age.

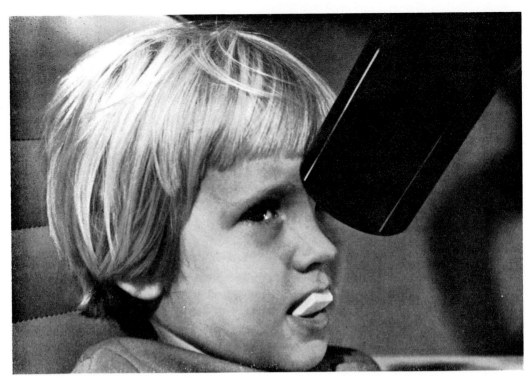

Figure 10-43. Maxillary anterior projection using the Stabe Film Holder in a child under 5 years of age. Since the paralleling technic is being utilized in this case, the x-ray beam is directed perpendicularly toward the film. This is not a short cone technic as it may seem in this illustration because the tube head has a recessed focal spot which extends the source-film distance.

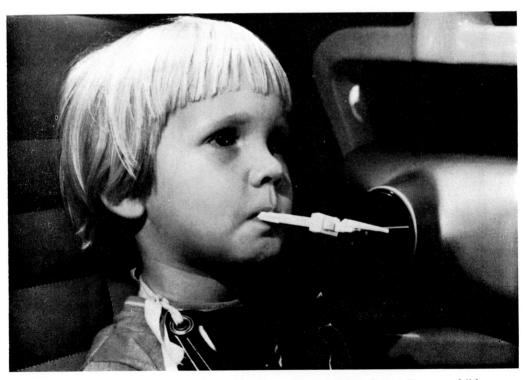

Figure 10-44. Mandibular posterior projection using the Rinn Snap-a-Ray on children under 5 years of age.

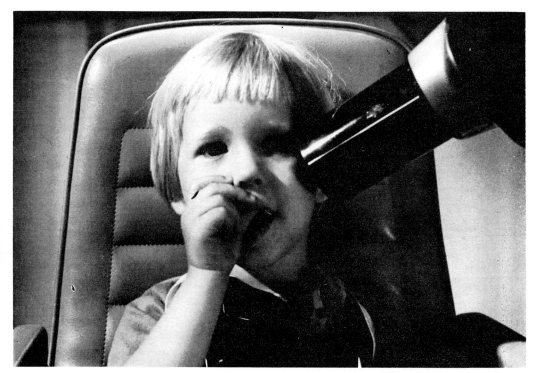

Figure 10-45. Maxillary primary molar projection using digital bisecting technic in a child under 5 years of age. Use the 0 child-size film in children under 5 years of age.

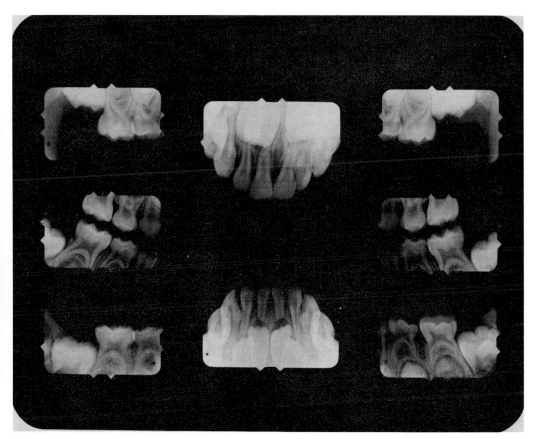

Figure 10-46. Complete radiographic survey in children under 5 years of age using #2 regular size film in anterior region with occlusal projection technic.

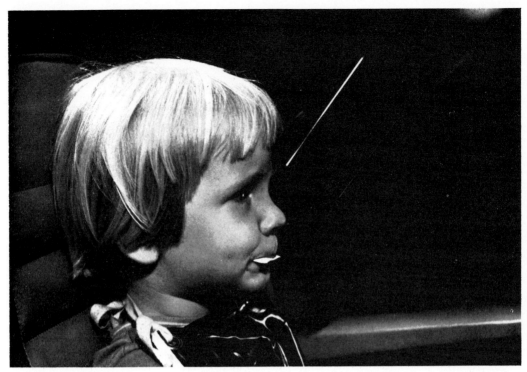

Figure 10-47. Maxillary occlusal projection in children under 5 years of age using #2 regular film.

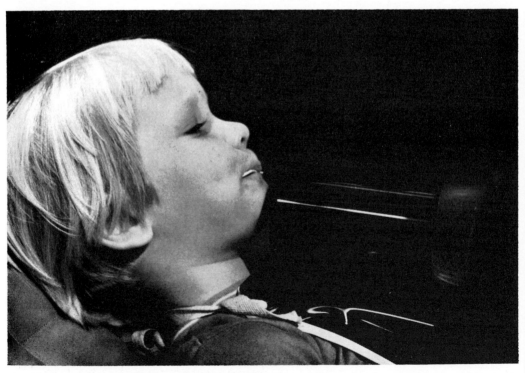

Figure 10-48. Mandibular occlusal projection in a child under 5 years of age using a #2 regular film.

Horizontal Angulation: The central beam is directed along the mid-sagittal plane.

Cone: Short (8″).

Entry of the Central Beam: The point of entry of the central beam will be about ½ inch above the tip of the nose directed at the apices of the central incisors.

b. Mandibular Pedodontic Anterior Occlusal (Age 2-6 years)

Purpose: Caries detection, supernumerary teeth, missing teeth, and injuries to the incisor teeth.

Head Position: The head is tilted back with the chin elevated. The mid-sagittal plane is vertical (See Figure 10-48).

FILM: #2 Adult Standard.

CONE: Short (8″).

FILM POSITION: The sensitive side of the film faces the mandibular teeth, symmetrical to the mid-sagittal plane with approximately ¼″ of the packet protruding labially to the central incisors. The child bites gently to secure the film.

TECHNIC:

Vertical Angulation: The central ray forms a 60 degree angle with the film packet, or use a −15 degree (cone upward) angulation and direct the central beam perpendicular to the line that bisects the angle formed by the lower central incisors and the film.

Horizontal Angulation: The central beam is directed along the mid-sagittal plane.

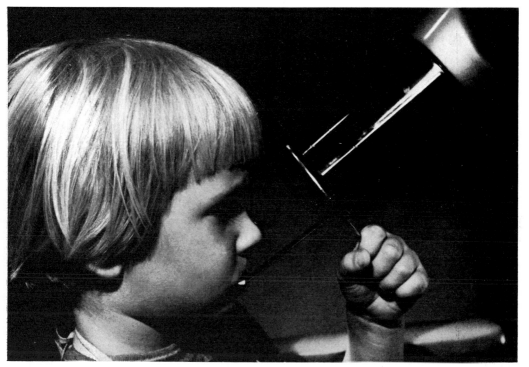

Figure 10-49. Maxillary occlusal technic in a child under 5 years of age using the Precision X-Ray Filmholder.

Entry of the Central Beam: At the apices of the lower incisors.

Medwedeff (1967) described an occlusal technic for preschool children using a flat **Precision** instrument (See Figure 10-49). The film is positioned parallel to the occlusal plane by the aid of a special occlusal instrument. The teeth hold the instrument in place while the x-ray cone is aligned with the flat surface of the instrument. While this technic does not produce the anatomical accuracy of the paralleling technic, it does give a full view of the developing dentition.

The Maxillary Posterior Occlusal Film (2-6 years)

Purpose: To reveal the apices and crowns of the maxillary posterior teeth, a portion of the antrum, and a portion of the palate. The lingual roots of the maxillary molars are elongated, and the primary molars and the developing premolars are not separated because of the high angulation of the central beam.

FILM: Adult #2 Standard.

FILM POSITION: The sensitive side of the film faces the maxillary teeth with approximately 1/4″ of the packet protruding bucally to the molars. The anterior edge of the packet is in line with the incisors. The child bites gently to secure the film.

TECHNIC:

Vertical Angulation: 60 degrees downward.

Horizontal Angulation: The central ray passes between the maxillary molars (Primary).

Entry of the Central Beam: At the apices of the primary molars.

Extra-Oral Lateral Jaw Films

Purpose: To view large areas of the body and ramus of the mandible, especially the mandibular posterior teeth. This technic is used when intraoral films are impossible. It is a poor substitute for the B-W film in the detection of interproximal caries.

FILM: 5 x 7 film.

TYPE OF HOLDER AND FILM: (1) No-screen film in cardboard film holder or (2) screen film in a cassette equipped with intensifying screen.

CONE: Short (8″).

FILM POSITION: The film holder is placed between the patient's face and the head rest. The film holder rests on the shoulder and is held by the patient along the anterior border. The chin is elevated and turned so that the side of the face is parallel to the film. The nose is positioned approximately 1/2″ from the holder.

TECHNIC:

Vertical Angulation: 17 degrees upward.

Horizontal Angulation: The central beam is directed at a right angle to the film.

Entry of the Central Ray: 1/2″ behind and below the angle of the jaw of the opposite side.

Panoramic Radiography

This technic is especially useful in children's radiography (See Figure 10-50 and 10-52). It produces a radiograph which reveals the entire mandibulofacial region on a single film. It is a useful diagnostic aid in studying (1) growth and development of the jaws, (2) eruption patterns, (3) the temporomandibular

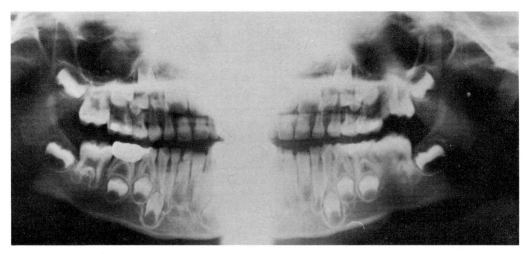

Figure 10-50. Panorex (Pennwalt) radiograph of six-year-old child.

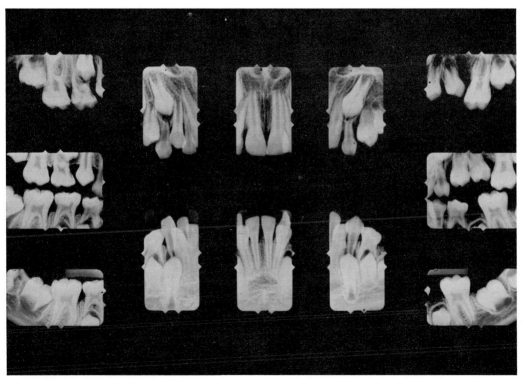

Figure 10-51. Complete radiographic survey (10 #1 films and 2 #2 bitewings) of a child between 6 and 9 years of age.

joint, (4) sinus and mastoid regions, (5) suspected fractures of the jaws, and (6) pathology of the teeth and jaws.

Mixed Dentition Group
(6-9 Years of Age)

The complete periapical survey recommended for the mixed dentition group (6-9 years of age) is the 10-periapical survey with two bitewing films (See Figure 10-51). The periapical films are of the #1 narrow type and the bitewing films are the #2 standard type. The panoramic survey is also a useful diagnostic tool in this age group (See Figure 10-52).

Preadolescent Group (9-12 Years of Age)

The complete periapical survey recommended for the preadolescent group (9-12 years of age) is the 12 periapical survey with two bitewing films. It is identical with the adult survey with the elimination of the molar projections.

Radiography for the Handicapped Patient

The handicapped child can be defined as a child who has a physical, mental or emotional problem. These children present challenging management problems to the radiographer.

Adelson (1961) uses three methods in radiographing a handicapped child: (1) parent assistance, (2) use of relaxant drugs, and (3) general anesthesia.

Many times the child with neuromuscular disorders may be radiographed intraorally with parent assistance. The parent and child should be draped with a lead apron if possible. While the child sits in the parent's lap, the parent holds the child's head steady with one hand. The child bites down on a bitewing tab or film holder, and the parent holds the jaws together with her other hand. Of course, the most rapid exposure factors should be used: 90 kVp—15 mA with ultra-speed film.

If intraoral radiography is impossible, lateral jaw radiographs should be tried. A 5 x 7 cassette with high speed screens should be used. The parent again holds the cassette and child's head steady during exposure. Sometimes a panoramic

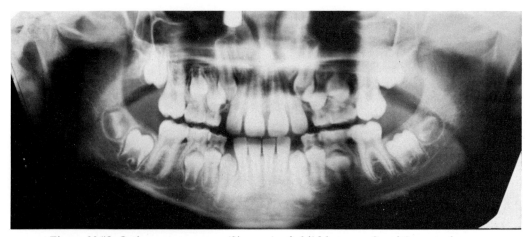

Figure 10-52. Orthopantomogram (Siemens) of child between 6 and 9 years of age.

radiograph can be taken with success; however, the exposure technic may take more time than the patient can remain motionless. A panoramic x-ray unit with a cephalostat is useful in these cases.

Sternberg (1961) recommended the use of a 5 x 7 cassette holder which is positioned on the child's head during exposure. Sometimes in very small children an occlusal film may be used as a lateral jaw.

Relaxant drugs and nitrous oxide analgesia may be used in patients with various behavior problems such as a hyperactive gag reflex or various neuromuscular problems. In some severely handicapped patients, their oral problems are treated under general anesthesia at one session. In these cases it is desirable to take the radiographs in the operating room after the patient has been anesthetized. Adelson (1961) has devised special equipment to facilitate the taking of radiographs while the patient is under general anesthesia.

Hand Radiography

Posteroanterior radiographs of the hand and wrist can be taken with non-screen film in 8 x 10 cardboard film holders. The exposure factors are 65 kVp—10 mA, 24-inch source film distance taken at ¾ second. The central ray should be perpendicular to the plane of the film to avoid distortion.

The handplate is an excellent index to skeletal maturation. This is determined by the number of centers of ossification in the wrist plus the stage of activity of the epiphysis. The epiphysis is that portion of bone which in early life is distinct from the shaft of the bone. If the skeletal age coincides with the chronological age (6-12 months), all is well. Investigators who have attempted to relate development (eruption age or root length) to carpal development have found that they are not strongly correlated. Therefore, dental age is not a good indication of bone age.

REFERENCES

Edentulous Survey

Barr, John H.: An effective and practical roentgenographic technique. *J Can Dent Assoc,* 21:30, 1955.

Cheppe, Erwin: Tabulation and analysis of the results of x-ray examinations of edentulous mouths. *Northwestern U D Res Grad Q Bull,* February 3, 1936, p. 12-15.

Cook, T. J.: Statistics obtained by clinical and roentgenographic examinations of 500 edentulous and partially edentulous mouths. *Dent Cosmos,* 69:349-351, April, 1927.

Eusterman, M. F.: Roentgenographic findings in 290 partially edentulous or edentulous mouths. *Dent Cosmos,* 63:901, September, 1921.

Gardner, B. S., and Stafne, E. C.: Incidence of failure in the removal of teeth. *Am Dent Surg,* 49:321-324, July, 1929.

Landa, J.: *Practical Full Denture Prosthesis,* 2nd ed. Brooklyn, Dental Items of Interest, Chap. 3, p. 23.

Logan, W. H. G.: Should all pulpless and impacted teeth be removed? *J Nat Dent Assoc,* 8:126-131, February, 1921.

Manual for Dental Radiology. Indiana University School of Dentistry, Revised in 1960.

McCall and Wald: *Clinical Dental Roentgenology,* 4th ed. Philadelphia, Saunders, 1957, p. 132.

Molt, F. F.: Value of roentgenograms in edentulous mouths. *J Am Dent Assoc,* 12:788-793, July, 1925.

Smith, E. S.: Findings in the roentgenograms of edentulous patients. *J Am Dent Assoc,* 33:584-587, May, 1946.

Swenson, H. M.: Roentgenographic examination of the edentulous mouth. *J Am Dent Assoc,* 31:475-478, April, 1944.

Waggener, D. T., and Austin, L. T.: Dental structures remaining in 1948 edentulous jaws: A statistical study. *J Am Dent Assoc,* 28:1855-1857, November, 1941.

Extraoral and Intraoral Occlusal Technics

Barr, John H.: *Dental Radiology.* Tufts University, School of Dental Medicine, 1971.

Baume: The direct analysis of cephalometric x-ray films. *Angle Orthodont,* 171-177, July, 1957.

Berry, Harrison M.: Lipiodol in roentgenographic interpretation. *Oral Surg,* 2:1474-1478, November, 1949.

Berry, Harrison M.: Roentgenographic examination. *Current Therapy in Dentistry.* St. Louis, C. V. Mosby, 1966, Vol. 2, pp. 331-365.

Berry, Harrison M.: Roentgenologic aspects of oral surgical problems. *J Oral Surg,* 10:194, July, 1952.

Blady, J. V., and Hocker, A. F.: Sialography, its technique and application in the roentgen study of neoplasm of the parotid gland. *Surg Gynecol Obstet,* 67:777-787, 1938.

Blady, J. V., and Hocker, A. F.: The application of sialography in non-neoplastic diseases of the parotid gland. *Radiology,* 32:131-141, 1939.

Blatt, I. M.: Diseases about the major salivary glands: differential diagnosis. *J Louisiana Med Soc,* 113:60-68, February, 1961.

Blatt, I. M.; Magrelski, J. E.; Maxwell, J. H.; and Holt, J. F.: Secretory sialography in diseases external to major salivary glands. *Annu Otol, Rhinol Laryngol,* 68:175-186, 1959.

Bloom, W. L., Hollenbach, John L., and Morgan, James A.: *Medical Radiographic Technic,* 3rd ed. Springfield, Ill., Charles C Thomas, 1969.

Brandrup-Wognsen, T.: A method of producing roentgenograms of the temporomandibular joint. *J Prosthetic Dent,* 5:93, 1955.

Broadbent, B. Holly: A new technique and its application to orthodontia. *Angle Orthodont,* 1:45-46, 1931.

Brodie, A. C., *et al.*: Cephalometric appraisal of orthodontic results. *Angle Orthodont,* 8:162-182, 261-351, 1938.

Caffey, John: *Pediatric X-ray Diagnosis,* 5th ed. Chicago, Year Book Medical Publishers, 1967.

Caldwell, Eugene W.: Skiagraphy of the accessory sinuses of the nose. *Am Q Roentgenol* (2), 27, 1906-1907.

Carlin and Seldon: Sialography: A useful aid in diagnosing parotid tumors. *J Oral Surg,* 25:139-146, March, 1967.

Castigliano, S. G.: Sialography of the submaxillary gland: A new technique. *Am J Roentgenol,* 187:385-386, February, 1962.

Chayes, C., and Finkelstein, G.: A technique for temporomandibular joint roentgenography. *J Prosthetic Dent,* 6:822, 1956.

Clark, C. A.: A method of ascertaining the relative position of unerupted teeth by means of film radiography. *Odonto Sec Royal Soc Med Trans,* 3:87-89, 1909-1910.

Clark, C. A.: *Bennett's Science and Practice of Dental Surgery.* New York, William Wood, 1914.

Crandell, Clifton: *Dental Radiology for Auxillary Personnel.* Chapel Hill, N. C. University of North Carolina Press, 1972.

Cook and Pollack: Sialography: Pathologic-radiologic correlation. *Oral Surg,* 21:559-573, May, 1966.

Doane, H. F.: Roentgenographic technic and interpretation in fractures of the jaws and facial bones. *J Oral Surg,* 12, April, 1954.

Dolan, Kenneth D.: Radiographic anatomy of nasal sinuses. *Otolaryngologic Clin North Am,* 4:13-24, February, 1971.

Donaldson, Robert G.: Lateral-jaw radiography (All posterior teeth on a single film), *Dent Radiogr Photogr,* 35:58, No. 3, 1962.

Donovan: Occlusal radiography of the mandibular third molars. *Dent Radiol Photogr,* 25:53, No. 3, 1952.

Downs, W. B.: Cephalometrics in orthodontic

case analysis and diagnosis. *Am J Orthodon,* 38:162-182, 1952.

Ennis, Leroy M.; Berry, Harrison M.; and Phillips, James E.: *Dental Roentgenology,* 6th ed. Philadelphia, Lea & Febiger, 1967, pp. 265-273.

Etter, Lewis E.: *Glossary of Words and Phrases Used in Radiology, Nuclear Medicine and Ultrasound,* 2nd ed. Springfield, Ill., Charles C Thomas, 1970.

Gallagher, Walter Neal: *Dental Roentgenology Review.* New York, The William-Frederich Press, 1967.

Gillis, Robert R.: X-rays reveal dysfunction. *Dent Surv,* 15:17-26, January, 1939.

Glasser, Otto (Ed.): *The Science of Radiology.* Springfield, Ill., Charles C Thomas, 1933.

Graber, T. M.: New horizons in case analysis: Clinical cephalometrics. *Am J Orthodont,* 38:603, 1952.

Grant, R., and Lanting, R. T.: Improved technic for roentgenographic examination of temporomandibular joint and condyle. *J Oral Surg,* 11:95, April, 1958.

Grewcock, R. J. G.: A simplified technique of temporomandibular joint radiography. *Br Dent J,* 94:152-154, 1953.

Gruelich, N. W., and Pyle, S. I.: *Radiographic Atlas of Skeletal Development of the Hand and Wrist,* 2nd ed. Stanford University Press, reprinted 1970.

Hanah, Ruhamah: Technique for lateral jaw radiographs. *Alumni Bulletin of the Indiana University School of Dentistry,* February 28, 1955, p. 11.

Hettwer, K. J., and Folsom, T. C.: The normal sialogram. *Oral Surg,* 26:790-799, 1968.

Hofrath, H.: Die Bedeutung der Rontgenfern und Abstrandsanfrauhe Fur die Diagnostiks der Kieferanomalien. *Fortschr Orthodont,* 1:232, 1931.

Jacobi, Charles A.: *X-ray Technology,* 2nd ed. St. Louis, C. V. Mosby, 1960.

Law, David B.; Lewis, Thompson M.; and Davis, John M.: *An Atlas of Pedodontics.* Philadelphia, W. B. Saunders, 1969.

Lewis, Granvelle R.: Temporomandibular joint radiographic technics: comparison and evaluation of results. *Dent Radiogr Photogr,* 37:No. 1, 1964.

Libequrst, B., and Welander, V.: Sialography, new application of substraction technique. *Acta Radiol* (Diag), 8:228-234, 1969.

Lindblom, G.: Technique for roentgenphotographic registration of the different condyle positions in the temporomandibular joint. *Dent Cosmos,* 78:1227-1235, 1936.

Lozier, Matthew: Significance of extraoral roentgenography of the mandible in general practice. *Oral Surg,* 1168-1171, September, 1950.

Lusted, Lee B., and Keats, Theodore: *Atlas of Roentgenographic Measurement.* Chicago, Year Book Medical Publishers, 1967.

Manson-Hing, Lincoln: Use of dental x-rays in roentgenography of the palatopharyngeal mechanism. *Oral Surg,* September, 1970.

Manson-Hing, Lincoln: Utilization of extraoral roentgenographic technics in general dental practice. *Dent Clin North Am,* 437, July, 1961.

Martini, Joseph: Maxillofacial radiography. *Oral Surg,* 3:1540, No. 12, December, 1950.

Matthews, George W.: Value of the occlusal roentgenogram in locating impacted mandibular third molars. *J Am Dent Assoc,* 42: 515-517, May, 1951.

McNeill, Clyde: *Roentgen Technique.* Springfield, Ill., Charles C Thomas, 1946.

McQueen, W. W.: Radiography of the temporomandibular joint articulations. *Minneapolis District Dent J,* 21:28-30, 1937.

Meine, Frederick, and Woloshin, Henry J.: Radiologic diagnosis of salivary gland tumors. *Radiol Clin North Am,* December, 1970, pp. 475-485.

Merill, Vinita: *Atlas of Roentgenographic Positions.* St. Louis, C. V. Mosby, 1949.

Meschan, I.: *Normal Radiographic Anatomy.* Philadelphia, W. B. Saunders, 1959.

Meschan, I.: *Roentgen Signs in Clinical Diagnosis.* Philadelphia, W. B. Saunders, 1956.

Mitchel, D., Jr.: Sialography. *J Oklahoma Med Assoc,* 56:316-321, July, 1963.

Norgaard, F.: *Temporomandibular Orthography.* Copenhagen, E. Mundsgaard, 1947.

Ohm, Morris: Device for roentgenographic localization of tooth remnants in edentulous jaws. *Dent Abstracts,* 3:523, September, 1958.

Ollerenshaw, R.: Sialography—a valuable diagnostic method. *Dent Radiol Photogr,* 29:37, No. 3, 1956.

Ollerenshaw, R., and Rose, S.: Sialography. *Dent Radiol and Photogr,* 33:93, No. 4, 1957.

Osmer, John C., and Pleasants, John E.: Distention sialography. *Radiology,* 86:116-118, July, 1966.

Pappas, Gus, and Wallace, William: Panoramic sialography. *Dent Radiol Photogr,* No. 2, 1970.

Park, William, and Mason, David: Hydrostatic sialography. *Radiology,* 86:116-118, July, 1966.

Poyton, H. G.: Radiographic technique for third molars. *Br Dent J,* April, 1958, p. 241.

Pucini, A. J.: Roentgen ray anthropometry of the skull. *J Radiol,* 3:231-322, 1922.

Richards, A.: Roentgenographic localization of the mandibular canal. *J Oral Surg,* 10: 325, October, 1952.

Richards: Technique for roentgenographic examination of impacted mandibular third molars. *J Oral Surg,* 10:138-141, April, 1952.

Richards and Alling: Extraoral radiography. *Dent Radiol Photogr,* 28:1, No. 1, 1955.

Ricketts, R.: Laminography in the diagnosis of temporomandibular joint disorders. *J Am Dent Assoc,* 46:620, 1953.

Ricketts, R.: The role of cephalometrics in prosthetics diagnosis. *J Prosthetic Dent,* 4: 488, 1956.

Riesner, S.: The T-M joint, its roentgenographic diagnosis and clinical importance. *Arch Clin Oral Pathol,* 4:19, March, 1940.

Schier, Mayer: Temporomandibular joint roentgenography: Controlled erect technics. *J Am Dent Assoc,* 65:456, October, 1962.

Shore, N.: *Occlusal Equilibration and T-M Joint Dysfunction.* Philadelphia, Lippincott, 1959, Chap. 8.

Spillman, R.: Early history of roentgenology of the sinuses. *Am J Radiol,* 54:643-646, 1965.

Thoma, K. H.: The use of radiopaque diagnostic media in roentgen diagnosis of oral surgical conditions. *Am J Orthodont,* 27: 64, February, 1941.

Thurow, Raymond C.: *Atlas of Orthodontic Principles.* St. Louis, C. V. Mosby, 1970.

Todd, T. W.: *Atlas of Skeletal Maturation.* St. Louis, C. V. Mosby, 1937.

Tolman, Dan E.: Roentgenographic techniques. *Stafne's Oral Roentgenographic Diagnosis,* 3rd ed. Philadelphia, W. B. Saunders, 1969.

Updegrave, W. J.: An evaluation of the T-M joint roentgenography. *J Am Dent Assoc,* 46:408-419, April, 1953.

Updegrave, W. J.: Practical evaluation of techniques and interpretation in roentgenographic examination of temporomandibular joints. *Dent Clin North Am,* July, 1961, p. 421.

Updegrave, W. J.: Interpretation of temporomandibular joint radiographs. *Clinics of North America.* Philadelphia, W. B. Saunders, 1966, pp. 567-586.

Updegrave, W. J.: Roentgenographic observations of functioning T-M joints. *J Am Dent Assoc,* 54:488, 1957.

Updegrave, W. J.: Temporomandibular articulation. *Dent Radiol Photogr,* 26:41, No. 3, 1953.

Vogt, E. C., and Vickers, V. S.: *Radiology,* 31: 441, 1938.

Waggener, Donald T.: Roentgenographic localization of unerupted teeth. *Oral Surg,* April, 1960, p. 439.

Waggener and Ireland: Intraoral roentgenography for children. *J Am Dent Assoc,* 47:133-139, August, 1953.

Waters, C. A., and Waldron, C. W.: Roentgenology of accessory nasal sinuses describing modification of occipit-frontal position. *Am J Radiol,* 1915.

Williams: Occlusal radiography. *Dent Radiol Photogr,* 27:50, No. 3, 1954.

Winter, George B.: *Impacted Mandibular Third Molars.* St. Louis, American Medical Book Co., 1926.

Wuehrmann, Arthur H.: *Radiation Protection and Dentistry* (the Postgraduate Dental Lecture Series), St. Louis, C. V. Mosby, 1960, p. 283.

Wuehrmann, Arthur H., and Chilcoat, Aaron: Extraoral techniques, the lateral jaw. *Oral Surg,* 12:1450-1457, 1959.

Wuehrmann, Arthur H., and Manson-Hing, L.: *Dental Radiology.* St. Louis, C. V. Mosby, 1965.

X-rays in Dentistry. Eastman Kodak Co., Rochester, N. Y., 1969.

Yune, H. Y., and Klatte, E. C.: Current status of sialography. *Am J Roentgenol,* 115:420-428, June, 1972.

Zech, Jerome M.: A comparison and analysis of 3 technics of taking roentgenograms of the T-M joint. *J Am Dent Assoc,* 59:725-732, October, 1959.

Zimmer, E. A.: *Schweiz Mschr Zahnheilk,* 51: 949, 1941.

Pedodontic Radiographic Procedure

Adelson, Jerry J.: Handicapped and problem patient: Radiodontic examination and treatment. *Dent Radiogr, Photogr,* No. 2, 1961, pp. 27-45.

Barber, Thomas K.: Roentgenographic techniques for children. *Dent Clin North Am,* November, 1961, p. 549.

Brauer, J. C., et al.: *Dentistry for Children,* 4th ed. Philadelphia, Blakiston, 1959, pp. 327-329.

Cohen, M. M.: *Pediatric Dentistry.* St. Louis, C. V. Mosby, 1957, pp. 249-253.

Ennis, L. M.: Roentgenographic examination of children. *N J State Dent Soc J,* 17:4-9, January, 1949.

Ennis, L. M., and Berry, H.: *Dental Roentgenology,* 5th ed. Philadelphia, Lea & Febiger, 1959, pp. 145-184.

Feasby, W. H.: The number and types of films necessary for a satisfactory radiological survey for children. *J Dent Child,* 2nd Quarter, 1960, p . 91.

Finn, S. B., et al.: *Clinical Pedodontics.* Philadelphia, W. B. Saunders, 1957, pp. 108-127.

Hayden, Jess, and Richards, Albert: Procedures for adequate radiographs of preschool children. *J Dent Child,* 2nd Quarter, 1955, p. 70.

Lozier, Matthew: Periapical roentgenography as applied in children. *Oral Surg,* 3:58-62, January, 1950.

McCall, J., and Wald, S.: *Clinical Dental Roentgenology,* 4th ed. Philadelphia, W. B. Saunders, 1959, pp. 149-179.

Medwedeff, Fred M., and Elcan, Paul D.: A precision technic to minimize radiation. *Dent Surv,* October, 1967.

Mink, John R.: Dental care for the handicapped child. *Current Therapy in Dentistry.* St. Louis, C. V. Mosby, 1966, Vol. 2, pp. 736-767.

Rapp, Robert: Radiographic technics for children. *J Ontario Dent Assoc,* December, 1959, p. 19.

Steinberg, Arnold D.; Braner, May L.; and May, Byron: *The Fortnightly Review,* 41: 9-11, March, 1961.

Updegrave, W. J.: Radiodontic technique for the child patient. *J N J State Dent Soc,* 22: 11, January, 1951.

Updegrave, W.: Simplifying and improving intraoral dental roentgenography. *Oral Surg,* June, 1959, p. 704.

Updegrave, W.: Supplementary radiographic examination for children. *Penn Dent J,* January, 1960, p. 3.

Waggener, D. T., and Ireland, R. L.: Intraoral roentgenography for children. *J Am Dent Assoc,* 47:133, August, 1953.

Wuehrmann, Arthur H.: The long cone technic. *Prac Dent Monogr,* July, 1957.

CHAPTER 11

PANORAMIC RADIOGRAPHY

THE VALUE of any diagnostic procedure is dependent upon the amount and validity of the information that can be obtained from it. The importance of the bite-wing and periapical radiograph as a diagnostic aid is well-documented. However, the periapical and bite-wing radiograph is somewhat limited in their overall coverage of the mandibulo-facial structures. Of course, occlusal and extra-oral radiographs can be used to obtain greater coverage, but these radiographs frequently contain distortion, lack of definition, and superimposition of anatomic structures.

Panoramic radiography overcomes many of these limitations and during the past decade it has become a valuable diagnostic aid to the dentist.

At present, there are five (5) panoramic x-ray units on the market. Four of these utilize the principle of *curved-surface tomography* in which anatomic structures are "blurred out."

Tomography is the radiographic demonstration of one chosen layer within an object by intentionally blurring the images above and below the point of interest (See Figure 11-1). In April of 1962, the International Committee of Radiological Units officially adopted the term "tomography" to describe all types of body section technics. This technic is also called laminagraphy (Kieffer, U. S. A.), planigraphy (Ziedses des Plantes, Holland) and stratigraphy (Vallebona, Italy).

Panoramic radiography combines the principles of tomography with scanography and applies them both to the curved surfaces of the jaws.

Scanography depends on a rotation of the x-ray tube on its focal axis, during exposure, so that the x-ray beam scans a larger area while the focus remains fixed in space (Watson, 1962). It is designed to measure the length of bone, but superior when used for peripheral angiography. Angiography is the demonstration of blood vessels utilizing radiopaque contrast medium.

The four panoramic units which apply the methods of tomography and scanography to curved surfaces are known commercially as the Panorex® (Pennwalt), Orthopantomograph® (Siemens), Panelipse (General Electric Medical Systems) and the PanographiX® (Moss).

Panorex

With the Panorex method, the patient's head remains stationary while the tube and film holder rotates around the head. The film also moves past a narrow exposure slot within the film holder as the tube and film holder rotates around the patient.

The film and tube rotate about two rotational axes which are located in the mandibular molar regions (See Figure 11-2). The axes of rotation is changed from one side to the other midway dur-

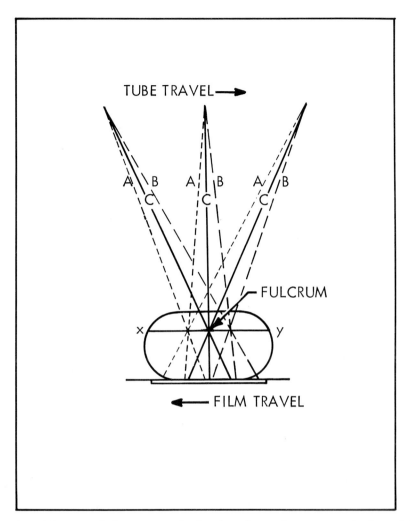

Figure 11-1. Diagram of the tomograph showing the stationary area (x-y) at fulcrum plane which is made by mechanical connection of travel of the tube with cassette holder with a rod or bar. At a prescribed distance on the cross bar or pivot, a fulcrum is established. The tube and the film holder travel in opposite directions during a continuous exposure of approximately one second. Central beam (C) and divergent ray (A & B) cross at a prescribed point and build up a plane which is recorded on the x-ray film—other structures being blurred. Width of plane is controlled by amplitude of tube travel. This technic is especially useful in TMJ radiography. (Courtesy of William R. Bloom, General Electric Co., Milwaukee, Wis.)

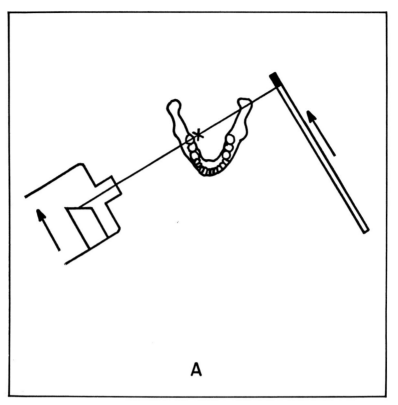

A

Figure 11-2A. Panorex radiography schematic drawings of movement of tube and cassette in opposite directions around patient's head. Patient is stationary, the x-ray source and the cassette holder rotate around patient's head. The arrow indicates the movement of the film past the slit in the cassette holder.

ing the exposure in order to symmetrically position the right and left sides of the patient with the film and to avoid the vertebral column. This is accomplished by a chair and patient shift of 4 inches. During this shift, the x-radiation shuts off, which causes a clear central portion of the resultant Panorex® film. Also, the right and left central incisors will be duplicated on the film. This will not effect the diagnostic value of the film (See Figure 11-4).

The Panorex unit (See Figure 11-3) consists of platform supporting a chair. Behind the chair is a vertical column which supports the x-ray tube and cas-

sette holder. A chair rest is provided on the chair to adjust the position of the patient's head. The control panel is separate and contains the kVp and mA settings. When the directional switch on the control panel is depressed, the cassette holder will start to rotate around the patient's head. The resultant film produced will be a panoramic view of the dental arches, sinuses and the temporomandibular joints (See Figure 11-4).

Orthopantomograph

The Orthopantomographic method is similar to the Panorex machine except that it has three axes of rotation and

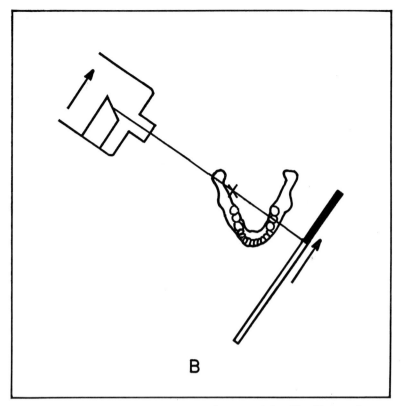

Figure 11-2B. Second movement phase on right side (Panorex).

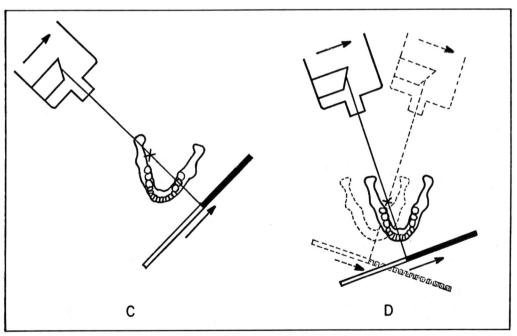

Figure 11-2C & D. Third phase (Panorex). Center of rotation "X" changes midway in the cycle by the automatic shifting of the chair. (Courtesy of Dr. William Updegrave, Temple University, Philadelphia, Pa.)

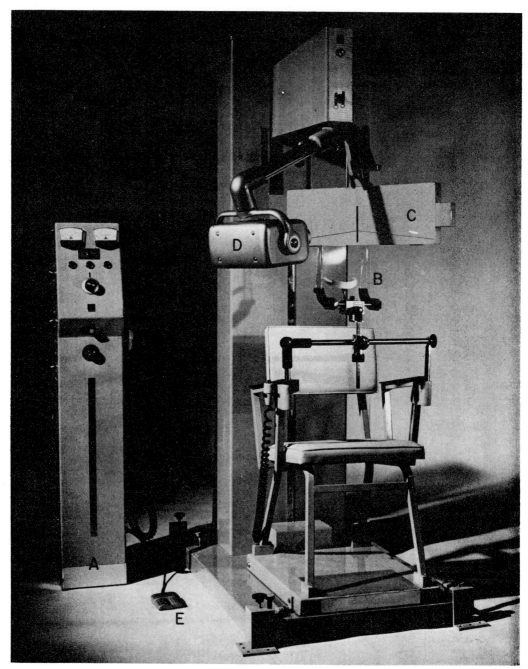

Figure 11-3. The Pennwalt Panorex. (A) Control panel. (B) Pancentric device with chin rest. (C) Cassette holder. (D) Tube head. (E) Foot control to raise and lower the tube head and casette holder. (Courtesy of Pennwalt Corp., Philadelphia, Pa.)

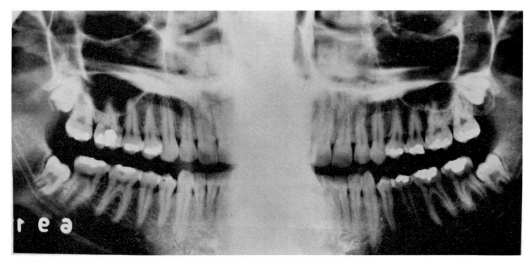

Figure 11-4. Panorex (Pennwalt) radiograph of adult. The condyles are usually shown in a Panorex radiograph. They are not shown in this radiograph.

the patient does not shift midway through the exposure. The orthopantomograph has two eccentric axes of rotation on the left and right sides of the mandible just behind the third molars and a concentric axes of rotation just behind the incisors in the region of the premolars (See Figure 11-5).

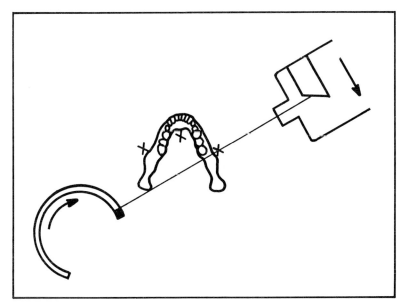

Figure 11-5. Orthopantomograph schematic drawing at start of exposure. Patient is stationary, and the x-ray tube and the film rotates around patient. (Courtesy of Dr. William Updegrave, Temple University, Philadelphia, Pa.)

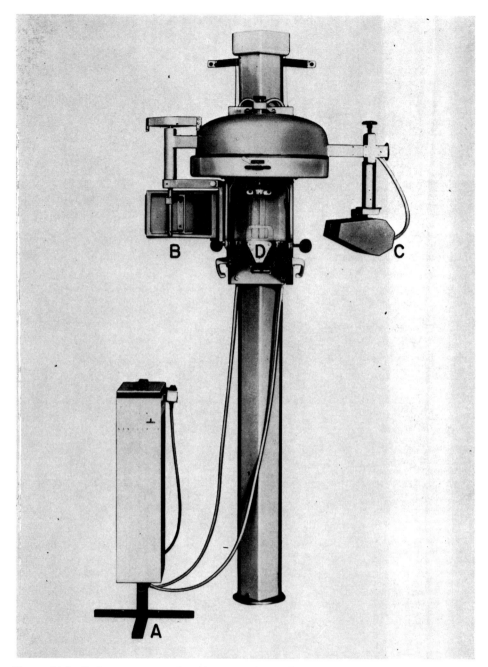

Figure 11-6. Orthopantomograph. (A) Control panel. (B) Cassette holder. (C) X-ray tube. (D) Chin rest. (Courtesy of Siemens Corp. of North America, Union, New Jersey.)

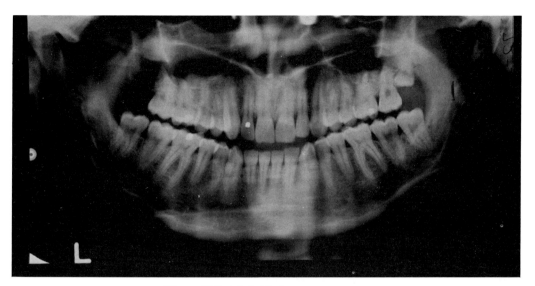

Figure 11-7. Adult Orthopantomogram.

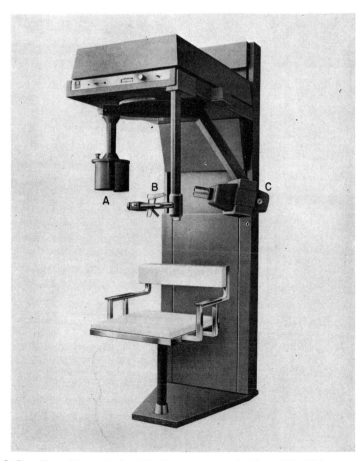

Figure 11-8. Panelipse X-ray Unit. (A) X-ray cassette holder. (B) Chin rest. (C) X-ray tube. (Courtesy of General Electric Co., Milwaukee, Wis.)

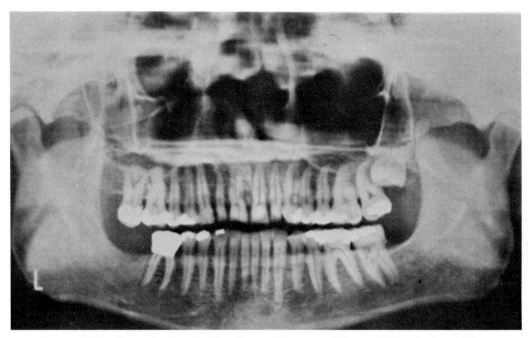

Figure 11-9. Radiograph taken by Panelipse. (Courtesy of General Electric Co., Milwaukee, Wis.)

The Orthopantomograph was developed by Paatero of Finland (1959). The patient sits immobile while the x-ray source and the curved film cassette circulates around his head. The film rotates around its own axes (See Figure 11-6). The resultant Orthopantomogram is a panoramic view of the dental arches, sinuses and the temporomandibular joints. The film does not have a clear center portion as the Panorex has. The radiograph is produced by exposing the film through the vertebral column, which is distorted out of proportion because it is outside the "focal layer" in the concentric axes of rotation (See Figure 11-7).

Panelipse

Like the Panorex and Orthopantomograph the patient is stationary while the tube head and the cassette holder assembly rotates around the patient's head. The Panelipse utilizes a continuously moving axis which follows the arch of the mandible and maxilla (See Figure 11-8).

The resultant radiograph reveals a panoramic view of the dental arches, sinuses and temporomandibular joints similar to the Orthopantomogram (See Figure 11-9).

PanographiX

The PanographiX incorporates one axis of the rotation. The patient is stationary with tube head and film cassette assembly rotating around the patient's head (See Figure 11-10). Images of both sides of the oral arches are obtained by shifting the patient at a time when the x-rays bisect the central anterior region.

The PanographiX automatically shuts off radiation when passing the spinal cord similar to the Panorex. This bypass can be adjusted to suit the patient and/or film requirement. A sample radiograph produced by the PanographiX can be seen in Figure 11-11.

Status-X

The Status-X employs a different method of radiography to produce the panoramic view of the mandible and maxilla. The x-ray source is introduced into the oral cavity and the film is positioned outside the teeth and jaws. In order to comply with the demands for maximum sharpness of the radiographic image, the focal spot of the anode must not be larger than approximately 0.2

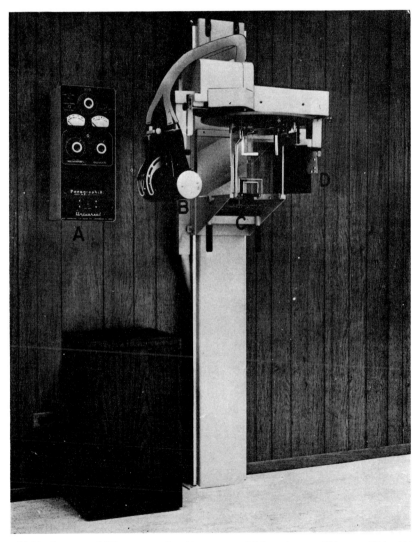

Figure 11-10. PanographiX x-ray unit. (Courtesy of Moss Corp., Chicago, Ill.) (A) Control panel. (B) X-ray tube. (C) Chin rest. (D) Cassette holder.

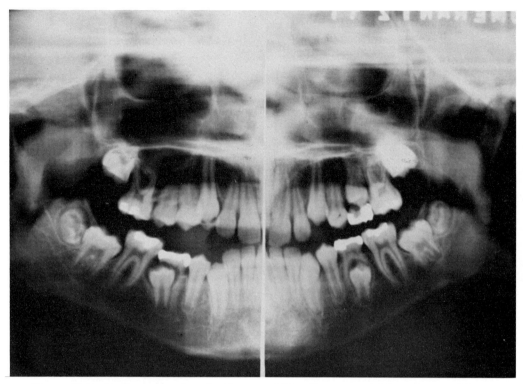

Figure 11-11. Radiograph taken by PanographiX. (Courtesy of Moss Corp., Chicago, Ill.)

mm. The x-ray tube which enters the mouth of the patient has a diameter of only 12 mm, so thin that no inconvenience is caused the patient. The x-ray unit delivers a tube current of approximately 1 mA at a tube voltage of 50 kV (See Figure 11-12).

The images of the teeth and supporting structures are projected onto a film in a flexible cassette that is adopted to the patient's face. The relatively short focal spot-film distance of 1½ to 2 inches causes a divergence of the x-ray beam which produces a magnification of more than twice the normal anatomic size. However, the extremely fine focal spot of 0.1 mm maintains the detail of the enlarged images (See Figure 11-13).

Advantages of Panoramic Radiography

1. *Comfort:* The procedure is quick and more comfortable than conventional radiography. The films are not placed within the mouth. The exposure time is 22 seconds for the Panorex and 13 seconds for the Orthopantomograph.

2. *Simple Technic:* It requires less physical cooperation of patient. This is especially helpful in handicapped patients, frightened children, patients with jaw fractures and edentulous patients. In some of the cases intraoral radiography would be impossible.

3. *Less Total Radiation:* Several stud-

ies have indicated that the total radiation received from panoramic radiography is considerably less than that received from a complete intraoral radiographic series. Jung (1965) concluded that a 15-film intraoral survey delivers a gonadal dose roughly from 0.7 to 1.21 mR or more than 3 times the amount received from panoramic examinations. Van Aken and Van der Lin-

der (1966) determined that the patient receives approximately $\frac{1}{7}$th to $\frac{1}{13}$th the amount of absorbed dosage from the Orthopantomograph as from a 14-film complete radiographic survey.

4. *Complete Coverage of Mandibulofacial Structures:* The panoramic radiograph reveals the anatomic structures of the jaws and face in their normal relationship without

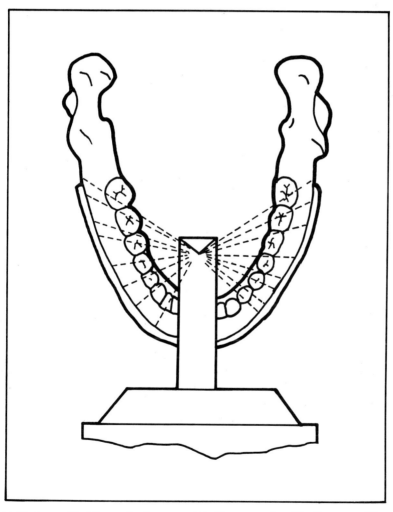

Figure 11-12. Status-X (Siemens) diagram. (A) X-ray anode. (B) Cassette. (Courtesy of Dr. William Updegrave.)

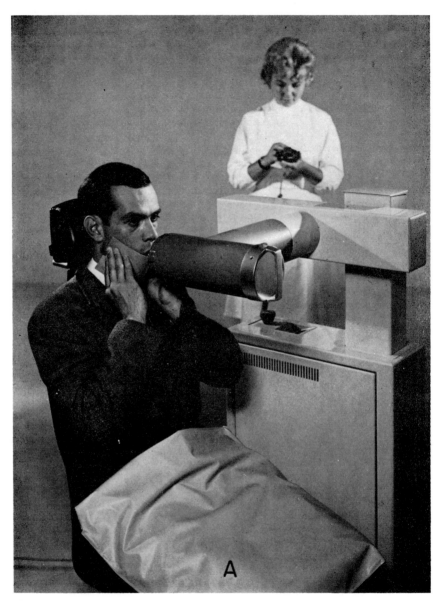

Figure 11-13A. Status-X x-ray unit. Mandibular projection.

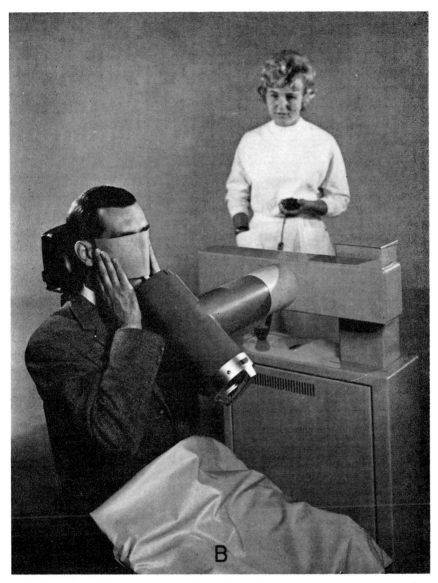

Figure 11-13B. Maxillary projection (Status-X). (Courtesy of Siemens Corp. of North America, Union, N.J.)

superimposition of intervening parts.

It is particularly valuable in locating neoplasms, cysts, supernumerary teeth, congenitally missing teeth, abnormal eruptive patterns, position of mandibular canal, proximity of sinuses, progress of root formation and impactions, many of which will not be seen in the intraoral survey.

The panoramic film provides good radiographic coverage of traumatic injuries of the jaws, particularly fractures of the ramus and condylar neck.

5. *Aid in Case Presentations:* The panoramic survey is an excellent aid in case presentation. The patient seems to understand the presentation in less time than usually is required when conventional methods are used. The mounted intraoral complete survey confuses the patient because of the many compartmentalized, duplicated views shown.

Disadvantages of Panoramic Radiography

1. *Lack of Detail and Definition:* The detail and definition of the panoramic survey are inferior to the intraoral periapical radiographs. This is because the panoramic method utilizes intensifying screens and a longer object-film distance, than intraoral radiography. However, it should be remembered that panoramic radiography is not intended to replace conventional intraoral radiography; it should be considered as a supplementary radiographic method only.

2. *Increases Distortion:* There is more distortion in panoramic radiographs than in conventional intraoral periapical radiographs. Distortion in panoramic radiographs is unavoidable for the following reasons:*

a. There is a fixed source-film distance.

b. The object-film distance varies in patients because of the differences in the size of the jaws and teeth, variations in arrangement of the teeth in the jaws and asymmetry between the right and left sides of the jaws. Magnification (size distortion) is controlled by the distance factors: object-film distance and source-film distance.

c. The x-ray beam is directed in an oblique direction toward the film rather than in the preferred right-angle direction. (This is to prevent superemposition of anatomic structures.) Alignment factors control shape distortion. In periapical radiography, shape distortion is minimized by proper adjustments in the placement of the film and angulation of the cone. In panoramic radiography adjustments in the position of the patient's head is the only compensatory factor available to the operator.

3. *Cost:* The initial cost of the panoramic unit could be called a disadvantage, since the unit does not replace the conventional x-ray ma-

---

* Updegrave, 1966.

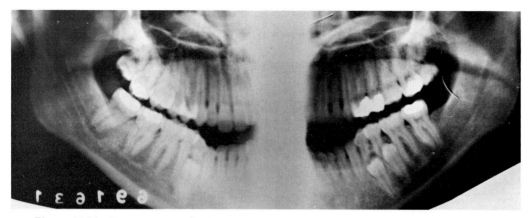

Figure 11-14. Common error in Panorex projection. The chin of the patient is placed too low.

chine. Of course, the initial cost factor would not be a great disadvantage to practices which find a daily use for the panoramic radiograph.

Common Errors in Panoramic Radiographs

There are certain common errors which interfere with the diagnostic quality of panoramic radiographs. The more common ones will be discussed separately.

1. *Head Positioning:* In positioning the head of the patient in the Panorex and the Orthopantomograph, the occlusal plane should be parallel to the floor.

   a. If the chin is placed so the occlusal plane is positioned in a downward position, the mesiodistance dimensions of all teeth will be narrower (See Figure 11-14).

   b. If the chin is placed so the oc-

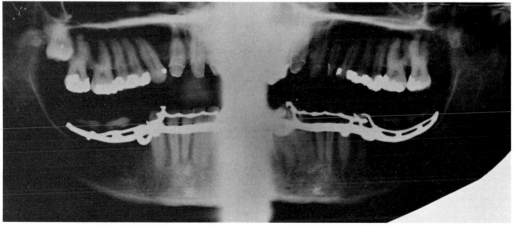

Figure 11-15. Common error in Panorex projection. The chin is placed too high, and metallic partial left in mouth.

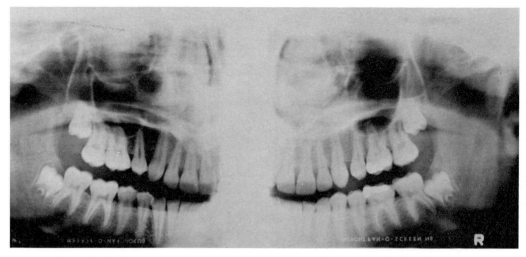

Figure 11-16. Common error in Panorex projection. The cassette is placed too high.

clusal plane is positioned in an upward position, the maxillary palate will be superimposed over the apices of the maxillary teeth (See Figure 11-15).

2. *Panorex Cassette Positioning:*

   a. If the Panorex cassette is not positioned inferiorly far enough, a partial image of the mandible will be produced (See Figure 11-16). This may happen in patients with thick, short necks.

   b. If the Panorex cassette has been positioned too low then the metal portion of the chin rest is seen on the radiograph (See Figure 11-17). This happens only on rare occasions.

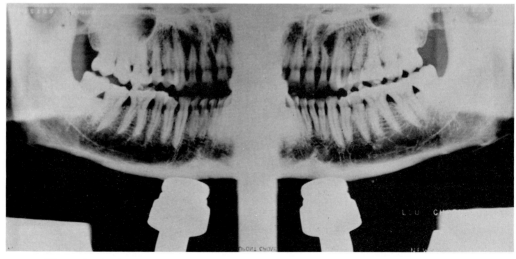

Figure 11-17. Common error in Panorex projection. The cassette is placed too low.

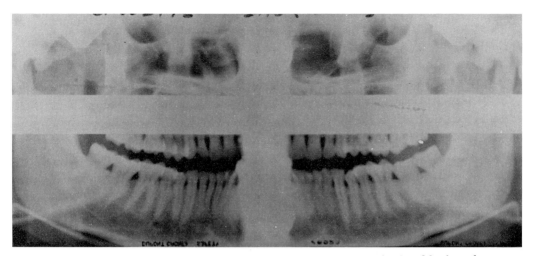

Figure 11-18. Common error in Panorex projection. The cassette is placed backwards.

c. When the Panorex cassette is positioned backwards in the cassette holder, the resultant radiograph has a thin density (See Figure 11-18).

3. *Midsagittal Plane Off Center:* If the midsagittal plane of the patient's head is not aligned with the vertical center line of the chin support, the image of the side of the man-

dible farthest from the tube-head will be enlarged on the film, while the opposite side will be reduced in size (See Figure 11-19). This is probably most common error.

4. *Metallic Objects Not Removed from Patient:* When metallic objects such as glasses, earrings, hair pins, and metal removable dental appliances are not removed from the pa-

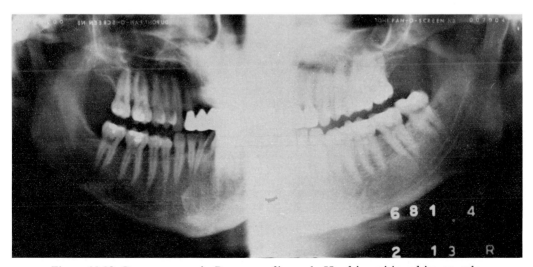

Figure 11-19. Common error in Panorex radiograph. Head is positioned improperly.

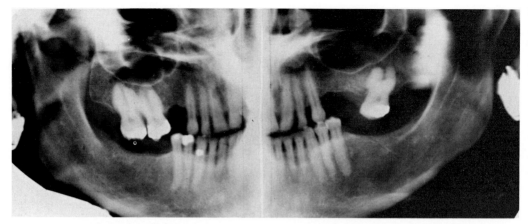

Figure 11-20. Common error in Panorex radiograph. Earrings not removed from patient.

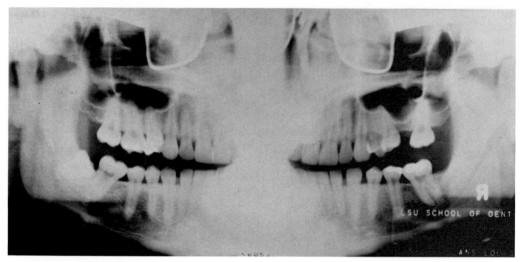

Figure 11-21. Common error in Panorex radiograph. Glasses were not removed before radiograph was taken.

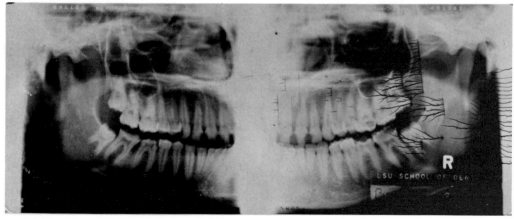

Figure 11-22. Common error in Panorex radiograph. Static electricity lines on radiograph.

tient prior to exposure, radiopaque images will be seen on the resultant radiograph (See Figures 11-20, and 11-21).

5. *Static Electricity:* Static electricity occurs in darkrooms which have a low relative humidity. A relative humidity of between 50 to 75 per-

cent is thought to be ideal. Most static markings are of the crown or tree types which are produced when the film is removed from the interleaving paper in a rapid motion, or when the film is touched by the finger of the operator (See Figure 11-22).

REFERENCES

Andrews, J. Robert: Planigraphy: introduction and history. *Am J Roentgenol,* 36:575-587, November, 1936.

Blackman, S.: Panoramic radiograph. *Br J Oral Surg,* 1:209-218, April, 1964.

Blackman, S.: Rotational tomography of the face. *Br Radiol,* 33:408-418, 1960.

Brueggemann, I. A.: Evaluation of the panorex unit. *Oral Surg,* 24:348-358, September, 1967.

Christen, A. G., and Segreto, V. A.: Distortion and artifacts encountered in Panorex radiography. *J Am Dent Assoc,* 77:1096-1101, November, 1968.

Graber, T. M.: Panoramic radiograph. *Angle Orthodont,* 36:293-311, 1966.

Graber, T. M.: Panoramic radiograph in dentistry. *J Can Dent Assoc,* 31:158-173, March, 1965.

Graber, T. M.: Panoramic radiograph in orthodontic diagnosis. *Am J Orthodontia,* 53:799, 1967.

Grossman, G.: Tomography I & II. *Fortsch A Geb Rontgenol,* 51:61-80, 191-209, 1935.

Hudson and Kumpula: Ionization chambers for radiation data during dental x-ray exposure. *U S Armed Forces M J,* 6:1131. 1955.

Hudson, D. C., Kumpula, J. W., and Dickson, G. A.: Panoramic x-ray dental machine. *U S Armed Forces M J,* 8:46-55, 1957.

Jung, Till: Gonadal doses resulting from panographic x-ray examinations of the teeth. *Oral Surg,* 19:745-753, June, 1965.

Kane, E.: *Missouri D A,* 44:15-18, June-July, 1964.

Kane, Ed G.: A cephalostat for panoramic radiography. *Angle Orthodont,* 31:325, October, 1967.

Karmiol, M., Walsh, R. F., and Loscalzo, L. J.: Panoramic radiography in a hospital dental service. *J Can Dent Assoc,* 36:184-188, May, 1970.

Keiffer: The laminograph and its variations, applications and implications of the planigraphic principles. *Am J Roentgenol,* 39:497-513, 1938.

Kite, Owen W., Swanson, Leonard T., and Levin, Samuel: Radiation and image distortion in the panorex x-ray unit. *Oral Surg,* 15:1201-1213, 1962.

Kraske, L. M., and Mazzurella, Maurice A.: Evaluation of a panoramic dental x-ray machine. *Dent Progr,* 1:171-179, 1961.

Kuba, R. K., and Becie, Jane O.: Radiation dosimetry in panorex roentgenography. *Oral Surg,* 25:380-392, March, 1968.

Kumpula, J. W.: Present status of panoramic roentgenography. *J Am Dent Assoc,* 63:194-200, 1961.

Langland, O. E.: The use of the orthopantomograph in the dental school. *Oral Surg,* 24:480-487, October, 1967.

Langland, O. E., and Sippy, F. H.: Anatomic structures as visualized on the orthopantomogram. *Oral Surg,* 26:475-484, 1968.

Littleton, J. T.: Polydirectional body-section rocntgcnography. *Am J Roentgenol,* 6:1197, June, 1963.

Littleton, J. T., Rumbaugh, C. C., and Winter, F. S.: Polydirectional body-section roentgenography—A new diagnostic method. *Am J Roentgenol,* 89:1179-1193, June, 1963.

MacLean: Current status of panoramic radiography. *J Can D A,* 32:346-353, 1966.

Manson-Hing, Lincoln R.: Advances in dental pantomography: The GE-3000, *Oral Surg.,* 31:430-438, March, 1971.

Masaph, F. W., Wickland, E. P., and Kim, H. H.: Principles and utilization of body section radiography in dentistry. *J Can Dent Assoc,* 37:370, October, 1971.

Mitchell, L. D., Jr.: Panoramic roentgenography, a classic evaluation. *J Am Dent Assoc,* 66:777-786, 1963.

Moore: Body section roentgenography with laminagraph. *Am J Roentgenol,* 39:514-422, 1938.

Morris, Charles; Marano, P. O.; Swinley, D. C.; and Runco, J. G.: Abnormalities noted on panoramic radiographs. *Oral Surg,* 28:772-782, November, 1969.

Nelson, R. and Kumpula: Panographic radiography. *J D Res,* 31:158, April, 1952.

Paatero, Y. V.: New tomographical method for radiographing curved outer surfaces. *Acta Radiol,* 32:177-184, 1949.

Paatero, Y. V.: Pantomography and orthopantomography. *Oral Surg,* 14:947-953, 1961.

Paatero, Y. V.: Pantomography orthoradial jaw. *Ann Med Int Fenn,* 48 (suppl 28) :222, 1959.

Paatero, Y. V.: Pantomography in theory and use. *Acta Radiol,* 41:321-335, 1954.

Paatero, Y. V.: *Suom Hamm-Seur Toim,* 48: 168-178, 1952.

Paatero, Y. V.: Use of mobile source of light in radiography. *Acta Radiol,* 29:221-227, 1948.

Pfeifer, J. S., and Dean, John: The value of panoramic radiography in periodontal diagnosis. *J Wis State Dent Soc,* 45:3-7, January, 1969.

Richardson, J. E., Langland, O. E., and Sippy, F. H.: A cephalostat for the orthopantomograph. *Oral Surg,* 27:642-646, May, 1969.

Rosenberg, H. M.: Laminagraphy: Methods and application in oral diagnosis. *J Am Dent Assoc,* 74:88-96, January, 1967.

Stewart, Jack L., and Bieser, Leo F.: Panoramic roentgenograms compared with conventional intraoral roentgenograms. *Oral Surg,* 39-42, July, 1968.

Stongman, William; Brodeur, Armand; and Brueggemann, I.: A new approach to the radiologic evaluation of the mandible. *Plast Reconstr Surg,* 39:376-381, 1967.

Tammisalo, E. H.: Observation of certain structural differences in orthopantomography of the jaws. *Suom Hammaslaak Toim,* 59:235-241, 1963.

Tammisalo, E. H.: Orthopantomographic roentgenography of the temporomandibular joint. *Suom Hammaslaak Toim,* 60:139-148, 1964.

Tammisalo, E. H.: The dimensional reproduction of the image layer in orthopantomography. *Suom Hammaslaak Toim,* 60:2-12, 1964.

Tammisalo, E. H., and Karhusaara, Y. S.: Radiation exposure in jaw orthopantomography. *Suom Hammaslaak Toim,* 60:128-137, 1964.

Tammisalo, E. H., and Nieminen, T.: The thickness of the image layer in orthopantomography. *Soum Ham Toim Finska Tand Fohr,* 60:119-126, 1964.

Updegrave, W. J.: Panoramic dental radiology. *Dent Radiogr, Photogr,* 36:75-83, 1963.

Updegrave, W. J.: The role of panoramic radiography in diagnosis. *Oral Surg,* 22:49-57, July, 1966.

Updegrave, W. J.: Visualizing the mandibular ramus in panoramic radiography. *Oral Surg,* 31:422-429, March, 1971.

Van Aken, J., and Van der Linden, L. W. J.: The integral absorbed dose in conventional and panoramic complete-mouth examinations. *Oral Surg,* 22:603-616, 1966.

Watson, W.: Rotoscanography. *Br J Radiol,* 35:847-851, December, 1962.

Zach, G. A., Langland, O. E., and Sippy, F. H.: The use of the orthopantomograph in longitudinal studies. *Angle Orthodont,* 39: 42-49, January, 1969.

Ziedes des Plantes, B. G.: Panigraphie. *Fortschr Rontgenstr,* 47:402, 1933.

CHAPTER 12

THE FUTURE OF DENTAL RADIOLOGY

T HE FIELD of dental radiology is expanding. This is the age of nuclear energy and electronics, and along with this are new and exciting discoveries which are influencing dental radiology. Although routine radiographic procedures in dentistry are important, the student of dentistry should inform himself of these new discoveries and perhaps participate in their development.

AREAS OF RESEARCH AND DEVELOPMENT

Polaroid® Film Packets

Polaroid packets with dental x-ray film in them can be used as self-containing processing packets. X-ray film then could be developed almost instantly without the use of a darkroom. Medical x-ray packets with Polaroid film was introduced in 1969. Mr. Land, the inventor of the Polaroid camera, has a patent recorded in Washington, D. C. on the use of dental film with Polaroid processing. Possibly Polaroid film packets for dentistry will be a reality someday as they are now used in medicine.

Cold Cathode Tube

Perhaps in the future we can operate the x-ray tubes on less current and therefore reduce the focal spot size which will give us better definition (sharpness) to the dental radiographic images. This may be accomplished by the use of the "cold cathode" tube. The cathode in this type of tube has a large number of needle points on its inner surface.

Panchromatic Film

Panchromatic film may be available for dental and medical radiography in the future. The film would contain three speeds of emulsion built on top of each other—high, medium, and slow. The film after exposure would be developed by a color processing system. The silver would be removed, but a silver dye image remains. The high speed emulsion would be yellow, the medium speed emulsion would be red or blood color, and the slow speed emulsion would be a blue color. By the use of different colors of filters on the viewbox various details of the film may be brought out. This would give the dentist a film with tremendous latitude.

Image Amplifiers

Image amplifiers of a fluorescent x-ray image which are tape-recorded by television cameras and played back on TV monitors at a later time. This equipment is used by the medical radiologist at the present time. Perhaps dentistry will find application of this type of equipment someday.

Cinefluorography

Cinefluorography (cineradiography) may be defined as the cinematographic recording of a fluoroscopic image formed on a conventional fluoroscopic screen or on the output screen of an image intensifier by means of a cinematographic camera optically coupled to the screen (Ter-Pogossian, 1967). Cinefluorography must be carried out with the use of some type of x-ray intensifier. The light output from a standard fluoroscopic screen is insufficient for the short exposure time ($\frac{1}{40}$ sec) required for cinematography. It would require an increase in x-ray exposure to the patient to overcome this difficulty, which would supersede the safety limitations for the patient. Therefore, the modern cinefluorography unit uses an x-ray image intensifier. An image intensifier tube is defined as a vacuum tube containing an input screen which converts an x-ray pattern into an electron pattern, and in which the electrons are accelerated and focused into an output screen which converts the electron patterns into a light image of higher intensity (NBS Handbook 89, 1963). Berry and Hofmann (1956, 1959, 1966) have applied the method of cinefluorography to the diagnostic study of the temporomandibular joint (See Figure 12-1).

Thermography

Thermography is the science of re-

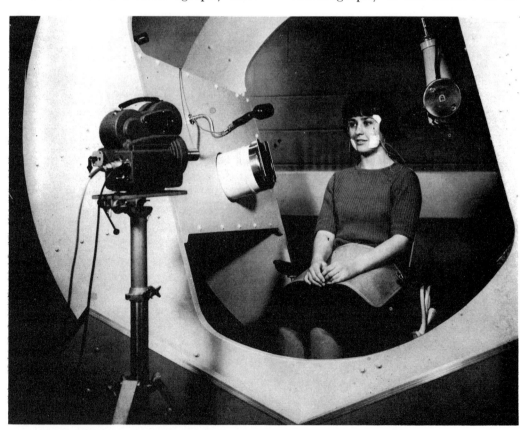

Figure 12-1. Patient prepared for temporomandibular study of joint function in cineradiographic circle unit. (Courtesy of Harrison Berry, Jr. and Allen Hofmann, University of Pennsylvania.)

cording graphically temperatures or changes of temperatures. Recently it has been used for diagnostic purpose in medicine. Gershon-Cohen, *et al.* (1965) have written an excellent monograph on the subject.

All objects give off infrared energy as a function of their temperature. In order that a thermal balance may be obtained in nature, invisible infrared radiation is being continuously emitted, absorbed, and remitted by everything in our environment. The human body normally gives off 3 to 20 microns of infrared radiation. Every patient would glow if our eyes could perceive infrared radiation. Since the infrared radiation emitted varies, some areas of the body will be dark while other portions of the body will be bright.

It is a well known fact that areas of the body with inflammation will emit more heat than usual, which can be determined by the sense of touch. However, there are minute increases in temperature in the body from increased cellular and metabolic activity which cannot be determined in the conventional manner.

The basic instrument used in thermography is the thermograph which records minute skin surface changes in temperature. The thermograms or temperature maps produced may be quantitatively analyzed. Thermograms are taken in total darkness and should not be confused with infrared photographs which are taken with an ordinary camera equipped with film sensitive to radiation in the infrared portion of the electromagnetic spectrum.

Duplicate thermograms of the same person should produce similar temperature patterns. When there are significant physiologic changes within the person, the thermograms will be different. Thermography has been used as a supplemental diagnostic aid to medical radiography with some success. There are possibilities that thermography could be used as a diagnostic procedure in dentistry (Irwin, *et al.*, 1971).

Ultrasound for Diagnostic Purposes

Sound at ultra-high frequencies (100 kilocycles to 20 megacycles) takes on properties similar to light. Sound at these frequencies can be focused with ultrasonic lenses and projected into long linear, pencil-like beams for diagnostic purposes (Howry, 1965). The method used is similar to SONAR used in World War II to locate submarines under water. High frequency sounds are transmitted through water and as the sound hit solid objects, the submarine SONAR would listen for their echoes.

Ultrasonic diagnostic equipment has been devised which transmit high frequency sounds by means of a transducer through the tissue fluids of the body. As the echoes travel back at various rates to a piezo-electric crystal, electrical charges develop which can be recorded or displayed on oscilloscopes and photographic film (Ennis, Berry and Phillips, 1967). Diagnostic ultrasonography has been used in the past to locate benign and malignant diseases of the liver, carcinoma of the breast, renal diseases, eye diseases and brain tumors (Elizondo-Martel and Gershon-Cohen, 1965).

Neutron Radiography

X-radiography and neutron radiography are similar except for the fact that the absorption of thermal neutrons in light and heavy materials is practically the opposite of that of x-rays. Images in neutron radiography are produced by thermal neutrons interacting with the atomic nucleus of the tissue cells while the x-ray image is produced by the interaction of x-radiation with the electrons of the atoms of the tissue (Boyne and Whittemore, 1971).

The sensitivity of conventional photographic emulsions is too low for practical use in neutron radiography (Herz, 1969). Therefore, special converter screens containing foils of certain elements which emit alpha, beta or gamma rays when exposed to thermal neutrons are used.

The drawback in using this type of radiography is the fact that the most suitable source for thermal neutrons comes from nuclear reactors. Only a few laboratories have nuclear reactors because of the high cost and their large size. However, other neutron sources could come from Van der Graaf accelerators or from isotopes.

In the future, it is possible that neutron radiography could be applied to the human jaws in suspected tumor cases (Boyne and Whittemore, 1971).

Autoradiography

An autoradiograph is a record of the structure of an object made on film by the object's own radioactivity (Etter, 1970). The specimen is placed in contact with a suitable photographic emulsion. The radioactive material within the specimen exposes the photographic emulsion, which in turn reveals the location of the radioactive material within the specimen.

Biologists now are able to study cells, nuclei and chromosomes by using tracer radioisotopes in conjunction with electron microscope autoradiography technics.

Scintillation Scanning

This is an extension of the autoradiographic technic utilizing a scanner. Scanning refers to the visual recording of the distribution of a radioactive substance within an organ (Horwitz, 1971). This requires the concentration of a suitable radioactive substance within the organ. The scanning device consists of a phosphor, photomultiplier tube and associated circuits for recording light emissions (scintillations) caused by the gamma radiation emitted from the organs in question. The scanner passes back and forth over the organ recording the radioactivity. The distribution of the radioactive material within the organ allows the clinician to evaluate the size, shape and position of the organ.

Also, it is possible to gain information on the physiological activity of the organ by the presense of high and low concentrations of the radioactivity within the organ.

The use of scintillation scanning with 85 Sr for the detection of bone involvement by squamous cell carcinoma of the oral mucosa was discussed by Mashberg, *et al.* in 1969.

Microradiography

Microradiography is a method of recording a photograph of the microscopic details in a thin specimen (under 100 microns) by means of soft x-rays generated by kilovoltage in the role of 10 to 40 kVp. Dental x-ray machines usually are not suitable because the x-rays are not soft enough. X-ray diffraction equipment is preferred (Herz, 1969).

Microradiography provides an excellent research tool for dental biologists to study the distribution of the mineral content in dental enamel and the microscopic carious lesion (Crabb and Mortimer, 1967).

Angiography

Angiography is the x-ray visualization of blood vessels filled with radiopaque material. This procedure is accomplished by the injection of contrast-material within the blood vessels followed by a radiograph of the region in question (Etter, 1970). This procedure can contribute to the diagnosis of neoplasms of the head and neck (Medellin and Wallace, 1970). The angiogram is particularly useful in the diagnosis of certain highly vascular tumors such as angiofibromas and hemangiomas. These neoplasms result in excessive blood loss at biopsy. Abrupt and irregular changes in the cali-

ber of the blood vessels and irregular pooling of contrast material seemingly outside the vessels are two reliable findings in malignant disease of the head and neck (Medellin and Wallace, 1970).

Xeroradiography

Xeroradiography is the technic of activating the xeroradiographic copying process with x-rays, rather than with ordinary light as is done in commercial copying machines (Rawls and Owen, 1972). This method produces a print of densities produced by x-rays on a specially-prepared selenium plate which has been exposed to x-rays (Etter, 1970).

The greatest disadvantage of xeroradiography seem to be its slow speed of producing an image. However, its improved image quality and resolution could surpass conventional dental radiography. Xeroradiography with future research and development has promising dental applications in the future (Rawls and Owen, 1972).

REFERENCES

Berger, H.: *Neutron Radiography*. New York, Elsevier, 1965.

Berret, A.: Value of angiography in the management of tumors of the head and neck. *Radiology*, 84:1952, 1965.

Berry, H. M., Jr., and Hofmann, F. A.: Cinefluorography with image intensification for observing temporomandibular joint movements. *J Am Dent Assoc*, 53:517-527, 1956.

Berry, H. M., Jr., and Hofmann, F. A.: Cineradiographic observations of T-M joint function. *J Prosthet Dent*, 21-31, January-February, 1959.

Berry, H. M., Jr., and Hogmann, F. A.: Cineradiographic circle unit. *Public Health Rep*, 81:470, 1966.

Boyne, P. J., *et al.*: Neutron radiography of os-

seous tumors. *Oral Surg*, 31:152-156, February, 1971.

Brown, M., and Parks, P.: Neutron radiography in biologic media. *Am J Roentgenol*, 106:472-485, 1969.

Charles, N. O., and Sklaroff, D. M.: The radioactive strontium photoscan as a diagnostic aid in primary and metastatic cancer in bone. *Radiol Clin North Am*, 3:499-509, 1965.

Cooper, H. K., and Hofmann, F. A.: The application of cinefluorography with image intensification in the field of plastic surgery, dentistry and speech. *J Plast Reconstr Surg*, 16:135-137, 1955.

Crabb, H. S. M., and Mortimer, K. U.: Two-dimensional microdensitometry: a preliminary report. *Br Dent J*, 122:337-343, April, 1967.

Elizondo-Martel, G., and Gershon-Cohen, J.: Medical ultrasources. *Am J Roentgenol*, 93: 791-802, 1965.

Ennis, L. M., Berry, H. M., and Phillips, J. E.: *Dental Roentgenology*, 6th ed. Philadelphia, Lea & Febiger, 1967.

Etter, Lewis E.: *Glossary of Words and Phrases Used in Radiology, Nuclear Medicine and Ultrasound*, 2nd ed. Springfield, Ill., Charles C Thomas, 1970.

Gershon-Cohen, J., Haberman-Brueschke, J. D., and Brueschke, E. E.: Medical thermography: A summary of current status. *Radiol Clin North Am*, 3:403-431, December, 1965.

Herz, R. H.: *The Photographic Action of Ionizing Radiations*. New York, Wiley-Interscience, 1969.

Horwitz, Norman H.: Scanning and scintigraphy. *Powsner and Raeside's Diagnostic Nuclear Medicine*. New York, Grune and Stratton, 1971, chap. 11.

Howry, Douglass H.: A brief atlas of diagnostic ultrasonic radiologic results. *Radiol Clin North Am*, 433-452, December, 1965.

Irwin, J. W., *et al.*: Intraoral thermography. *Oral Surg*, 32:724-730, 1971.

Landman, G. H. M.: *Laryngography and Cinelaryngography*. Baltimore, Williams and Wilkins, 1970.

Lapinskas, V. A., and Lapinskene, A. V.: Xeroradiography and the progress of its use in dentistry. *Stomatologiia (Mosk)*, 47:35-38, 1968.

Loveland, Roger P.: *Photomicrography*. New York, John Wiley & Sons, 1970.

Mashberg, A., *et al.*: Use of the scintillation scanning for the early detection of bone involvement by squamous cell carcinoma of the oral mucosa: Preliminary report. *J Am Dent Assoc*, 79:1151-1159, November, 1969.

Medellin, H., and Wallace, Sidney: Angiography in neoplasms of head and neck. *Radiol Clin North Am*, 8:307-321, December, 1970.

Methods of Evaluating Radiological Equipment and Materials. NBS Handbook 89, Washington, D. C., U. S. Government Printing Office, 1963.

Powsner, E. R., and Radside, D. E.: *Diagnostic Nuclear Medicine*. New York, Grune and Stratton, 1971.

Rawls, H. R., and Owen, W. D.: The dental programs for xeroradiography. *Oral Surg*, 33:476-480, March, 1972.

Ricketts, R. M.: Present status of laminagraphy as related to dentistry. *J Am Dent Assoc*, 65:55-64, 1962.

Ter-Pogossian, M. M.: *The Physical Aspects of Diagnostic Radiology*. New York, Hoeber Medical, Harper & Row, 1967.

Wolfe, J. N.: Xeroradiography of bones, joints and soft tissues. *Radiology*, 93:583-587, 1969.

CHAPTER 13

LEGAL ASPECTS OF DENTAL RADIOGRAPHY

Ownership of the X-rays

WHEN THE PATIENT pays for a set of radiographs, he is paying for the dentist's ability to interpret the radiographs and arrive at a diagnostic opinion based on his radiographic and clinical findings. X-rays are a part of the dentist's records and do not rightfully belong to the patient.

One of the most important decisions by a higher court concerning ownership of radiographs was handed down by the Supreme Court of Michigan in 1935 (McGarry versus J. A. Mercier Co.).

In this case, the plaintiff was a physician who was employed by a construction company (J. A. Mercier Company) to treat their employees in case of injury on the job. J. A. Mercier Company had refused to pay the physician for services rendered one of their employees because the physician failed to deliver to them radiographs taken of the employee during treatment.

The court ruled in favor of the physician stating that the radiographs were legal property of the physician. They further declared that "it is a matter of common knowledge that x-ray negatives are practically meaningless to the ordinary layman. But the retention by the physician or surgeon constitutes an important part of his clinical record in the particular case, and in the aggregate these films may embody and preserve much of value incident to a physician's or surgeon's experience. They are as much a part of the history of the case as any other case record of the physician or surgeon. In a sense they differ little, if at all, from microscopic slides of tissue made in the course of diagnosis or treatment of the patient, but it would hardly be claimed that such slides were the property of the patient."

Care in Billing

If the radiographs are billed separately from the diagnosis and treatment, the dentist may run the risk that the court may render a verdict in favor of the patient saying the patient owns the radiographs because he paid for them.

Always include the radiographs in services rendered for diagnosis and treatment when billing a patient. Do not itemize a separate charge for radiographs.

Precautions in Loaning Radiographs

The dentist should never give radiographs to the patient. The dentist should realize that the radiograph is greatest protection against a possible claim of negligence he has. It is sad when a dentist is sued for malpractice and the radiographs which would have proved his competence have been misplaced or lost.

There are times when the dentist may want to lend the patient's radiographs to another dentist for viewing. When lending radiographs to another dentist, the following suggestions are given: (Miller, 1970).

1. Have the second dentist request the radiographs in writing. Place this letter in the patient's folder.
2. Send the radiographs by registered or certified mail.
3. Request that the dentist retain the radiographs in his files for six years, or send them back to you after he is through with them. Even though the patient may move to another city, the dentist is not legally bound to send the patient's radiographs to a second dentist. The radiographs are still his legal property.
4. A copy of the cover letter sent with the radiographs and the postal receipt should be kept in the patient's folder.
5. The patient's records should be kept for at least six years.

Liability Arising Out of Failure to Use Radiographs

It depends upon the dentist's professional judgement whether he should use radiographs as a diagnostic procedure or not. Certainly there are instances when radiographs are not necessary to render a diagnosis. However, one of the most common causes for malpractice suits is the failure of the dentist to use radiographs in his diagnosis or after treatment of cases involving pain, swelling or infection.

Consider this case cited by Sarner (1963). A dentist in Kentucky refused to radiograph a patient's jaws when there was a question whether he had left a root tip in the patient's jaws after an extraction. The patient visited a second dentist, who found a root tip in the jaws by means of a radiograph. It is now considered a dental principle that a dentist who fails to radiograph in some circumstances constitutes malpractice (Agnew vs. City of Los Angeles, 97 Cal. App. 557, 218 P. 2d 66—1950). Therefore, if there is any doubt in the mind of the dentist whether he should use radiographs or not, he should do so. The use of radiographs has been so embedded in the minds of the public, that a jury in most cases will find the dentist negligent if he fails to use x-rays. For sure, a radiograph should be taken before and after each extraction.

There are times when a patient will refuse radiographs for some reason or another. In such a situation, Miller (1970) suggests two alternative procedures for the dentist to take to minimize a malpractice suit at a later date.

1. Record the refusal in the patient's record and have patient sign it.
2. Offer to take the radiographs at no charge for his records.

Either one of these procedures would lessen the possibilities of a malpractice suit against the dentist for the failure to use radiographs.

Radiographs as Evidence

In the court of law one must remember that the best evidence is that which is factual. Radiographs are factual evidence. Of course, the radiographs must be of good diagnostic quality or they could reflect the competency of the dentist. Radiographs of inferior quality should not be kept and retaken for two reasons: (Miller, 1970).

1. These radiographs will be of no use as evidence.

2. They will reflect on the dentist's ability as a practitioner and could cause irreparable harm to the dentist's reputation.

If a dentist retains radiographs of inferior quality in his records, they will only prove his incompetence as a dentist if he produces these radiographs as evidence in court. There is no substitute for good radiographs, and the ability of the dentist to interpret the radiographs accurately according to his clinical findings.

Unquestionably, the most important legal aspect of dental radiographs is that it constitutes in itself invaluable malpractice insurance. Any attorney will hesitate to bring a suit of malpractice against a dentist who has taken preoperative and postoperative radiographs. The lawyer will know in advance that the case will be difficult to win and probably will try to settle out of court. However, if a dentist has done his treatment competently and has taken comprehensive radiographs he should not be concerned, because he has irrefutable evidence in his possession.

REFERENCES

Carnaham, C. W.: *The Dentist and the Law.* St. Louis, C. V. Mosby, 1955.

Donaldson, S. W.: Ownership of radiographs. *Radiogr Clin Photogr,* 17:27-29, 1941.

Ennis, L. M.; Berry, H. M.; and Phillip, J. E.: *Dental Roentgenology.* Philadelphia, Lea & Febiger, 1967, p. 330.

Miller, Sidney L.: *Legal Aspects of Dentistry: A Programmed Course in Dental Jurisprudence.* New York, G. P. Putnam, 1970.

Rabe, Richard T.: Who owns the x-ray films? *Oral Hygiene,* 37-39, July, 1957.

Sarner, Harvey: *Dental Jurisprudence.* Philadelphia, W. B. Saunders, 1963.

Sweet, Porter: The legal aspects of dental roentgenograms. *J Am Dent Assoc,* 25:1687-1697, October, 1938.

Wuehrmann, Arthur H.: *Radiation Protection and Dentistry.* St. Louis, C. V. Mosby, 1960.

GLOSSARY

A

abscess (ab'ses): A localized collection of pus in a cavity formed by the disintegration of tissues.

absorption: 1. The process whereby the total number of particles or quanta emerging from a body of matter is reduced relative to the number entering, as a result of interaction of the particles with the body. 2. For particulate radiation, energy is lost by collisions with electrons or nuclei. For protons, the reduction is due to the transfer of the energy to electrons by scattering and photoelectric processes and, at voltages greater than a million, by pair production.

Note: In the above sense this term is used interchangeably with attenuation. More specifically absorption refers to processes by which the radiation disappears or is transformed and not merely scattered.

acanthion (ah-kan'the-on): A point at the base of the anterior nasal spine.

accelerator, developer: An accelerator in a developer is an alkaline chemical (sodium carbonate, sodium hydroxide, or sodium metaborate) that makes possible the activity of the developing agents. It softens the gelatin to permit the reducing agents' easy access to the exposed silver bromide contained in the emulsion.

acid: An acid is a solution containing less hydrogen ions than water. Its pH is less than 7. The H ions can be replaced by metals and can form salts. Test for acidity: blue litmus paper turns pink when immersed in the acid solution.

acidifier: The acidifier in a fixer provides an acid medium for proper fixation of the radiograph. It also serves to neutralize carryover of alkaline developer. The usual acids employed are acetic and citric.

actinic: A type of radiation which is capable of producing a chemical change. That portion of light which affects photographic emulsion, and is generated by action of x-rays on a fluorescent intensifying screen, or on a fluoroscopic screen.

acute (adj.): Having a sudden onset and short course.

agent, clearing: the clearing agent in the fixing bath is a chemical (sodium, or ammonium thiosulfate) whose function is to remove unexposed and undeveloped silver bromide crystals in the x-ray film emulsion.

agent, developing: Developing or reducing agents in a developer are chemicals that change the exposed silver bromide crystals to black metallic silver. Substances commonly employed are elon and hydroquinone.

agent, hardening: The fixing bath hardener is a chemical (potassium alum) used to harden and shrink an x-ray film emulsion after the unexposed and undeveloped silver bromide crystals have been removed.

agent, wetting: A wetting agent is a solution used following the washing process to accelerate the flow of water from both film surfaces and to hasten the drying of radiographs.

air-bells: Small spherical clear areas on the finished x-ray film due to bubbles of air adhering to the emulsion during processing and preventing the action of the developer and fixer on these areas.

ala (pl. alae, n.): A wing-like process or structure such as the ala of the nose.

alkali: An alkali is a solution containing more hydrogen ions than water. Its pH is greater than 7. Alkali can react with acids to form salts. It reacts with red litmus paper and turns it blue.

alopecia (al-o-pe'she-ah): Baldness, deficiency of hair, natural or abnormal.

alpha particle: 1. A positively charged particle emitted from a nucleus and composed of two protons and two neutrons. It is identical in all measured properties with the nucleus of a helium atom. 2. By extension, the nucleus of a helium atom $(Z = 2, A = 4)$, especially when it is in rapid motion as when artificially accelerated.

alpha ray: A synonym for alpha particle.

alternating current: The flow of electrons in one direction immediately followed by a flow in the opposite direction.

aluminum equivalent: The thickness of aluminum affording the same attenuation, under specified conditions, as the material in question.

aluminum filter: Various thicknesses of aluminum used as filtration in the x-ray beam to absorb the longer, ineffective rays.

ammeter *(n.):* An instrument for the measurement of the quantity of an electric current.

ampere: The unit of intensity of an electric current, being the current produced by one volt acting through a resistance of 1 ohm.

angle-board: A device used in certain radiographic procedures enabling the technician or dentist to place the patient's head in particular angles.

angstrom: An angstrom is a unit employed in expressing the length of light waves. It is equal to one ten-thousandth of a micron. Symbol: Å.

anion: An ion carrying a negative charge.

ankylosis: Stiffness of a joint resulting from either traumatic or intentional union of the joint surfaces.

anode, x-ray tube: An x-ray tube anode is a heavy copper bar containing a tungsten target (focal spot) at the end facing the cathode that can be bombarded by an electron stream from the cathode resulting in x-ray production. The face of the target in stationary tubes is cut to an angle of 18-20°; in rotating anode tubes the face is 13-15°. It is the positive electrode in the x-ray tube.

anterior (an-te're-or) : situated in front of or in the forward part of, affecting the forward part of an organ, toward the head end of the body; in official anatomical nomenclature, used in reference to the ventral or belly surface of the body.

a-p: Abbreviation for anteroposterior position or projection.

atlas (at'las) : The 1st cervical vertebra.

atom: The atom is the smallest unit of matter (element) remaining unchanged in chemical reactions. It consists of a central positively charged nucleus surrounded by enough electrons to produce an equivalent negative charge to make the atom electrically neutral. The number of positive charges on the nucleus (atomic number) and thus the number of electrons around the nucleus determines the properties of the atom.

atomic number (Z) : It is the number of electrons outside the nucleus of a neutral atom and, according to present theory, the number of protons in the nucleus.

atomic weight (A) : A weighted mean of the masses of the neutral atoms of an element expressed in atomic-weight units.

atrium (a'tre-um): A chamber; used in anatomical nomenclature to designate such a chamber affording entrance to another structure or organ.

attenuation: 1. (Radiation theory) The reduction in the flux density, or power per unit area with distance from the source; it may be due to absorption, to scatter—or to both processes. 2. (Nuclear physics) The reduction in the intensity of radiation upon passage through matter; in general, it is due to a combination of scattering and absorption. The term is best used in a sense that excludes the geometric decrease of intensity with distance from the source (inverse-square effect) ; the attenuation then depends only on the nature of the radiation and of the material traversed.

B

background radiation (background) : Background can take various forms, depending on the nature of the measurement. In electrical measurements of radioactivity and nuclear phenomena, the term usually refers to those undesired counts or currents that arise from cosmic rays, local contaminating radioactivity from the environment and in the laboratory, insulator leakage, amplifier noise, power line fluctuations, and so on. For the dentist, background implies radioactivity arising from nature. This includes cosmic rays and radioactive elements in the earth and air. It does not include any type of man-made radiation.

beam, x-rays: An unidirectional or approximately parallel flow of electromagnetic rays (x-rays). It is the bundle of x-rays that emerge from the portal of an energized tube. It comprises primary radiation and remnant radiation when an object is in its path.

benign (be-nin'): Not malignant, not recurrent, favorable for recovery.

beta particle: Negatively charged electrons in rapid motion and is a particulate form of radiant energy. Most beta radiation is more penetrating than alpha particles and the particles have an average "path" or penetration in tissues of a few millimeters up to a cm or more before they are absorbed.

betatron, induction accelerator: A device for accelerating electrons by means of magnetic induction.

bilateral (bi-lat'er-al): Having two sides, or pertaining to both sides.

biologic effectiveness or relative biologic effectiveness (RBE): Ability of all ionizing radiations to produce biologic effects. Certain types of radiation are more effective than others in that smaller absorbed doses of these radiations are required to produce a particular effect. A comparison between one type of radiation and another with respect to this ability is known as the relative biologic effectiveness (RBE) of that type of radiation. Relative biologic effectiveness is expressed in numerals, usually from 1 to 10.

bitewing radiographs: A paper or cardboard wing or tab is attached to the center of the film, parallel with the long axis of the film. The patient bites on the cardboard wing to hold the film in the proper place. It records shadow images of crown, necks, and coronal 1/3rds of the roots of both upper and lower teeth and dental arches.

body-section radiography: General term for a technic that provided a distinct image of any selected plane through the body while the images of structures that lie above and below the plane are blurred. The name "body-section radiography" has been applied to the procedure, although the several ways of accomplishing it have been given distinguishing names such as laminagraphy, planigraphy, tomography, stratigraphy, and vertigraphy.

brachycephaly *(n.):* Unusually short skull; one having a short AP diameter.

bregma *(n.):* A topographic point on the skull at the junction of the coronal with the sagittal suture and the site of the metropic fontanelle.

bremstrahlung (bremsthrahlen) *(n.)* (German): Deceleration of charged particles as they pass through matter producing secondary photon radiation. This is often referred to as continuous or white radiation since, like white light, it consists of a continuous range or wavelength.

bucky diaphragm: Invented in 1909 by Dr. Gustav Bucky. It is an ingenious piece of radiographic apparatus consisting of a grid of parallel strips of lead arranged on the radius of curvature of a cylinder whose center is at the focal spot of the x-ray tube. The purpose of this is to reduce the effects of scattered radiation.

C

Caldwell projection: A P.A. oblique position of the skull for radiography of the frontal and anterior ethmoid sinuses made with an angle of 23 degrees toward the feet. Named for Dr. Eugene W. Caldwell who devised the position.

cancellous bone: Bone having a reticular, spongy, or latticelike structure.

cancer: Any malignant neoplasm.

canthus: The angle, either temporal (outer) or nasa (inner) formed by the junction of the eyelids.

capacity, tank: Tank capacity is the volume of solution held in an x-ray processing tank. It is computed by multiplying the width, depth (minus 1 inch) and length, in inches and dividing the product by 231. The answer is in gallons.

cardboard holders: A lightproof holder made of cardboard used for holding certain types of x-ray films. The back side has a thin sheet of lead which prevents a backscatter. It is used to produce high contrast and detail in extremity radiographs.

cassette: A device for holding x-ray films during exposure. Cassettes are made in several sizes. The front size is composed of bakelite or aluminum and the back side contains a thin lead sheet. The back is hinged and fits into the front or tube side, sealing out all light. Two intensifying screens are mounted inside, one each side, between which the film is sandwiched.

cathode rays: Streams of electrons passing from the hot filament of the cathode to the target or anode in an x-ray tube with approximately 1/3rd of the speed of light, depending on the impressed potential.

cathode, x-ray tube: An x-ray tube cathode contains a spirally wound filament that can become incandescent and produce electrons when a low voltage electric current is passed through it. It is so designed that it can focus an electron beam on the focal spot of the anode. It is the negative electrode in the x-ray tube.

caudad: Toward the tail or cauda; in man, downwards.

cell: A minute protoplasmic mass which in the aggregate makes up organized tissue. The cell consists of a circumscribed mass of cytoplasm in which is a nucleus. In some of the low forms of life such as bacteria and viruses, a morphological nucleus is absent, but nucleoproteins (and genes) are present.

central ray: The central ray is the center of the x-ray beam. The term is employed to designate the direction of the x-rays in a given projection. The central ray may be considered to extend from the focal spot of the x-ray tube to the x-ray film. The symbol is CR.

cephalad: Toward the head.

cephalometric radiographs: Lateral and posteroanterior head films used in orthodontics and to a lesser extent in prosthodontics. Usually a five-foot distance is used between the focal spot and the midline of the patient's head.

cephalometry *(n.):* Measurement of the head of the living subject without removal of soft parts.

cervical *(adj.):* Pertaining to the neck or cervical vertebrae.

chamber, ionization: An instrument designed to measure a quantity of ionizing radiation in terms of electricity associated with ions produced within a defined volume.

characteristic (discrete) radiation: The specific type of secondary radiation resulting when rays from an x-ray tube strike an inorganic substance of greater atomic weight than aluminum. The wavelength of the emitted radiation is specific for the element used.

chemical fog: A blurred appearance of the radiograph produced by contaminated developer or other chemicals, not by light or x-rays.

chromosome: One of the definite number of small dark-staining and more or less rod-shaped bodies situated in the nucleus of a cell. Chromosomes are especially prominent at the time of cell division at which time they divide and distribute equally to the daughter cells. They contain genes arranged along their length. The number of chromosomes in the somatic cells of an individual is constant (diploid number), whereas just half of this number (haploid number), appears in germ cells; the number of chromosomes or diploid number, etc., within a species is usually constant.

chromosome aberration: Any rearrangement of chromosome parts as a result of breakage and reunion of broken ends.

cine-fluorographic examination (cine-fluorography): A moving picture camera used with an image amplifier to record a moving study of the fluoroscopic observations. This recording of the opacified heart and great vessels was achieved as early as 1935 by Stewart *et al.* and independently in 1941 by Sussman and his group.

collimator, diaphragm: Terms used interchangeably to refer to devices or mechanisms by which the x-ray beam is restricted in size.

collision: Encounter between two subatomic particles (incl. photons) which changes the existing momentum and energy conditions. The products of collision need not be the same as the initial systems.

collision, elastic: A collision in which there is no change either in the internal energy of each participating system or in the sum of their kinetic energies of translation.

collision, inelastic: A collision in which there are changes in both the internal energy of one or more in the colliding systems and in the sums of the kinetic energies of translation before and after collision.

compact bone or cortical bone: It is a dense lamellar structure. The layers are a three-dimensional system. Cortical or compact bone composes the hard surface of all bones. It varies in thickness in different bones.

Compton effect (Compton scatter): Interaction of a photon of x or gamma radiation with an orbital electron of the absorber atom producing a recoil electron and a photon of energy which is less than that of the incident photon. Compton scattering photons carry away a fraction of the incident photon energy, ranging from an average of about 85 percent of the initial energy for a 0.1-mev photon to an average of about 30 percent for a 10-mev photon. Sometimes referred to as incoherent scattering.

concrete equivalent: The thickness of concrete based on a density of 2.35 gm per cubic centimeter (147 lbs per cubic foot) affording the same attenuation, under specified conditions, as the material in question.

cone distance: Refers to the distance between the focal spot and outer end of the cone usually expressed in inches or centimeters. Modern dental x-ray units usually have a cone distance of 7 inches or 14 inches.

cones: Restrict the beam of x-radiation to the immediate part of the object under examination and thus minimizing the secondary radiation by limiting the volume of the exposed area. Of course the cone would have to restrict the rays to do this. The result is increased contrast which makes roentgenographic detail more plainly visible.

contaminated: Made radioactive by the addition of minute (sometimes) quantities of radioactive material.

contrast: Is the relative degree of blackness of the black of the film as compared with the whiteness of the white portions. As contrast is decreased, the percentage of difference

between these various densities on the film is reduced, and vice versa. The controlling factors are: (1) KvP, (2) Development, and (3) Fog from light, secondary radiation, chemical factors, age of the film and character of the tissue being examined.

contrast emulsion: Emulsion contrast refers to the ability of the emulsion to affect the contrast of the radiograph under specific conditions of exposure, development, and type of tissue being examined. Different emulsions can produce different contrasts despite the same exposure and development.

contrast, long scale: Long scale contrast is recognized by the large number of translucent densities that make possible the visualization of an abundance of image details. The transition between image densities is small. Silver deposits representative of both thick and thin parts are usually present. It is produced by relatively short wavelength x-radiation.

contrast medium (media): Various forms of radiopaque substances used to delineate anatomical structures roentgenographically.

contrast, short-scale: Short-scale contrast characterizes an image produced by long wavelength x-radiation. The transition between densities as to silver content is large and exaggerated. The range of densities in an image is small. Silver deposits (details) representative of both thick and thin parts are seldom shown. Detail visibility in these image areas is diminished and in most instances is diagnostically worthless. Opacities and absence of image silver denotes short-scale contrast.

contrast, tissue: Tissue contrast refers to the relative differences in tissue density and thickness of the components of an anatomic part with respect to their x-ray absorbing properties. Radiographically, tissue contrast is evidenced by the variations in radiographic densities caused by the differences in absorbing power of the different kinds of tissue traversed by an x-ray beam resulting in reduced intensities that reach the film.

Coolidge tube: An x-ray tube which has the gas

pressure purposely made so low that it plays no role in the operation of the tube, and the operation depends upon the emission of electrons by the heated filament of the cathode. This is the basis of the modern x-ray tubes.

cortex (kor′teks) : The outer layer of an organ or other body structure, as distinguished from the underlying substance.

cortical (kor′ti-kal) : Pertaining to or of the nature of a cortex.

cosmic rays: Radiation that has its origin outside of the earth's atmosphere. Cosmic rays are of extremely short wavelengths. They are able to produce ionization as they pass through the air and other matter and are capable of penetrating many feet of material such as lead and rock. The primary cosmic rays probably consist of atomic nuclei, mainly protons, some of which may have energies of the order of 10^{10} to 10^{15} electron volts. Secondary cosmic rays are produced when the primary cosmic rays interact with nuclei and electrons, for example in the earth's atmosphere. Secondary cosmic rays consist mainly of mesons, protons, neutrons, electrons, and photons that have less energy than the primary rays. Practically all of the primary cosmic rays are absorbed in the upper atmosphere. Almost all cosmic radiation observed at the earth's surface is of the secondary type.

coulomb: The unit of quantity of current electricity. The quantity afforded by 1 ampere of current flowing 1 second against 1 ohm of resistance with a force of 1 volt.

crepitus (krep′i-tus) , **bony:** The crackling sound produced by the rubbing together of fragments of fractured bone.

cumulative dose (radiation): The total dose resulting from repeated exposures to radiation of the same region or of the whole body.

current, alternating: Alternating electric current is a type that reverses its direction at regular intervals. Symbol: AC.

current, direct: Direct current is electricity flowing in one direction only. Symbol: DC.

current, electric: An electric current is a flow of electrons through a conductor.

current, high tension: High tension current possesses high voltage and relatively low amperage.

current, unidirectional: Unidirectional, as applied to a current of electricity, is a current that flows only in one direction.

D

darkroom: A room which can be completely darkened so that x-ray or photographic film may be processed using only safelights.

definition: Definition is the degree of distinctness with which radiographic details are recorded on an x-ray film. It is dependent upon optimum image sharpness.

densitometer: A devise for determining amount of radiation delivered by exactly measuring the degree of blackening of x-ray or photographic film by the photoelectric principle.

densitometer, photographic: Instrument for measuring photographic density.

density (radiographic): The degree of gradation of blackness in roentgenogram. It is due to a silver deposit which remains on the film after processing. For practical purposes, density refers to the percent of light transmission through the film and it is defined mathematically as the logarithm to the base of the ratio of the intensity of the light incident on the film to the intensity of light transmitted equals $\log_{10} (I_1 / I_t)$. Example: Density or $\log_{10}10 = 1$ or $10^1 = 10$. Controlling factors of density are mAs (Milliampere-seconds) , kVp, and local film distance. The densities range from about 0.4 (more light transmitted) in the relatively clear areas, to more than 3.0 in the very blackest areas (less light transmitted) .

density, decreased: A radiographic term used to denote a part relatively more permeable to x-rays.

density, increased: A radiographic term used to denote less permeability to x-rays, hence, producing a whiter shadow on the x-ray film or one of less brightness on the fluoroscopic screen.

density, regulation of: When a fixed kilovoltage is employed, the radiographic density is regulated by increasing or decreasing the mAs to a correct value so that the remnant radiation will be sufficiently intense to produce a satisfactory image.

density, tissue: Tissue density may be considered as the resistance of the tissues to the passage of x-rays.

dermatitis, roentgen-ray: Inflammation of skin from exposure to roentgen-rays.

detail: Detail refers to the sharpness of various contour lines and the clean-cut, clearly defined lines of cancellous structure of the bones. The sharper and more distinct such contour lines, the better the detail. Detail can be considered a visual quality and depends first, upon sharpness (definition) and secondly upon radiographic contrast. Five factors which have the most to do with the production of detail sharpness are: (1) the size of the tube focal spot, (2) the source-film distance, (3) the distance of the object from the film, (4) motion of the part during exposure, and (5) type of intensifying screens. Diffusion of detail, or geometric unsharpness is loss of definition. The formula for geometric unsharpness is:

$$\text{Geometric unsharpness} = \frac{\text{Focal Spot Width} \times \text{Object-Film Dist.}}{\text{(mm)} \qquad \text{(in)}}$$
$$\frac{}{\text{Source} - \text{Object distance (in)}}$$

detail, radiographic: Radiographic detail comprises a multitude of deposits of black metallic silver of varying translucency to the light of an x-ray illuminator and represents the structural configuration of body tissues in the form of a radiographic image. Visibility of detail is dependent upon optimum image sharpness and radiographic contrast.

developer: The solution in which films are developed. It brings out the latent image. The developer solution oxidizes the silver bromide that has been affected by exposure. In other words, it changes the latent image of an exposed film to a visible image composed of minute masses of metallic silver. An x-ray developer contains four basic types of ingredients: (1) developing agents or reducing agents, (2) accelerator or an alkali, (3) an antioxidant preservative, and (4) restrainers.

developer, constituents: There are 6 chemicals found in an x-ray developer solution. These chemicals and their functions are as follows:

1. Water—solvent.
2. Elon—reduces the exposed silver emulsion.
3. Hydroquinone—reduces the exposed silver emulsion.
4. Sodium carbonate—accelerates rate of development.
5. Sodium sulfite—preserves developer, controls solution oxidation.
6. Potassium bromide—restrains or controls rate of development.

developer, dilution: The effect of dilution of a developer beyond that recommended is to cause the film to be underdeveloped when a standard time-temperature development is employed. Frequently, the capacity of tanks is incorrectly estimated and insufficient developer chemicals are dissolved in the solution.

developer, rapid: A rapid developer is one in which a strong alkali such as Kodalk or potassium hydroxide is employed as the accelerator.

developer, regular: A regular developer is one in which sodium carbonate is employed as the accelerator. It possesses less developing speed than rapid developer and tends to produce gas when neutralized by the fixing bath.

developer, temperature of: The temperature of the developer solution influences the rate of development. The higher the temperature, the greater the rate and vice versa.

development: Development is the chemical process of converting exposed silver bromide (latent image) to black metallic silver (silver image). The rate of development is influenced by the time and temperature of the developer and its chemical activity. The optimum temperature range of development is 60°-75°F.

development, degree of: The degree of development depends on development time, temperature, amount of agitation and activity of the developer.

development, over: The gain in density or contrast obtained with development of a correctly exposed radiograph beyond five minutes at 70°F is relatively small. The slight density gain is largely due to development of unexposed silver bromide crystals that show as fog. There is little or no increase in film speed by such practice. Prolonged development of the properly exposed film may cause chemical fogging of the image. Over-development cannot produce silver deposits (detail) on the radiograph if the x-rays employed do not reach the emulsion to expose it.

diagnosis: Is the art of recognizing the presence of disease from its symptoms and deciding as to its character; the determination of a type or condition through case or specimen study; the conclusion arrived at through critical perception of the many diagnostic aids known and used in the field of medicine and dentistry.

diaphragms: Usually lead sheets with apertures of various sizes and shapes. The diaphragm limits the size of the primary beam to the area of interest thereby minimizing patient exposure to the primary beam and materially reducing the amount of secondary radiation. For safety the primary beam of dental x-ray machines should be collimated in order to reduce the diameter of the beam to 2.75 inches as the radiation strikes the skin.

distal (dis'tal): Remote; farther from any point of reference; opposed to proximal.

distance factor: Distance as referred to in radiography means that distance between the focal spot of the tube and the film. It is to be remembered that when varying the distance factor, to maintain the density of the film it will be necessary to increase the time of exposure of the penetration (kVp) accordingly. The law to follow is: "the time of exposure will vary inversely as the square of the distance." To determine exposure with a given film at varying distances use the following formula:
Distance-Time Rule:

$$\frac{T_1}{T_2} = \frac{D_1{}^2}{D_2{}^2} \text{ or } T_2 = T_1 \frac{(D_1{}^2)}{D_2{}^2}$$

T_1 and D_1 are respectively the exposure time and source-film distance of the old technic, and T_2 and D_2 stand for the corresponding respective quantities in the new technic.

distortion: A change in the size or shape of the resulting image upon the film. It is due to improper alignment of the object, the film, and/or to a disproportionate ratio between the object-film and source-film distance.

(a) Size distortion: (magnification) results when the film-object distance (the distance between a plane of the object under consideration and the film) is great in proportion to the source-film distance. It is possible to have magnification with little or no shape distortion. On the other hand, it is very difficult to have shape distortion without magnification.

(b) Shape distortion: the unequal magnification of various portions of a plane of the object under consideration. Can be produced from a malalignment of the tube in relation to the film and object.

dorsal (dor'sal): 1. Pertaining to the back or to any dorsum. 2. Denoting a position more toward the back surface than some other object of reference; same as posterior in human anatomy.

dose or dosage: In recent years there has been an increasing tendency to regard a dose of radiation as the amount of energy absorbed by tissue at the site of interest per unit mass. (See rad.)

absorbed dose: The quantity of energy imparted to a mass of material exposed to radiation (See rad.)

air dose: X-ray or gamma-ray dose expressed in roentgens delivered at a point in free air. In radiologic practice it consists of the radiation of the useful beam and that scattered from surrounding air.

cumulative dose (radiation): The total dose resulting from repeated exposures to radiation of the same region, or of the whole body.

dose rate: (dosage rate): Radiation dose delivered per unit of time.

dose, RBE: The unit of RBE dose is the rem, which is that dose having a biological effect equivalent to that of one rad of x- or gamma radiation of a given energy (about 250 Kev). Numerically, the dose in rems equals the dose in rads times the RBE. (Relative biological effectiveness.)

exit dose: Dose of radiation at surface of body opposite to that on which the beam is incident.

integral dose or volume dose: A measure of the total energy absorbed by a patient or any object during exposure to radiation. According to British usage the integral dose of x- or gamma rays is expressed in gram-roentgens.

maximum permissible dose (MPD): Maximum dose of radiation which may be received by persons working with ionizing radiation.

median lethal dose (LD-50): Dose of radiation required to kill, within a specified period, 50 percent of the individuals in a large group of animals or organisms.

skin dose: Dose at center of irradiation field on skin. It is the sum of the air dose and backscatter.

threshold dose: The minimum dose that will produce a detectable degree of any given effect.

dosimeter: Instrument used to detect and measure an accumulated dosage of radiation; in common usage it is a pencil size ionization chamber with a built-in self reading electrometer, used for personnel monitoring.

drying process: The drying process is the removal of water from the emulsion of an x-ray film so that it may be freely handled.

dyne: The unit of force which, when acting upon a mass of one gram, will produce an acceleration of one centimeter per second.

E

effective kilovoltage: A sort of average kilovoltage in an alternating current cycle, between the peak and zero kilovoltages. The effective kilovoltage ordinarily equals .707 multiplied by the peak kilovoltage.

electricity: As a source of power, electricity is a flow of electrons through a closed conducting circuit. The flow is governed by an excess of electrons at one point and a deficiency at another point. The flow is in the direction of least electron concentration (lower potential).

electricity, static: Static electricity is stationary electricity as opposed to electricity in motion as an electric current.

electrode: A terminal of a conductor of electricity, usually of metal or carbon.

electrolyte: An electrolyte is a chemical compound that can be ionized.

electromagnetic wave: A wave produced by the oscillation of an electric charge.

electromotive force: Potential difference across electrodes tending to produce an electric current.

electron: An elementary particle which is constituent of every neutral atom. Most frequently it is a unit of negative electricity called a negatron which is equal to 4.8×10^{10} electrostatic units or 1.6×10^{-9} coulombs. Its mass is $\frac{1}{1845}$ of an atomic mass unit.

electron volt: The kinetic energy gained by an electron in falling through a potential difference of 1 volt. It is equivalent to 1.6×10^{-12} ergs. Kev and Mev refer to a thousand and million electron volts respectively.

electrostatic unit (E.S.U.): Quantity of charge which produces a force of one dyne on an equal charge at a distance of 1 cm.

element: A substance all of whose atoms have the same atomic number (i.e. same number of orbital electrons). This is a distinguishing characteristic. The atomic weight (mass) of an element may vary (this has to do with the number of neutrons in the nucleus) and thus produce a mixture of isotopes of the same element.

elon, function: Elon is a reducing agent that starts action on the exposed emulsion within a few seconds and the entire image appears rapidly. Fine detail is produced but the contrast is low.

elongation: An elongated image is one that is longer than the object radiographed. In the bisection of the angle technic it is caused by directing the x-ray beam perpendicular to the plane of the tooth instead of the plane of the bisector, or the vertical angulation is "too flat."

emesis (em'e-sis) **vomitus:** The act of vomiting.

emulsion, film: Composed of minute particles of sensitive silver bromide or silver chloride suspended in special gelatin. This silver halide emulsion is coated evenly on one or both sides of a blue-tinted, transparent cellulose acetate base.

energy: Capacity for doing work.

energy, ionizing: The average energy lost by ionizing radiation in producing an ion pair in a gas. For air, it is about 33.73 eV.

energy, radiant: The energy of electromagnetic radiation, such as radiowaves, visible light, x- and gamma rays.

erg: Unit of work done by a force of one dyne acting through a distance of one cm. Unit of energy which can exert a force of one dyne through a distance of one cm; C.G.S. units: dyne-cm or $gm\text{-}cm^2/sec^2$.

erythema (er-e-the'mah): A redness of the skin following exposure to certain irritants. It is due to congestion of the capillaries.

erythema dose. The minimum quantity of x- or gamma radiation which will produce the appearance of erythema to a particular part of the integument. The quantity of the dose will vary from part to part on the same individual and among different individuals.

(a) *TED (Threshold Erythema):* (250 r) is the dose that would produce reddening of the skin in the most sensitive person. 400 MAS is the limit TED for a third of the face.

(b) *AED (Average Erythema Dose):* (500 r) would produce reddening in majority of individuals.

(c) *Maximum Erythema Dose:* (750 r) would produce reddening in even the most radioresistant person.

(d) *Erythema Dose:* (165 to 300 r or more) 1200 MAS at the target skin distance of 8″ or 4800 MAS at 16″.

(e) *Safety Dose:* 100 roentgens, or ¼ of an erythema dose to same skin area within a period of 3 weeks. The roentgen output using 8″ SFD and 65-10 is 1 roentgen/second.

exostosis: An abnormal bony or osseous outgrowth from a bone surface (cortex).

exposure: Condition of being in the path of radiations.

exposure acute: Radiation exposure of short duration, usually of an intense nature.

exposure, chronic: Radiation exposure of long duration, usually by fractionation or protraction in the case of therapy or of small daily doses in the case of radiation workers (including dentists).

exposure, MAS: When a fixed kilovoltage is employed, the radiographic density is regulated by increasing or decreasing the mAs to its correct value so that the remnant radiation will be sufficiently intense to produce a satisfactory image.

exposure, over-: An overexposure is evidenced in a radiograph after incorrect exposure and full development and the image contains excessive silver deposits, many of which are opaque to transmitted light.

exposure, under-: An underexposure is evidenced in a radiograph when the image displays insufficient silver deposits following full development.

F

fallout: The radioactive particles or dust that falls to earth after an atomic explosion.

filament: The filament of an x-ray tube is a coiled tungsten wire which when heated to incandescence emits electrons. The temperature of the wire, and hence the rate of emission of electrons, is controlled by a low voltage heating current in a process termed thermionic emission. The filament is part of the cathode.

film badge: Appropriately packaged photographic film worn on a person and used for approximate measurement of radiation exposure for personnel monitoring purposes.

film base: X-ray film base is the cellulose supporting medium for the radiographic emulsion. It is transparent, slightly blue in color, is slow-burning and approximately 8/1000-

inches thick. Its stiffness and flatness satisfies the purpose of handling.

film, direct-exposure: Direct-exposure film is highly sensitive to the direct action of x-rays but has low sensitivity to screen fluorescence. It has a greater silver content. It should not be employed with screens.

film, emulsion: An x-ray film emulsion is a light and x-ray sensitive coating on both sides of a transparent film base, consisting of crystals of silver bromide, chloride or iodide held in suspension and apart in gelatin. The emulsion is $\frac{1}{1000}$-inch thick. X-ray film emulsions vary as to contrast, speed, fogging characteristics and rate of development. In these respects, films of different manufacture vary quite widely and from an exposure and processing standpoint cannot be considered interchangeable.

film, screen-exposure: Screen-exposure film is sensitive to the fluorescent light of intensifying screens and not so sensitive to the direct action of x-rays. It may be employed with or without screens.

filter: Usually a 1 or 2 mm thick sheet of aluminum, placed in the tube housing aperture. It is used to filter out the softer rays and reduce the amount of radiation to the patient's skin.

filter, inherent: Filtration introduced by the glass wall of the x-ray tube, and oil used for tube immersion, and any permanent tube enclosure in the path of the useful beam. Some definitions include the pointed plastic cone on the dental x-ray machine, but this seems unjustified since open-ended cones are often used instead of pointed cones (i.e. it is not permanent).

filter, total: Sum of inherent and added filters.

filtration: Filtration of the x-ray beams alters its intensity and quality. As filtration is increased, radiographic contrast decreases.

fission: The splitting of a nucleus into two fragments. Fission may occur spontaneously or may be induced by man-designed methods. In addition to the fission fragments, particulate radiation energy and gamma rays are usually produced during fission.

fission, products: The nuclides produced by the fission of a heavy element nuclide.

fixation: Fixation is the chemical removal of unexposed and undeveloped silver bromide crystals from an x-ray film, after the exposed crystals have been reduced to silver by the development process. It occurs in an acid medium. This is the clearing function of the fixer. The second function of fixation is to harden and shrink the emulsion so that the film may be dried and handled safely.

fixation, clearing time: The clearing time is the period begun by immersion of the films in the fixer and ending with the disappearance of all undeveloped and unexposed crystals (milkiness). It is during this interval that the fixer dissolves the unexposed silver salts and removes them from the emulsion.

fixation, rate: The rate of fixation is determined by the:
1. Concentration and nature of the fixer chemicals.
2. Temperature of the solution.
3. Degree of agitation in the fixer.
4. Tank volume in relation to size and number of films fixed.

fixation, time: The general rule for applying the fixation time is to leave the films in the fixing bath twice the length of time it takes to clear them.

fixer: The solution, commonly called "hypo," in which the manifest image is fixed and hardened. It is a chemical solution that removes from the exposed film the silver halide crystals that have been unexposed or unaffected by the action of the x-radiation. The solution is acid to stop the action of the developer.

fixer, constituents: There are 5 chemicals usually found in an x-ray fixing bath. The chemicals and their functions are as follows:
1. Water—solvent.
2. Sodium, or ammonium thiosulfate—removes unexposed and undeveloped silver bromide.
3. Sodium sulfite—preservative.
4. Potassium alum—hardener.
5. Acetic acid—acidifier.

fluorescence: The emission of electromagnetic radiation by a substance as a result of an absorption of energy from some other source of radiation, either electromagnetic or corpuscular (particulate). Such radiation is characterized by the fact that it occurs only as long as the stimulus responsible for it is maintained.

fluorescent screen: A surface coated with zinc sulfide (formerly platinobarium cyanide) which fluoresces when irradiated by x-rays. Used for visual examination by x-rays in a darkened room. To protect the operator from the effects of the x-rays during this process, the outer surface is covered with lead glass. For radiography, screens are composed of calcium tungstate crystals that fluoresce only as long as they absorb x-rays. These screens are known as intensifying screens because they augment the x-ray exposure effect 20-30 times.

focal spot: The focal spot of a tube is that area of the anode or target which is bombarded by the electron stream when the tube is in action. All other factors being equal, the smaller the size of the focal spot, the finer the definition.

fog: A general or local deposit of silver or silver compound, formed as the result of exposure to extraneous radiation or by chemical action; it is in addition to the legitimate image. Light fog is produced by light striking the x-ray film. Chemical fog is caused by faulty darkroom technic. Age fog is the result of using outdated x-ray film. Radiation fog is caused by secondary radiation. Fog refers to the generalized darkening of a processed x-ray film.

foreshortening: A foreshortened image is one that is shorter than the object roentgenographed. In the bisection of the angle technic this is accomplished when the x-ray beam is directed perpendicular to the plane of the film instead of the plane of the bisector. The vertical angulation is too steep.

frequency: Number of cycles, revolutions or vibrations completed in a unit of time.

G

gamma rays: Short-wavelength electromagnetic radiation of nuclear origin with a range of wavelengths from about 10^{-8} to 10^{-11} cm, emitted from the nucleus.

gelatin: Gelatin is a jelly-like protein substance obtained from animal tissues by boiling. It is used in x-ray film manufacture as a means for suspension of the sensitive silver salts on the film base.

gene: Fundamental unit of inheritance, which determines and controls hereditary transmissible characteristics. Genes are arranged linearly at definite loci in chromosomes.

genetic effects: Genetic effects of radiation are those changes produced in an individual's genes and chromosomes of all nucleated body cells, both somatic and gonadal. The more frequent meaning relates to the effect produced in the reproductive cells. It is believed that any amount of radiation received by the gonads before the end of the reproductive period is likely to add to the number of undesirable genes present in the population. Such mutated genes may have no recognizable effect for a number of generations, but, potentially, practically all will eventually result in untoward changes in the form of spontaneous genetic abnormalities.

genial tubercle: A small bony prominence on the posterior surface of the mandible on either side of the symphysis.

glabella: A point midway between supraorbital ridges.

glenoid fossa: The depression in the temporal bone for articulation with the condyle of the mandible.

gnathion: The lowest point on the medial line of the lower jaw.

gonad: An ovary or a testis, site of origin of eggs or spermatozoa.

gonion: The center of the symphysis of the mandible used as a radiographic landmark.

Granger projection: A PA radiograph of the skull made with the head at an angle of 17° with the tabletop, for showing the frontal and sphenoid sinuses.

grenz waves: Soft x-rays of long wavelengths produced at voltages of 5 to 20 кV; but more usually from 8-12 кV.

grid: A grid is a device which consists of a series of alternate radiopaque and radioparent strips deeper than wide which when interposed between patient and film allows primary rays to pass through the radiopaque strips; but secondary radiation is absorbed by the radiopaque strips. There are two general types of grids—stationary and moving. The efficiency of a grid ranges from 80-95 percent in the elimination of secondary radiation, thereby enhancing contrast and increasing detail visibility.

grid cassette: One with a grid fitted into the cover of the cassette. Also known as the Camp grid cassette, and was devised by Dr. John D. Camp of Los Angeles.

grid ratio: The ratio of a grid is expressed as the relation of the depth of the lead strips to the width of the radiolucent separators between lead strips. For example—if the depth of the lead strips of a grid is eight times greater than the width of the separating strips, the grid is said to have a ratio of 8:1.

H

half-life, radioactive: Time required for a radioactive substance to lose 50 percent of its activity by decay. Each radionuclide has a unique half-life.

half-value, layer (HVL): Used in radiation physics and therapy as an indicator of the average penetrability of the beam of x-rays coming from an x-ray tube; its value is determined by finding the thickness of a given filter, such as aluminum or copper, which will reduce the ionizing effect of the primary x-ray beam to one-half of its value. The HVL is a measure of the "hardness" or penetrating ability of radiation; the thickness of any given absorber that will reduce the intensity of a beam of radiation to one-half its initial value.

hanger, processing: A processing hanger is a stainless steel frame containing film clips at each corner that hold the x-ray film firmly during the processing procedure.

hard, x-rays: X-rays of short wavelengths of high-penetrating power.

hardener, fixing bath: The fixing bath hardener is a chemical (potassium alum) used to harden and shrink the x-ray film emulsion after development.

heal effect: Actually, the intensity of radiation varies over the area covered by the primary beam. The variation in intensity is due to the angle at which x-rays are emitted from the focal spot. This is the "heal effect," and this is why the cathode end of the x-ray tube has a slightly visible tendency to make a sharper image than has the anode end. This phenomenon is used by medical radiologists in obtaining balanced densities in radiographs of heavier parts of the body.

health physics: A term in common use for that branch of radiological science dealing with the protection of personnel from harmful effects of ionizing radiation.

Heberden's nodes: Enlargements of the distal interpharyngeal joints of the hands in hypertropic osteoarthropathy (osteoarthritis).

hertzian wave: Electromagnetic waves of long wavelength and frequency; radio waves.

holder, exposure: An exposure holder is a radioparent cardboard and envelope device used to hold an x-ray film for exposure purposes. The back of the holder is lined with a thin sheet of lead to protect the film from radiation back-scatter. The envelope mounted between the cardboard covers is to enclose the x-ray film.

hydroquinone, function: The function of the chemical hydroquinone in a developer is to build up contrast in the image so that the detail becomes readily visible.

hypo: A common name for sodium or ammonium thiosulfate, the chemicals used in fixing baths.

I

illuminator: X-ray is a device before which radiographs are viewed. It consists of a metal box containing two fluorescent tubes that emits light of standard color (daylight) and intensity. The face of the illuminator consists of a sheet of blue-tinted opal glass or plastic to diffuse the transmitted light.

image: Used in radiography and photography to designate the impression made on an x-ray or photographic film by x-rays or light.

image, latent: The latent image refers to the atomic changes that occur in the silver bromide crystals in the emulsion of an x-ray film upon x-ray exposure which renders the crystals reducible to metallic silver upon development.

image, radiographic: A radiographic image is a pictorial record of the internal structural elements of a part of the body as projected by x-rays on an x-ray film. It consists of deposits of black metallic silver of varying concentration on the radiograph.

impulse: In A.C. current there are 120 impulses. Each impulse has a time span of $\frac{1}{120}$ second. The number of impulses in a span of $\frac{1}{20}$ second would be 6.

inferior (in-fe're-or): Situated below, or directed downward; in official anatomical nomenclature, used in reference to the lower surface of an organ or other structure.

inherent filtration: Refers to the filtration effect of the materials (such as glass and oil) making up the wall of the modern, shock-proof x-ray tubes.

intensifying screen: A screen composed of fluorescent material placed in close contact with an x-ray film to intensify the action of x-rays in radiography. First developed in 1896 by Dr. Michael Pupin of Columbia University in collaboration with Thomas Edison.

intensity: This is the quantity of x-rays generated at the target of an x-ray tube and varies directly with (1) number of electrons impinging on target per second (mA), (2) with character of target material (tungsten), and (3) with square of the voltage. The intensity of the emergent x-ray beam after it penetrates the object depends on the (1) intensity of x-rays generated at target and (2) the thickness, density and atomic number of the object and (3) distance of target from object. The lightest areas on a film indicate the least intensity of radiation, hence, the greatest absorption by the particular tissues. The darkest tones on the film indicate the greatest intensity of radiation as a result of least absorption by tissues. By increasing kVp from 65 to 90 will cause a "leveling out" of the differences in light and dark areas because the tissues will not absorb as much of the radiation as before.

intensity of radiation: Energy flowing through a unit area perpendicular to the beam per unit of time. It is expressed in ergs per square centimeter or in watts per square centimeter. This is not synonomous with dose rate in air.

interpretation (x-ray film): The explanation of what is obscure; it is used to show the meaning of, to explain, to elucidate, or to translate. When an x-ray examination of any part of the body is made for diagnostic purposes, it becomes necessary to study the roentgenogram and interpret the film in order to integrate these findings of other examinations, such as case history and clinical examinations, to arrive at a final diagnosis. Therefore, the dentist does not "diagnose" the roentgenogram; he "interprets" and studies the obscure shadows on the roentgenogram. Radiographs themselves do not lie, but the interpreter can overlook important details when he fails to take into consideration certain factors such as film properties and the projection used in making a given radiograph.

inverse square law: The law which is applied to all point sources of radiation, that the intensity of radiation is inversely proportional to the square of the distance. Example: If the intensity is 16 r at 10 inch target-part distance, then at 20 inches it will be $16 \times (10/20)^2 = 16/4 = 4$ r.

ion: A charged atom or molecularly bound group of atoms; also a free electron or other charged subatomic particle. An ion pair consists of a positive ion and a negative ion (usually an electron) having charges of the same magnitude and formed from a neutral atom or molecule by the action of radiation.

ion pair: Formed during the interaction of radiation and matter and usually considered as two particles of opposite charge, the electron and a positive atomic or molecular residue.

ionization: The making of an electrically stable atom unstable by displacing or adding one or more units of electrical charge. Any process by which a neutral atom or molecule loses or gains electrons, thereby acquiring a net charge.

ionizing radiation: Electromagnetic radiation (i.e. x-rays or gamma rays) or particulate radiation (i.e. electrons, neutrons, protons, etc.) usually of high energy, but in any case, capable of ionizing air directly or indirectly.

isotopes: One of several nuclides having the same number of protons in their nuclei (and electrons in the orbits outside the nucleus) and hence belonging to the same element, but differing in the number of neutrons and therefore in mass number (A), or in energy content (isomers). In common usage, a synonym for nuclide.

irradiation: Exposure to radiation.

J

joule: The unit for work and energy equal to one newton expended along a distance of one meter ($1 = 1N \times 1m$). (Newton: the unit of force, which when applied to a one kilogram mass will give it an acceleration of one meter per second per second) ($1N = 1 \text{ kg} \times 1m/ 1s^2$.)

K

Kev: Thousand electron volts.

kilovoltage (1,000 volts): As an exposure factor is used in radiography to influence radiographic density, contrast, production of secondary radiation, fog, penetration of tissues and exposure latitude. Electrically, it is the potential applied to an x-ray tube to drive the electrons emitted by the cathode toward the tungsten target located on the face of the anode. It directly influences the qualitative characteristics of the x-ray beam (wavelength). Symbol kVp.

kilovoltage, optimum: An optimum or fixed kilovoltage is one that, for a given projection, will always penetrate the body part irrespective of size and will produce an image of satisfactory contrast when the mAs employed is practical in value.

kilovoltage, peak (kVp): The crest value of the potential wave in kilovolts in an A.C. cycle. When only one half of the wave is used, the value refers to that of the useful half of the wave.

L

lambda: The point at the site of the posterior fontanel where the lambdoidal and sagittal sutures meet.

lambdoid: A suture between the Occiput, Parietal and Temporal bones.

lamella: A small plate or thin layer.

lamina dura: The thin plate of dense or compact bone that lines the tooth sockets which show in the roentgenogram as a fine radiopaque line passing around the tooth.

lateral: 1. Denoting a position farther from the median plane or midline of the body or of a structure. 2. Pertaining to a side.

latitude, exposure: Exposure latitude is the range (exposure spread) between the minimum and maximum exposure that will provide a scale of translucent densities of a body part acceptable for diagnostic purposes. It is influenced by the scale of contrast, hence by kVp. The lower the kVp, the less the exposure latitude, and vice versa. Exposure latitude improves as the kilovoltage is increased until a point is reached where the scale of contrast becomes too long.

Law position for mastoid process: 15° caudad and 15° toward the face, with the sagittal plane of the skull parallel with the cassette.

lead apron: A lead-impregnated rubber apron to protect patient and personnel from radiation.

leakage (direct) **radiation:** The radiation which escapes through the protective shielding of the x-ray unit tube head. This radiation is detected at the sides, top, bottom, or back of the tube head.

logEtronics: An electronic device for reproducing radiographs and automatically compensating for under or overdeveloped areas. This method of printing is called "log Etronic" because exposure (log E) of a photographic material is not only controlled, but also generated by purely electronic means.

luminescence: Radiation coming from a substance as a result of previous action of some form of energy in the substance; for instance, the luminescence of phosphorus after exposure to sunlight.

M

magnification, image: Magnification is the degree of image enlargement of body tissues.

malar bone (zygomatic bone): One of the bones of the face producing the prominence of the cheek.

mAs, mA.s: Abbreviation for milliampere-seconds, the product of millamperage multiplied by the number of seconds. With all other factors being held constant, the film density is related to the mAs; and the density will remain constant even though the mAs, and the seconds of time are varied, so long as they vary reciprocally and their products remain unchanged.

mass: The material equivalent of energy—different from weight in that it neither increases nor decreases with gravitational force.

maximum permissible dose (MPD): Dose of ionizing radiation that, in the light of the present knowledge, is not expected to cause detectable bodily injury to the average person at any time during his lifetime. Maximum permissible limits for exposure either to primary or scatter radiation are expressed for practical purposes as a quantitative measure of radiation intensity in air at a given location, expressed in units known as roentgens (r) or milliroentgens (mr). It should be borne in mind that the roentgen is not a unit of absorbed dose even in air. The rad is the unit of absorbed dose, and the rem is a unit of biological dose. In general, for x-radiation, the biological dose in rems for soft tissue is equal to the absorbed dose in rads and it is roughly equal to the exposure dose in roentgens. MPD for whole-body exposure for occupational workers is .1 or 100 mr per week. Maximum 13-week dose is 3 r and maximum accumulated dose for a year is approximately 5 roentgens governed by formula for maximum accumulated dose to age 30. 5 (n-18) N equals the age of worker. In addition, it is recommended that 10 r to the gonads during the first 30 years of life is the limit from all sources of man-made radiation.

meatus (me-a'tus): An opening or passage.

media, contrast: Contrast media are employed to render high contrast in viscus that normally has very low tissue contrast. Barium sulfate is a common contrast medium for visualization of the alimentary tract.

medullary bone: Actually, this is largely the marrow cavity which is continuous with the inner surfaces of the cancellous bone. It is simply nontrabeculated expansion of the central area of tubular bone.

mega electron volt (MeV): One million electron volts, 10^6 eV.

mesial: Toward the middle line, especially of the dental arch.

milliampere: Milliampere (mA) is a radiographic exposure factor that regulates the intensity of radiation emitted by the x-ray tube. It directly influences the radiographic density. Electrically, the milliampere is $\frac{1}{1000}$ of an ampere of electric current.

milliampere seconds: Milliampere seconds are the product of milliamperes and seconds of time. Its symbol is mAs and is an important exposure factor in the regulation of the amount of silver deposit in the radiographic image.

milliroentgen (mr): A submultiple of the roentgen (equal to $\frac{1}{1000}$th of a roentgen).

molecule: A molecule is composed of one or more particles known as atoms. It is the smallest quantity of matter (compound) which can exist by itself and retain its chemical properties.

monitoring: Periodic or continuous determination of the dose rate in an occupied area (area monitoring) or the dose received by a person (personnel monitoring).

monochromatic x-rays: X-rays having a single or extremely narrow band of wavelengths.

mutant (mu'tant): A variation from the parent stock which breeds true in future generations.

mutation: An individual showing a permanent change in his characteristics from those of his parents.

N

naris: The nostril.

nasal: The bone of the nose.

nasion (na'ze-on): An anthropometric landmark, the point at which a horizontal line tangential to the highest points on the superior palpebral sulci is intersected by the midsagittal plane.

negative charge: An unstable condition of the atomic structure in which electrons are increased beyond the normal number.

neoplasm: A new growth of cells which is more or less unrestrained and not governed by the limitation of normal growth.

Benign: some degree of growth restraint and no spread to distant parts.

Malignant: invasive growth into the tissues of the host, probably with spreading to distant parts.

neutron: A neutron is an electrically neutral particle having an atomic weight equal to one. Its mass is approximately equal to the hydrogen atom. Neutrons are constituents of atomic nuclei (except hydrogen). Being uncharged, neutrons are able to penetrate nuclei and are, therefore, used for bombardment in nuclear disintegration experiments.

no-screen film: An x-ray film with a different and faster speed emulsion than that emulsion of plain or screen film. It is used in cardboard holders for radiographing thin parts (less than 13 cm) where great detail and high contrast are desired.

nucha: The nape of neck.

nucleus: The nucleus is the compact central portion of an atom. It is characterized by the number of its positive charges and its mass. The nucleus contains about 99.97 percent of the mass of the atom.

nuclide: A species of a given atom characterized by the constitution of its nucleus. (The make-up of the orbital electron arrangement remains constant.) The nuclear constitution is specified by the number of protons (Z), number of neutrons (N), and energy content. The terms nuclide and isotope tend to be used interchangeably.

number, atomic: The atomic number is the number of protons or positive charges on the nucleus of an atom and serves to identify an element. It is also equal to the number of electrons surrounding the nucleus.

O

object-film distance: Distance between object (tooth or jaw) and the film.

oblique: Angular view of a surface or object, not a true anteroposterior or lateral position; toward midsagittal plane.

occiput: A bone of the cranial section of the skull, forms the posterior portion and base of the skull.

occipital bone: The flat bone which forms the back of the head.

occlude (o-klood): To fit close together; to close tight, as to bring the mandibular teeth into contact with the teeth in the maxillae.

occlusal film: Film placed between the occlusal surfaces of the teeth, with the x-ray beam directed caudad or cephalad to record the dental arches in occlusion.

occlusal plane: The plane of the masticating surfaces of the molar and bicuspid teeth of the maxilla and mandible when the jaws are closed.

occlusal roentgenograms: Made for recording shadow images of incisal edges and occlusal surfaces of teeth, and cross section of dental arches.

Ohm: The electrical unit of resistance; it is the unit of resistance to be overcome by a potential of 1 volt driving a current of 1 ampere through a conductor.

Ohm's law: I (current) =
$$\frac{V \text{ (Electromotive force)}}{R \text{ (Resistance)}}$$

oocyte: Immature ovum.

opalescence, fixation: opalescence in a radiograph sometimes occurs in freshly-made fixer but soon disappears after washing and drying. The transient condition is caused by the reaction of the gelatin to the high concentration of sodium thiosulfate in the fresh fixer. There is little tendency for opalescence to appear when ammonium thiosulfate is used as a clearing agent.

opaque: Impenetrable by light or x-rays of diagnostic quality range (cf. radiopaque).

osteoradionecrosis or radiation osteonecrosis: A curative dose of radiation in the treatment of a malignant disease or nonmalignant diseases or bad technique and/or ignorance of the effects of radiation may cause damage and death of normal tissue. First, the mucosa or periosteum will become devitalized and the bone will become exposed. Exposure of bone leads to infection which spreads through and around the bone and may cause extensive cellulitis of face and neck. The infection may go on until whole jaw is separated from periosteum and osteomyelitis follows.

oxidation: Oxidation occurs in a chemical reaction when an electron is removed from an atom of a substance. The development of an exposed x-ray film is basically a matter of oxidation of the silver bromide emulsion. Oxidation signifies a loss of electrons.

$$\text{Silver atom} - \text{electron} =$$
$$\text{Silver ion}^+ + \text{electron}^-$$

It is any process which increases the proportion of oxygen or acid-forming element or radical in a compound.

P

P-A: Abbreviation for posteroanterior position or projection.

paralleling technic: By paralleling the long axis of the object and the plane of the film packet with the central beam directed perpendicular to the two parallel planes, a truer profile and relative level registration of the shadow images are the result on the roentgenogram. This technic also employs a slightly increased object-film distance and an increased focal spot-film distance (cone distance) that is greater than that commonly used.

patent (pa'tent): Open or exposed.

peak kilovoltage (kVp): The highest kilovoltage attained at any time in any electrical cycle.

penetration, tissue: The penetration of tissue is a function of x-radiation wavelength and is controlled by the applied kilovoltage.

pentrometer: (Stepped wedge) A roentgenographic testing device usually made of aluminum and built up in steps of varying thickness. It is used in testing the roentgenographic efficiency of x-ray equipment and for roentgenographic calculations, since minor changes in roentgenographic density can readily be detected and the proper compensation or adjustment can be made.

penumbra: The secondary shadow that surrounds the periphery of the primary shadow. Umbra pertains to shadow proper. A penumbra is the ill-defined margin or shadow produced by light. In radiography, it is the blurred margin of an image detail.

periapical roentgenograms: Roentgenograms made for recording shadow images of the outline, position and mesiodistal extent of the teeth and surrounding tissue. It is the best means available whereby the apices of the teeth and their contiguous tissues are disclosed.

periphery: The outside surface, or around the circumference of a part of the body.

pH: A value that expresses the hydrogen ion concentration of a solution—degree of acidity or alkalinity. Pure water is neutral and its pH is 7. Solutions with pH values less than 7 are acid in reaction; those above 7 are alkaline. A rapid developer is strongly alkaline and might have a pH of 14. A strong fixer is exceedingly acid in reaction and might have a pH value of about 3.

phantom: A phantom is a device that absorbs and scatters x-ray in approximately the same way as the tissues of the body. It may be made of a balloon full of water, a set of masonite or presswood sheets, a sack of rice, a coconut, or other similar substances. Readings taken without a patient or phantom in the examining position are meaningless for personnel protection purposes because they do not take into account the effect of the patient's body in scattering radiation throughout the room.

phase: The period of progress of electrical vibration of an electric current cycle.

phosphorescence: Ability of a substance to emit light without sensible heat or luminescence caused by exposure to light or other forms of radiation, and lasting after exposure has ceased.

photoelectric effect: A process by which a photon ejects an electron from an atom. All the energy of the photon is absorbed in ejecting the electrons and in imparting kinetic energy to it.

photoelectron: An electron emitted from a substance under the stimulus of light or other radiation of appropriate wavelength.

photography: Photography is the art or process of obtaining images on sensitized surfaces by the action of light or other radiant energy.

photon: A quantum of gamma radiation or light; also used in reference to x-ray.

photoradiography: Photoradiography is the technic of photographing the x-ray fluorescent screen image on 35 or 70 mm roll film or 4″ × 10″ cut film.

Planck's constant (h): A universal constant h that has the value 6.624×10^{-27} erg/sec. It is the proportionality factor that relates the energy E of a photon to its frequency v, that is, $E = hv$.

planes (skull) (True planes not lines):
Sagittal: Divides the skull in right and left halves.
Horizontal: Plane passes through the inferior margins of orbit and superior margins of external acoustic meatuses.
Vertical: Plane passes through the center of both external acoustic meatuses, and is perpendicular to the horizontal plane.
Frankfort Horizontal: Plane through orbitales and through superior borders of external auditory meatuses.

pocket chamber: A small pocket-sized ionization chamber used for monitoring radiation exposure of personnel. Before use, it is given a charge and the amount of discharge is a measure of the quantity of radiation received.

posterior: Situated in back of, or in the back part of, or affecting the back part of an organ; in official anatomical nomenclature, used in reference to the back or dorsal surface of the body.

Potter-Buckey diaphragm (Bucky): A device comprising a grid and the mechanism for

moving it. The grid absorbs a large part of the secondary radiation because it is composed of alternating strips of lead and radiotransparent material, such as wood or aluminum, so arranged that when the focal spot is centered over the grid, the plane of each lead strip is in line with primary beams. It is used on thick, heavy parts of the body which produce a much higher proportion of scattered radiation.

preservative: A preservative is a chemical placed in an x-ray developer and employed to reduce the amount of oxidation of the reducing agents by air. Sodium sulfite is the chemical usually employed. Due to its slight alkalinity, it contributes to the alkalinity of the developer. Sodium sulfite is also used in the fixer to prevent decomposition of the sodium thiosulfate by acid.

primary circuit: The first winding of the core of a transformer constitutes the primary circuit.

primary radiation (direct radiation): The useful beam of x-radiation that emanates directly from the focal spot.

processing: The chemical treatment of an exposed x-ray film that results in the production of a radiographic image. It involves the processes of development, rinsing, fixation, washing and drying.

projection: A term for the position of a part of the patient with relation to the x-ray film.

prone (pron). Lying with the face downward.

proximal (prok-si-mal): Nearest; closer to any point of reference; opposed to distal.

Q

quality, radiographic: A radiograph may be said to possess radiographic quality when by reason of existing contrast and definition all required anatomical details within the body part being examined become visible in the image.

quality, x-ray: A property determined by the distribution of intensity among the various wavelengths.

quantum: The amount of energy associated with a photon; the x-ray energy reacting with or affecting a single atom or ion. A quantum is an elemental unit of radiant energy (x-rays). The term is almost synonymous with the term of photon.

quantum theory: Originally promulgated by Planck and since extended and confirmed, that in the emission or absorption of energy by atoms or molecules the process is not continuous, but takes place by steps, each step being the emission or absorption of an amount of energy (hv), called quantum, where h is Planck's constant and v is a frequency associated with the atom or molecule.

R

RAD (radiation absorbed dose): Unit of absorbed dose, that is, energy absorbed by material, such as tissue, 1 rad is 100 ergs per gram. With x-rays, 1 roentgen of exposure will usually produce about 1 rad of absorbed dose in soft tissue.

radiation: Energy propagated through space. For our purposes, radiation refers to x-rays.

Leakage radiation: All radiation coming from within the tube housing except the useful beam.

Scattered radiation: All radiation that, during passage through matter, has been deviated in direction. It may also have been modified by a decrease in energy. Scattered radiation is produced by materials lighter than aluminum, and from organic substances (patient). Other sources of scattered radiation are materials beyond the image plane. Radiation arising from such sources may be scattered back to image.

Secondary radiation: Radiation emitted by any irradiated material. It is dependent upon the quality and quantity of the primary radiation and the atomic number of its tissue source. Light elements such as water, tissue, and wood generate large quantities of secondary radiation. The primary factor influencing the production of secondary radiation is kVp.

Stray radiation: Radiation not serving any useful purpose. It includes leakage and secondary radiation.

Characteristic radiation: When primary rays become incident upon a metal heavier than aluminum, the primary radiation energy is transformed into a new radiation of relatively longer wavelength, which is known as characteristic radiation of that metal.

Primary radiation: Radiation coming directly from the target of the x-ray tube. Except for the useful beam, most of this radiation is absorbed in the tube housing. The useful beam is that part of the radiation which passes through the window aperture, cone, or other collimating device of tube housing.

Background radiation: Cosmic Rays, together with radiation given off by radioactive elements.

Remnant radiation: The energy which forms the latent image.

radiation hazard: The hazard that exists in any area to which a person has access while x-ray equipment is in operation and the dosage rate is greater than the permissible dosage rate.

radiation, heterogeneous: Heterogeneous radiation contains a mixture of many different x-ray wavelengths as it leaves the portal of the x-ray tube.

radiation, homogeneous: Homogeneous radiation is one consisting of x-rays of the same wavelengths; that is, monochromatic.

radiation, hygiene: The art and science of protecting human beings from injury by radiation. Since any amount of radiation is harmful in some degree, the ideal objective is to prevent the exposure of any person without a definite purpose.

radiation, primary: Primary radiation (PR) comprises the x-rays that emerge from the portal of an x-ray tube. The quality and quantity are influenced by the exposure factors kVp and mAs.

radiation, remnant: Remnant radiation (RR) is the emergent radiation from a body part which has been selectively diminished in intensity by the various tissues traversed by the primary radiation. It is the radiation that produces the radiographic image and is influenced largely by the absorption characteristics of the tissues examined.

radioactivity: The property possessed by certain elements of spontaneously emitting x-rays or gamma rays.

radiobiology: That branch of biology which deals with the effects of radiation on biological systems.

radiograph: A radiograph contains the image of the internal structures of an object produced by the passage of x-rays and recorded by an x-ray film.

radiography: Radiography is that procedure which depends on the differential absorption of x-rays traversing an object 'to emerge to expose an x-ray film and produce a radiographic image.

radiology: Term employed to designate the broad subject of the medical use of roentgen-rays for diagnostic and treatment purposes and the therapeutic uses of radium.

radiolucent: Permitting the passage of radiant energy or waves.

radiopaque: Not permitting the passage of radiant energy or waves.

radioparent: Offering no barrier to the roentgen-ray.

reaction, chemical: A chemical reaction is an exchange of atoms between molecules to form molecules of a different kind. The result of a chemical reaction is illustrated by an equation:

$$NaCl + AgNo_3 \rightarrow NaNO_3 + AgCl\downarrow$$

reciprocity: The reciprocity law is an important law formulated by Bunsen and Roscoe. It states that the reaction of a photographic emulsion to light is equal to the product of the intensity of the light and the duration of the exposure. The law is valid for direct x-ray exposures but fails for exposures with intensifying screens.

rectification: The restriction of the flow of A.C. current to a particular direction: i.e. the flow of current in each half cycle or each full cycle is in a direction useful in the production of x-rays. Rectification may be achieved by use of the x-ray tube alone. In such an instance, the rectification is called self-rectification and the flow of current is produced in each half cycle.

reduction: Reduction occurs in a chemical reaction when an electron is added to an ion of a chemical to form an atom. Reduction signifies a gain in electrons.

Silver ion$^+$ + electron$^-$ = Silver atom

Reduction is any process which increases the proportion of hydrogen or base-forming elements or radicals in a compound.

Reed's base line: The base line of the skull, also called the infraorbital-meatal line; a line from the infraorbital ridge to the external auditory meatus and the middle line of the occiput.

REM (roentgen equivalent unit): The unit of RBE. The REM takes into account the biological effect of the particular nuclear radiation absorbed.

Dose in rem = RBE $\times$ Dose in rads

In general for x-radiation: 1 rem = 1 rad = 1 roentgen.

replenisher: Solutions for replenishing and strengthening and prolonging the life of the developer and fixer. There is a specific replenisher for each of the solutions.

replenishment systems: The replenishment system of development or fixation makes possible the use of a constant development or fixing time by constant chemical replenishment of the solutions to maintain a standard strength.

restrainer, developer: A restrainer is a chemical (potassium bromide) used in a developer to check development of the unexposed silver bromide and to control the working speed of the developer with respect to the exposed silver bromide.

reticulation: A network of corrugations produced accidentally or intentionally by treatment producing rapid expansion and shrinkage of the swollen gelatin in processing. It is the result of too great a difference in temperature between any two of the three darkroom solutions.

rinsing: After development the film is saturated with alkali. When the film is placed in the fixer, development continues until the alkali is neutralized by the acid fixer. This causes artifacts on the film, hastens exhaustion of the fixer and destroys its hardening properties. To maintain the correct chemical balance in the fixer, all films after removal from the developer should be thoroughly rinsed in flowing water or an acid rinse bath for at least 30 seconds.

roentgen or x-rays: Electromagnetic radiations which have been produced by rapidly changing electric and magnetic fields. They have no mass, no electrical charge, and can be considered as quanta or "packets" of energy traveling in wave motion at the speed of light. X-rays are a form of radiant energy having both a wave nature and a quantum nature.

roentgen (unit): The quantity of x- or gamma radiation such that the associated corpuscular emission per 0.001293 grams of air produces, in air, ions carrying 1 electrostatic unit of quantity of electricity of either sign. It is a unit of exposure dose which is based upon ionization of air; it is not a unit of ionization, nor is it an absorbed dose in air. A milliroentgen is $\frac{1}{1000}$th part of one roentgen.

roentgenograms: Essentially a shadowgram in which x-rays emanating from the focal spot of the tubes through the object and are recorded on photographic film. Often called radiographs.

roentgenology: Can be defined as the study and use of the rays discovered by Roentgen as applied to medical science for photographic and therapeutic purposes.

rule, heel effect: Align the long axis of the tube and the long center axis of the part and film, and direct the cathode portion of the x-ray beam toward the anatomic area of greatest tissue density or thickness.

S

sagittal (saj′i-tal): Shaped like or resembling an arrow; straight. Situated in the direction of the sagittal suture, said of an anteroposterior plane or section parallel with the long axis of the body.

sarcoma (sar-ko′ma): A tumor made up of substance like the embryonic connective tissue; tissue composed of closely packed cells embedded in a fibrillar or homogeneous substance. Sarcomas are often highly malignant.

scattering: Change of direction of subatomic particle or photon as a result of a collision or interaction:

Compton Scattering: The inelastic scattering of a photon through interaction with atomic electrons, accompanied by ejection of a recoil electron from the atom with which the interaction occurred. Compton-scattered photons carry away a fraction of the incident photon energy, ranging from an average of about 85 percent of the initial energy for a 0.1 Mev photon. Sometimes referred to as incoherent scattering.

Elastic Scattering: Scattering effected through the agency of elastic collisions and therefore with conservation of kinetic energy of the system.

Inelastic Scattering: Scattering effected by inelastic collision.

scintillation: A flash of light produced in a phosphor by an ionizing event.

scintillation counter: The combination of phosphor, photomultiplier tube, and associated circuits for counting scintillations.

sella turcica (sel′ah tur′si-ka): A transverse depression crossing the midline on the superior surface of the body of the sphenoid bone and containing the hypophysis.

shield: A body of material to prevent or reduce the passage of particles or radiation.

sickness: Radiation (Radiation Therapy). A self-limited syndrome characterized by nausea, vomiting, diarrhea, and psychic depression, particularly to the abdominal region.

soft x-rays: Soft x-rays are x-rays of low penetrating power.

somatic: Body cells exclusive of germ cells.

speed: The term speed in roentgenography is used to refer to the relative amount of darkening produced on a film from a given amount of radiation.

stereoradiography: A single radiograph lacks the third dimension of depth, but the effect can be created by stereoradiography. Two radiographs are made, one from each of two positions of the x-ray tube of the same area. When viewed through a pair of lens, each eye sees one picture and the brain fuses them into one picture having the impression of depth.

superior (su-pe're-or): Situated above, or directed upward in official anatomical nomenclature, used in reference to the upper surface of an organ or other structure, or to a structure occupying a higher position.

survey instrument: A portable instrument used for detecting and measuring radiation under varied physical conditions. The term covers a wide range of devices utilizing most of the detection methods defined elsewhere.

T

target: That part of the anode which faces the cathode and is bombarded by the high speed electrons.

target-angle: The target angle is the angle away from perpendicular at which the electron stream from the cathode strikes the anode target.

target-film distance (TFD): The distance in inches between the x-ray tube anode and the film.

technic, optimum kVp: The optimum kilovoltage technic is based upon standardization of the processing procedures and the reduction of all exposure factors to constants for a given projection with the exception of one variable mAs. The kilovoltage is fixed for a given projection and the mAs is the variable.

thermionic emission: Release of electrons from the cathode filament by heat.

tissue (tish'u): An aggregation of similarly specialized cells united in the performance of a particular function.

tone: A tone (or brightness) value represents the amount of light transmitted through a radiographic density from a conventional x-ray illuminator; all tones are translucent. The x-ray absorption differences of tissues are rendered as differences in density or tones. The light transmission is dependent upon the silver concentration in the image.

total filtration: Refers to the total filtration of the x-ray beam provided by both the inherent filtration and the added filtration.

tragus: The small prominence of cartilage projecting over the meatus of the external ear.

transformer: It is a device used to transfer alternating current electrical energy from one current to another and from one voltage level to another. Voltage is induced in the secondary winding when energy is applied to the primary. The x-ray machine has three types of transformers, step-down or low voltage transformer for the filament, a high voltage or step-up transformer for the cathode, and an auto-transformer to adjust the line voltage.

translucent: A material that is translucent admits the passage of light, but does not permit objects to be distinctly seen through it.

transparent: A material is transparent when it has the property of transmitting rays of light so that objects can be seen through it.

transverse (trans-vers'): Placed crosswise; situated at right angles to the long axis of a part.

tube, x-ray: An x-ray tube is a highly evacuated glass container in which two electrodes—cathode and anode—are mounted and designed to produce x-rays.

tumor (tu'mor): 1. A swelling, one of the cardinal signs of inflammation; morbid enlargement. 2. Neoplasm, a mass of new tissue which persists and grows independently of its surrounding structures, and which has no physiologic use.

U

umbra: An umbra is a complete shadow produced by light, with sharply demarcated margins. In radiography, it is a sharply delineated image detail.

underexposure: An underexposure is evidenced in a radiograph when the image displays insufficient silver deposits.

useful beam: That part of the primary radiation which passes through the aperture, cone, or other collimator.

V

valence: The valence of an element (or radical) is measured by the number of atoms of hydrogen with which it can combine or by the number of atoms of hydrogen that it can replace by reaction with an acid.

volt: A volt is the electrical unit of pressure that moves or tends to move electrons.

W

washing: Washing is the terminal part of the processing procedure. The film saturated with fixing bath and soluble silver salts is washed until these salts are removed. The rate of washing is dependent upon the temperature of the water and the rate and volume of the water flow.

watt: The unit of power equal to one joule per second $(1W = J/1S)$.

wavelengths: Distance between any two similar points of two consecutive waves (λ) for electromagnetic radiation. The wavelength is equal to the velocity of light (c) divided by the frequency of the wave (v) ($\lambda = c/v$).

weight, atomic: The number of protons and neutrons found in the nucleus of the atom is known as the atomic weight.

X

x-chromosome: The differential sex chromosome carried by half the male gametes and all the female gametes in human beings.

x-rays: Electromagnetic radiation of very short wavelength possessing the properties of (1) penetration of matter, (2) exposure of photographic materials, (3) excitation of fluorescence, and (4) ionization of matter. The useful band of wavelengths employed for medical radiography is 0.50 to 0.100 angstrom units.

Y

Y chromosome: The differential sex chromosome carried by half the male gametes in human beings.

Z

zygoma (zi-go'mah): The zygomatic process of the temporal bone. Also the malar bone.

zygote (zi'gote): 1. The cell resulting from the fusion of two gametes; the fertilized ovum. 2. The individual developing from a cell formed by the union of two gametes.

REFERENCES

1. Etter, Lewis E.: *Glossary of Words & Phrases Used in Radiology, Nuclear Medicine and Ultrasound,* 2nd ed. Springfield, Ill., Charles C Thomas, 1970.
2. Fuchs, Arthur W.: *Principles of Radiographic Exposure and Processing,* 2nd ed. Springfield, Ill., Charles C Thomas, 1969.
3. *Dental Radiological Health Course Manual.* Robert A. Taft, Sanitary Engineering Center, Cincinnati, Ohio, U. S. Department of Health, Education and Welfare, January, 1961.
4. *Radiological Health Handbook,* revised ed. U. S. Department of Health, Education and Welfare, Consumer Protection and Environmental Health Service, Rockville, Md., January, 1970.
5. Blatz, Hanson: *Radiation Hygiene Handbook,* 1st ed. New York, McGraw-Hill, 1959.
6. Meschan, Isadore: *Radiographic Positioning and Related Anatomy.* Philadelphia, W. B. Saunders, 1968.
7. Wuehrmann, Arthur H.: *Radiation Protection and Dentistry.* St. Louis, C. V. Mosby, 1960.
8. Jacobi, Charles: *Intro to Anatomy and Physiology in Radiologic Technology.* St. Louis, C. V. Mosby, 1968.

APPENDIX A

FILM BADGE SERVICE

THE AMOUNT of x-ray radiation that reaches the body of the dentist or of the auxiliary dental personnel can be measured economically with a film badge. The film badge is worn on the clothing for one or two weeks or for one month and is then returned by mail to the laboratory where it was purchased originally. At the laboratory, the film in the badge[1] is carefully processed, and its exposure is evaluated. The amount of radiation recorded by the film badge is a measure of the exposure of the wearer. He is notified by mail of the amount of his exposure.

Film badges can be obtained on a weekly, biweekly, or monthly basis. Some laboratories require contracts which state that film badges will be accepted for a minimum of 13 consecutive weekly, biweekly, or monthly periods. Other laboratories set no limit on the minimum length of time for which the service is desired.[2]

Following is a list of commercial companies and organizations known to have a program for film badge monitoring. The list does not necessarily include all organizations which have a film badge program. This does not constitute an endorsement or a recommendation of the companies listed.

Applied Health Physics, Inc.
Bethel Park, Pennsylvania 15102

Atomic Energy Industrial
   Laboratory of the Southwest
6413 South Main
Houston, Texas 77025

Controls for Radiation, Inc.
130 Alewife Brook Parkway
Cambridge, Massachusetts 02140

Eberline Instrument Corporation
805 Early Street
Santa Fe, New Mexico 87501

Gardray Film Badge Service
P. O. Box 117
Burlington, Massachusetts 01803

Nuclear Consultants Corp.
Box 6172, Lambert Field
St. Louis, Missouri 63145

Nuclear Service Laboratories
Box 1885
Knoxville, Tennessee 37901

Nucleonic Corporation of America
196 De Graw Street
Brooklyn, New York 11231

R. S. Landauer, Jr., & Co.
3920 216th Street
Matteson, Illinois 60443

Radiation Detection Company
385 Logue Avenue
Mountain View, California 94040

---

1. *Physical Survey Manual*, Dental X-Ray, U. S. Public Health Service, April, 1967.
2. Barr, J. H.; Silha, R. E. and Richards, A. G.: Effective use of x-ray radiation in dentistry. *Oral Surg,* 16:299-300, March, 1963.

Health Physics Service, Inc.
1109-13 Low Street
Baltimore, Maryland 21202

Nuclear Chicago Corporation
333 East Howard Avenue
Des Plaines, Illinois 60018

Technical Associates, Nuclear
    Instrumentation
140 West Providencia Avenue
Burbank, California 91502

Tracerlab, A Division of Laboratory
    for Electronics, Inc.
1601 Trapelo Road
Waltham, Massachusetts 02154

St. John X-Ray Laboratory
Califon, New Jersey 07830

T. M. Gaines Company
845 University Avenue
Berkeley, California 94710

United States Testing Company, Inc.
1415 Park Street
Hoboken, New Jersey 07030

Westinghouse Radiation Monitor
Westinghouse X-Ray Dept.
2519 Wilkens Avenue
Baltimore, Maryland 21223

APPENDIX B

LEAD APRONS, PROTECTIVE BARRIERS, AND PROTECTIVE BARRIER MATERIALS[1]

FOLLOWING ARE LISTS of commercial companies and organizations known to sell lead aprons, protective barriers, and protective barrier materials. The lists do not necessarily include all organizations handling these articles. These lists do not constitute an endorsement or recommendation of the organizations listed.

Lead Aprons and Sheeting

Bar-Ray Products, Inc., 209 25th Street, Brooklyn, New York 11232

LeadX Protective Aprons	Office Personnel
	Patients' Aprons
Sheeting	.25 mm lead equivalent
	.50 mm lead equivalent
	1.00 mm lead equivalent

General Electric Co., X-Ray Department, 4855 Electric Avenue, Milwaukee, Wisconsin 43219

Lead Protective Aprons	Office Personnel
	Patients' Aprons
Sheeting	.50 mm lead equivalent

Picker X-Ray Corporation, 25 South Broadway, White Plaines, New York 11580

Lead Protective Aprons	Office Personnel
	Patients' Aprons
Sheeting	.50 mm lead equivalent
	1.00 mm lead equivalent

Buck-X-Ograph, 87 Xograph Avenue, St. Louis, Missouri 63136
Buffalo Weaving & Belting Co., 300 Chandler, Buffalo, New York 14207
Halsey X-Ray Products, Inc., 1425 37th Street, Brooklyn, New York 11218
J. Palmero Sales Co., P. O. Box 368, Westport, Connecticut 06880
Wolf X-Ray Products, Inc., 93 Underhill Avenue, Brooklyn, New York 11238
Rinn Corporation, 2929 N. Crawford Avenue, Chicago, Illinois 60646
Bar-Ray Products, 209 25th Street, Brooklyn, New York 11232

Floor Screen (Shield)	1.5 mm lead-lined;
	8″ x 10″ lead glass window

---

1. *Physical Survey Manual.* Dental X-Ray, U. S. Public Health Service, April, 1967.

General Electric Company, X-Ray Department, 4855 Electric Avenue, Milwaukee, Wisconsin 43219

Floor Screens   1.5 mm lead-lined;
8″ x 10″ lead glass window

Picker X-Ray Corporation, 25 South Broadway, White Plains, New York 11580

Floor Screens   1.5 mm lead-lined;
8″ x 10″ lead glass window

Campbell X-Ray Transformer Company, 146 Exchange Street, Malden, Massachusetts 02148

Wolf X-Ray Products, Inc., 93 Underhill Avenue, Brooklyn, New York 11238

Protective Barrier Materials

Ameray Corp.
Route 46
Kenvil, New Jersey 07847

Andel & Co., Inc.
5218 N. Kedzie Ave.
Chicago, Illinois 60625

Bar-Ray Products, Inc.
209 25th St.
Brooklyn, New York 11232

Division Lead Co.
7742 W. 61st St.
Summit, Illinois 60501

Duro Metal Spinning Co.
207 Oster St.
Glenolden, Pennsylvania 19030

General Electric Co.
X-Ray Department
4855 Electric Ave.
Milwaukee, Wisconsin 43219

General Lead Construction Corp.
1800 Harrison Ave.
Kearney, New Jersey 07032

Keleket Division
(Laboratory for Electronics, Inc.)
Medical X-ray Apparatus
1601 Trapelo Road
Waltham, Massachusetts 02154

Keller Products, Inc.
37 Union
Manchester, New Hampshire 03103

O. G. Kelley & Co.
105 Taylor St.
Boston, Massachusetts 02148

Maryland Metal Spinning Co.
604 W. Fairmount Ave.
Baltimore, Maryland 21201

Met-L-Wood Corp.
6755 W. 65th St.
Chicago, Illinois 60638

Picker X-Ray Corp.
1273 Mamaroneck Ave.
White Plains, New York 11580

Ray Proof Corp.
843 Canal St., P.O. Box 1454
Stamford, Connecticut 06902

Westinghouse Electric Corp.
X-Ray Department
2519 Wilkins Ave.
Baltimore, Maryland 21223

Wolf X-Ray Products, Inc.
93 Underhill Ave.
Brooklyn, New York 11238

APPENDIX C

SUPPLIERS OF ELECTRONIC TIMERS

Electronic Control Corp.
1573 E. Forest Ave.
Detroit, Michigan 48207

Hanau Engineering Co., Inc.
1233 Main St.
Buffalo, New York 14209

Pennwalt Corporation
S. S. White Dental Health Prod.
Three Parkway
Philadelphia, Pennsylvania 19102

Liebel Flarsheim Co.
111 E. Amity Road
Cincinnati, Ohio 45237

APPENDIX D

SUPPLIERS OF LONG OPEN END CONES

R. Margraf, Fab.
27 Woodhill Dr.
Willow Grove, Pennsylvania 19090

General Electric Co.
4855 Electric Ave.
Milwaukee, Wisconsin 53201

Ritter Equipment Co.
P. O. Box 848
Rochester, New York 12603

Weber Dental Mfg. Co.
2206 13th St., N.E.
Canton, Ohio 44705

Pennwalt
S. S. White Dental Health Prod.
Three Parkway
Philadelphia, Pennsylvania 19102

APPENDIX E

MANUFACTURERS OF DENTAL X-RAY EQUIPMENT*

Presently making equipment:

General Electric Co., 4855 Electric Ave., Milwaukee, Wisconsin 43219

North American Philips Co., Inc. Norelco Medical and Dental Division, 100 East 42nd St., New York, New York 10017

Ritter Company, Inc., Rochester, New York 12603

Litton Medical Products, Profexray Division, 515 E. Touhy Ave., Des Plaines, Illinois 60018

Siemens America Inc., Dental Division, 10-39 44th Drive, Long Island City, New York 11101

Universal, 1138 North Western Ave., Chicago, Illinois 60622

Weber, 2206 13th, N.E., Canton, Ohio 44705

Pennwalt, S. S. White, Dental Health Products, Three Parkway, Philadelphia, Pennsylvania 19102

No longer making dental x-ray equipment:

Adams

A. S. Aloe Company, Continental Pace Maker MX-F-8435, St. Louis, Missouri

Edwards

Englen

H. G. Fischer, Franklin Park, Illinois

Grenz-Ray

Humphrey

Internation

Liebel Flarsheim Co., Cincinnati, Ohio

Mattern

G. M. McFedrier

Meyer, Chicago, Illinois

Pengelly

Philberg

Picker X-Ray Corp., Waite Mfg. Div., Inc., Cleveland, Ohio

Pony

Professional Equipment Co.

Standard, Chicago, Illinois

Thomas Plaster Co.

X-Cell-Ray

Waite and Bartlett

Wappler

Westinghouse, Baltimore, Maryland

---

* Addresses given where known.

AUTHOR INDEX

SUBJECT INDEX